AF703616

Copyrights©

ISBN
Paperback: 979-8-90190-438-1
Hardcover: 979-8-90190-439-8

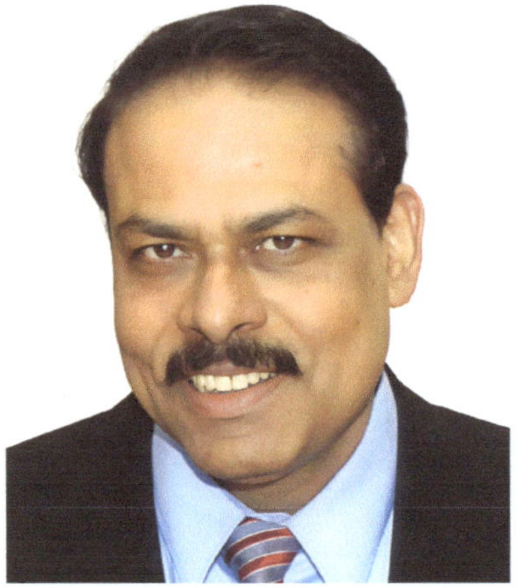

Dr. Eapen Daniel

About the Author

Dr. Eapen Daniel is a renowned Botanist who received his master's degree in Botany/Biochemistry from the University of Kerala and taught at the same University until migrating to the USA. He got his Doctorate in Health Administration and has been deeply involved in seminars and writings on life practices in relation to nature, diet, and ancient practices of Yoga & Meditation. This two-part book is a brief introduction to possible life habits changes and common spices used in culinary cooking, worldwide. Currently, Eapen is employed at PENN MEDICINE, the Health System side of the University of Pennsylvania, as a senior Information Systems Analyst with a focus on Laboratory Sciences, and latest Information technology Applications.

Making meaningful improvements to your health doesn't require drastic overhauls—small, consistent changes often yield the best results. Prioritizing 7-9 hours of quality sleep each night helps your body recover and supports mental clarity. Incorporating regular physical activity, such as 30 minutes of walking most days, strengthens your cardiovascular system and boosts your mood. Eating more whole foods, such as fruits, vegetables, lean proteins, and whole grains while reducing processed foods and added sugars, provides essential nutrients your body needs. Managing stress through techniques such as meditation, deep breathing, or spending time in nature can help lower inflammation and improve overall well-being. Finally, staying socially connected with friends and family, limiting alcohol consumption, and avoiding smoking are foundational habits that significantly reduce disease risk and enhance longevity. The key is choosing one or two changes to start with rather than trying to transform everything at once, allowing new habits to become sustainable parts of your daily routine.

Dedication

I dedicate this book to my late parents, Mr. T N Daniel and Mrs. Annamma Daniel, my loving wife, Gracey, and my loving children, Angela and Benjamin,and Holly, and my precious grandchildren, Theo, Lucas, and Max.

INTRODUCTION TO THE BOOK

INDRANILL BASU-RAY, MD, DNB (CARD), D Sc (Honoris Causa), FACP, FACC.

As a practicing cardiologist with decades of experience treating cardiovascular disease, I have witnessed firsthand how dietary choices profoundly impact our health trajectories. It gives me immense pleasure to introduce this comprehensive guide that brilliantly bridges the gap between culinary tradition and evidence-based medicine.

The ancient wisdom of using spices as both flavor enhancers and therapeutic agents has been validated by modern scientific research. Turmeric's curcumin reduces inflammation and supports cardiovascular health. Cinnamon helps regulate blood sugar levels. Garlic and ginger possess powerful cardioprotective properties. These aren't merely culinary ingredients; they are nature's pharmacy, available in every kitchen.

This book's approach to healthy longevity practices resonates deeply with my clinical philosophy. True wellness isn't achieved through restrictive diets or temporary interventions, but through sustainable lifestyle choices that nourish both body and soul. The author masterfully demonstrates how incorporating simple behavioral practices and diverse herbs and spices into a daily diet can transform health, making daily living both enjoyable and disease-free. What particularly impresses me is the book's inclusive approach to longevity practices for all ages. From children developing healthy taste preferences to seniors managing chronic conditions, these principles apply universally. The connection between flavorful, spice-rich cuisines and the longevity observed in Blue Zones worldwide is not coincidental; it's scientific.

I encourage readers to embrace these time-tested practices. Your heart, your taste buds, and your family will thank you for generations to come.

Dr. Basu-Ray is a Cardiologist & Interventional Cardiac Electrophysiologist, Director of Cardiovascular Research, Director of Clinical Cardiology Electrophysiology Laboratory, Lt. Col. Luke Weathers, Jr. VA Medical Center, Memphis, Tennessee.

Adjunct Professor; School of Public Health, University of Memphis, Adjunct Associate Professor of Medicine (Cardiology), University of Tennessee Health Sciences Center. G 401 A, 4th floor, Bed Tower; 1030 Johnson Ave, Memphis, TN 38104

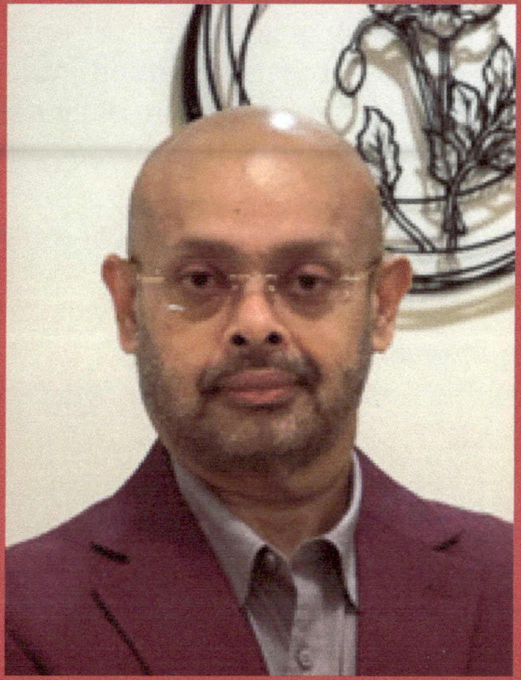

Dr. Indranill Basu-Ray, MD, FACC
Interventional Cardiologist

INTRODUCTION

HEALTH WISE

Welcome to the world of healthy living and the listing and properties of common cooking spices! In this book, we embark on a journey to explore how simple, everyday actions and food ingredients can transform our health and well-being. From the aromatic allure of cinnamon to the fiery zest of turmeric, each spice holds unique properties that enhance the flavor of our meals and offer remarkable health benefits.

Our modern lifestyle often leads us to overlook the natural remedies that have been cherished for centuries. This book aims to reconnect you with these timeless treasures, providing insights into their nutritional value, medicinal uses, and practical applications in your daily diet.

Example - Health Benefits of a couple of Common Cooking Spices

Turmeric : Known for its anti-inflammatory and antioxidant properties, turmeric can help reduce inflammation, improve brain function, and lower the risk of heart disease.

Cinnamon : This sweet spice can help regulate blood sugar levels, reduce the risk of heart disease, and has potent antioxidant properties.

Ginger : Ginger is excellent for digestion, reducing nausea, and has anti-inflammatory effects that can help with muscle pain and soreness.

Garlic : Garlic boosts the immune system, reduces blood pressure, and has antibacterial and antiviral properties.

Cumin : Cumin aids in digestion, boosts the immune system, and has antioxidant properties that help fight free radicals.

Black Pepper : Known as the "king of spices," black pepper enhances nutrient absorption, improves digestion, and has anti-inflammatory properties.

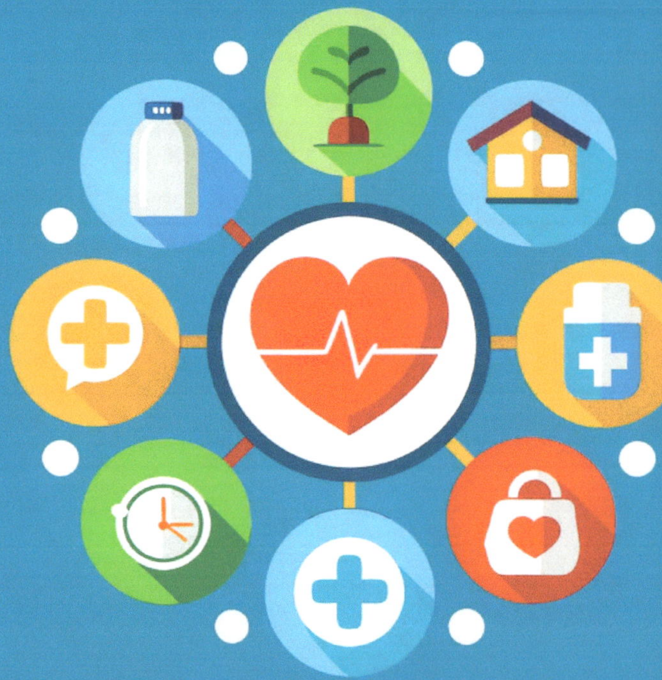

CONTENT

Eastern Traditions

The Five Elements and Vital Energy

While Western traditions focused on four elements, many Eastern cultures developed five-element systems with equally profound implications for understanding the human body. Traditional Chinese Medicine (TCM) presents perhaps the most sophisticated example, with its Wu Xing theory of wood, fire, earth, metal, and water.

In TCM, these elements don't represent literal substances but rather dynamic processes and qualities that manifest throughout nature and the human body. Wood embodies growth, flexibility, and the liver's functions of planning and vision. Fire represents expansion, circulation, and the heart's role in consciousness and emotional expression. Earth signifies nourishment, transformation, and the spleen's digestive and metabolic processes. Metal governs contraction, purification, and the lungs' respiratory and eliminative functions. Water symbolizes storage, conservation, and the kidneys' role in reproduction and fundamental life essence.

This system emphasizes the interconnectedness of all elements through cycles of generation and control. Wood feeds fire, fire creates earth (ash), earth produces metal (minerals), metal collects water (condensation), and water nourishes wood. Simultaneously, each element controls another: wood depletes earth, earth absorbs water, water extinguishes fire, fire melts metal, and metal cuts wood. Health depends on maintaining harmony among these elemental energies.

Traditional Chinese medicine also incorporates the concept of qi (vital energy) flowing through meridian channels that connect organ systems to elemental correspondences. Acupuncture, herbal medicine, and other therapeutic modalities aim to balance elemental energies and ensure smooth qi circulation throughout the body.

Similar five-element traditions developed in other cultures. Ayurveda, India's ancient medical system, builds upon the Vedic foundation by recognizing how these five elements (panchamahabhuta) - Prithvi, Apas, Agni, Vayu, and Akasha - combine to form three constitutional types (doshas). Japanese traditions adapted Chinese elemental theory while incorporating indigenous beliefs about natural forces and spiritual energies.

HUMAN BODY
Life Elements and Ancient Beliefs

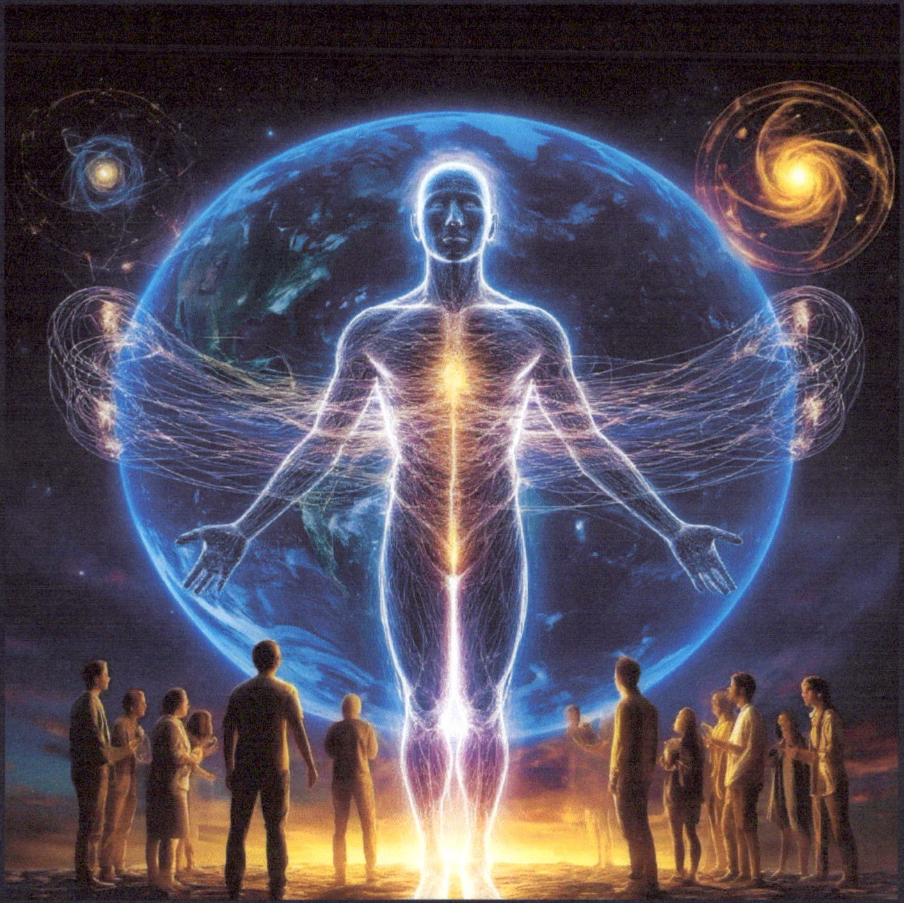

Hippocrates, often called the father of medicine, developed the theory of the four , directly linking bodily functions to elemental qualities.

Historical Background

Throughout human history, civilizations have sought to understand the mysteries of the human body and the forces that animate life itself. Long before modern anatomy and physiology, ancient cultures developed sophisticated theories connecting the human form to fundamental elements of nature, creating holistic worldviews that integrated physical, spiritual, and cosmic dimensions of existence. These elemental theories not only shaped medical practices but also influenced philosophy, religion, and our understanding of humanity's place in the universe.

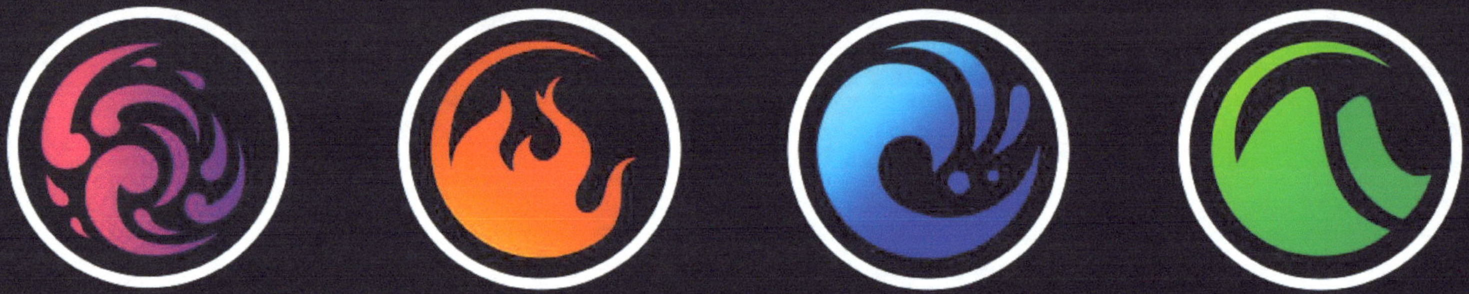

THE FOUR CLASSICAL ELEMENTS

Foundation of Western Thought

The ancient Greeks established one of the most enduring frameworks for understanding the human body through their theory of four classical elements: earth, water, air, and fire. This system, refined by philosophers like Empedocles and later Hippocrates, proposed that all matter, including the human body, consisted of these fundamental components in various combinations.

Hippocrates, often called the father of medicine, developed the theory of the four humours, directly linking bodily functions to elemental qualities. Blood corresponded to air and was considered hot and moist, governing cheerful and optimistic temperaments. Yellow bile represented fire, characterized as hot and dry, associated with choleric or irritable dispositions. Black bile aligned with earth, cold and dry, linked to melancholic or depressive states. Finally, phlegm embodied water, cold and moist, connected to phlegmatic or calm personalities.

This humoral theory suggested that health resulted from balanced humors, while illness arose from their imbalance. Physicians prescribed treatments based on elemental principles: cooling foods for excess fire, warming remedies for excess water, drying treatments for too much moisture, and moistening therapies for excessive dryness. This approach dominated Western medicine for over two millennia, influencing everything from dietary recommendations to surgical procedures.

The Greeks also believed that these elements connected humans to the cosmos. Each element corresponded to celestial bodies and seasonal cycles, creating an intricate web linking individual health to universal rhythms. This holistic perspective viewed the human body not as an isolated biological system but as a microcosm reflecting the macrocosm of the universe.

Spiritual Dimensions

Elements as Divine Essence

Ancient beliefs consistently viewed bodily elements not merely as physical components but as expressions of divine or spiritual forces. Many traditions taught that human bodies contained spark of cosmic consciousness, with elements serving as vehicles for soul expression and spiritual evolution. Egyptian cosmology described the human body as a temple housing multiple spiritual aspects, each corresponding to different elemental qualities. The ka represented life force energy associated with air and breath, the ba embodied individual personality linked to fire and animation, and the akh symbolized enlightened consciousness connected to celestial light and ether.

Hindu philosophy presents the most detailed exploration of elements as spiritual principles. According to the Indian Vedas, believed to be written between 1200 to 1500 BCE, the five main elements of human life are: Prithvi (Earth), Apas (Water), Agni (Fire), Vayu (Air), and Akasha (Aether or space). These ancient texts describe how cosmic consciousness (Brahman) manifests through increasingly dense elemental layers: Akasha provides the field for manifestation and pure space, Vayu enables movement and breath, Agni governs transformation and metabolism, Apas maintains fluidity and circulation, and Prithvi creates solid structure and form.

This tradition teaches that spiritual evolution involves understanding and transcending elemental attachments. Yoga practices work with elemental energies through breathwork (pranayama), physical postures (asanas), and meditation techniques designed to balance and purify elemental influences within the body-mind complex.

Indigenous shamanic traditions worldwide maintain similar perspectives, viewing the human body as a confluence of elemental spirits that must be honored and balanced for optimal health and spiritual development. Healing ceremonies often involve calling upon elemental powers to restore harmony between individual constitution and natural forces.

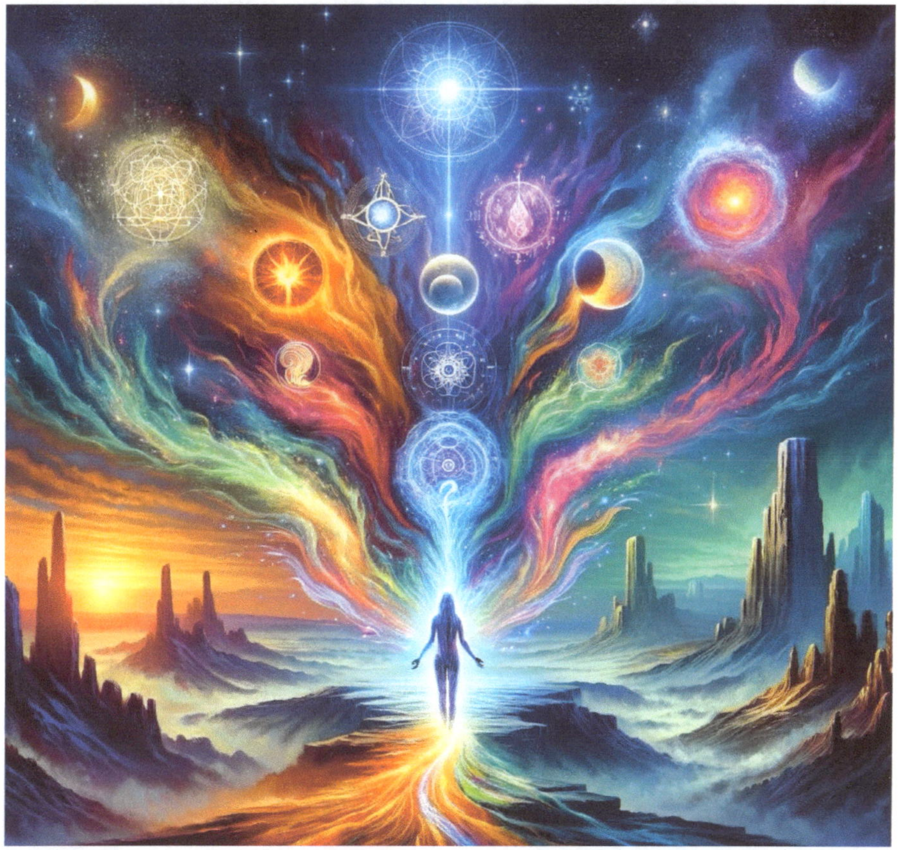

Modern Reflections

Ancient Wisdom in Contemporary Context

While modern science has revealed the molecular and cellular basis of human physiology, ancient elemental theories continue to offer valuable insights into holistic health and wellbeing. Many contemporary healing modalities draw upon traditional elemental frameworks, recognizing their psychological and energetic validity even when their literal interpretations have been superseded.

Research in psychoneuroimmunology demonstrates how mental and emotional states significantly influence physical health, validating ancient observations about temperamental connections to bodily functions. Studies of circadian rhythms and seasonal affective patterns confirm traditional beliefs about human synchronization with natural cycles.

The growing field of integrative medicine increasingly incorporates elemental concepts, particularly from TCM and Ayurveda, recognizing their effectiveness in treating chronic conditions that conventional medicine struggles to address. Acupuncture, herbal therapies, and constitutional treatments based on elemental typologies have gained scientific validation and mainstream acceptance.

Environmental medicine also echoes ancient wisdom by recognizing how elemental imbalances in our surroundings affect human health. Air pollution, water contamination, soil depletion, and electromagnetic radiation represent modern versions of elemental disharmony that ancient physicians would readily recognize.

Perhaps most significantly, ancient elemental theories offer frameworks for understanding human beings as integral parts of natural systems rather than separate from or superior to the environment. This perspective becomes increasingly relevant as we face ecological crises requiring fundamental shifts in how we conceptualize the relationship between human health and planetary wellbeing.

The enduring appeal of elemental theories suggests they address deep human needs for meaning, connection, and holistic understanding that purely reductionist approaches cannot fully satisfy. By honoring both ancient wisdom and modern knowledge, we can develop more comprehensive approaches to health that integrate physical, psychological, spiritual, and environmental dimensions of human existence.

In conclusion, ancient beliefs about life elements and the human body represent sophisticated attempts to understand the fundamental nature of existence and our place within the cosmic order. While scientific advances have expanded our knowledge far beyond these early frameworks, the underlying insights about interconnectedness, balance, and the spiritual dimensions of embodied existence continue to offer profound wisdom for contemporary seekers of health and understanding.

In today's pursuit of life, liberty, and happiness, everything we do is to attain some pleasure, which can be material possessions, physical happiness, or even mental satisfaction and soothing effects, including consuming food that you like. We want to avoid something you do not like or do not want. But circumstances and situational aspects take you to such unpleasant areas and feelings. Instead of looking within, we seek the comforts outside, trying to attain that comfort zone, which is kind of a dream. I remember reading the quote of a famous Psychiatrist who said, "one who looks outside dreams and one who looks within awakens".

Living with nature and taking care of nature is part of critical human responsibility, as our thoughts and deeds are also influenced by changes in nature, including climatic changes due to pollution. Pleasant natural surroundings help humans develop happier moods and clear thinking, and unpleasant surroundings do the opposite to our body and mind.

The human body is a complex machine with a lot of continually functioning systems, including organs and tissues related to each system. There is a constant energy flow throughout your body that varies based on your age and health conditions. The major systems that are constantly at work include our Respiratory System, Circulatory System, Nervous System, Muscular System, and Digestive System. Various organs assist with these system functions. It's important to keep these systems in good shape. Your surroundings, food intakes, mental stability, and clear thinking has a lot to do with the smoother and better functioning of these essential systems.

I grew up in a small village in the Southernmost state of India – Kerala, where the old traditions, Ayurvedic Medicine, Religious Cultures of many religions, and simple life/living were prominent. As my family home was situated on the banks of Manimala River, I used to watch Hindu Swamies and other temple devotees engaged in their early morning Yoga and Meditation near the quietness of the river, on the vast sand banks, after cleansing themselves using the crystal-clear waters of that river. I have also watched them leading healthy, long lives, some even into their late nineties, and many over 100 years. I am talking about a time and space where there was no electricity in the village, no running water, only rare automobiles, and no phones or TVs. In other words, the distractions and wants were minimal. The village dwellers mostly depended on agriculture – rice fields, black pepper, cardamom, sugar cane, coconut plantation, banana plantations, tapioca cultivations, and similar tropical staples. Everything consumed was purely organic and freshly made. A drastic difference from today's world. We still have many such villages existing in South India where modernity and technology are unfamiliar terms.

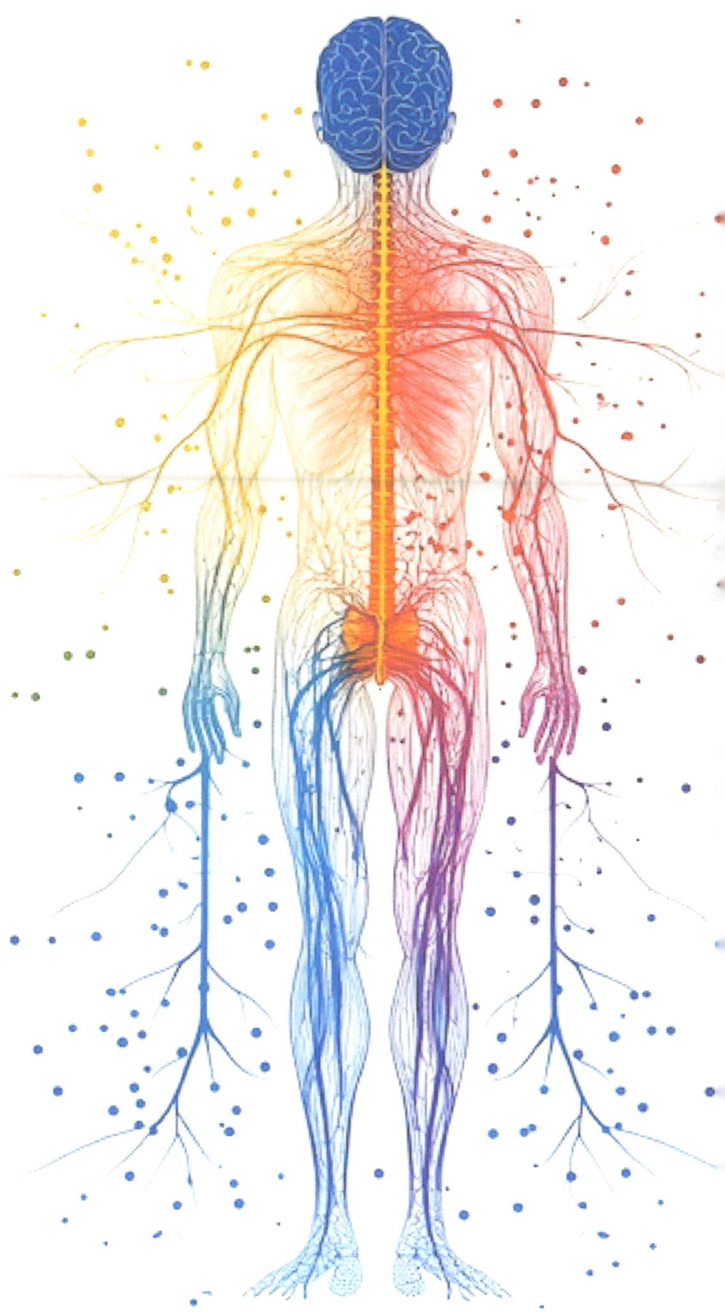

The 4 Major and Critical Aspects of the Human Body

whichmust be attended to and always maintained for better health.

Although there are various ways to explain the normal functioning of a human body, the basic structure and functioning are controlled by one prime system and three subordinate systems. The primary system is the Musculoskeletal System, which plays a pivotal role in almost everything we do, such as our breathing, heartbeat, digestion, and general body movements. Anything we do on any given day impacts these critical systems.

1. **MUSCULAR SYSTEM** (primary system that controls our movements and posture)
2. **BREATHING** (controlled by the Diaphragm and Lungs)
3. **BLOOD CIRCULATION** (Controlled by the Heart Muscles
4. **DIGESTION** (Controlled by the smooth muscles of the digestive tract.

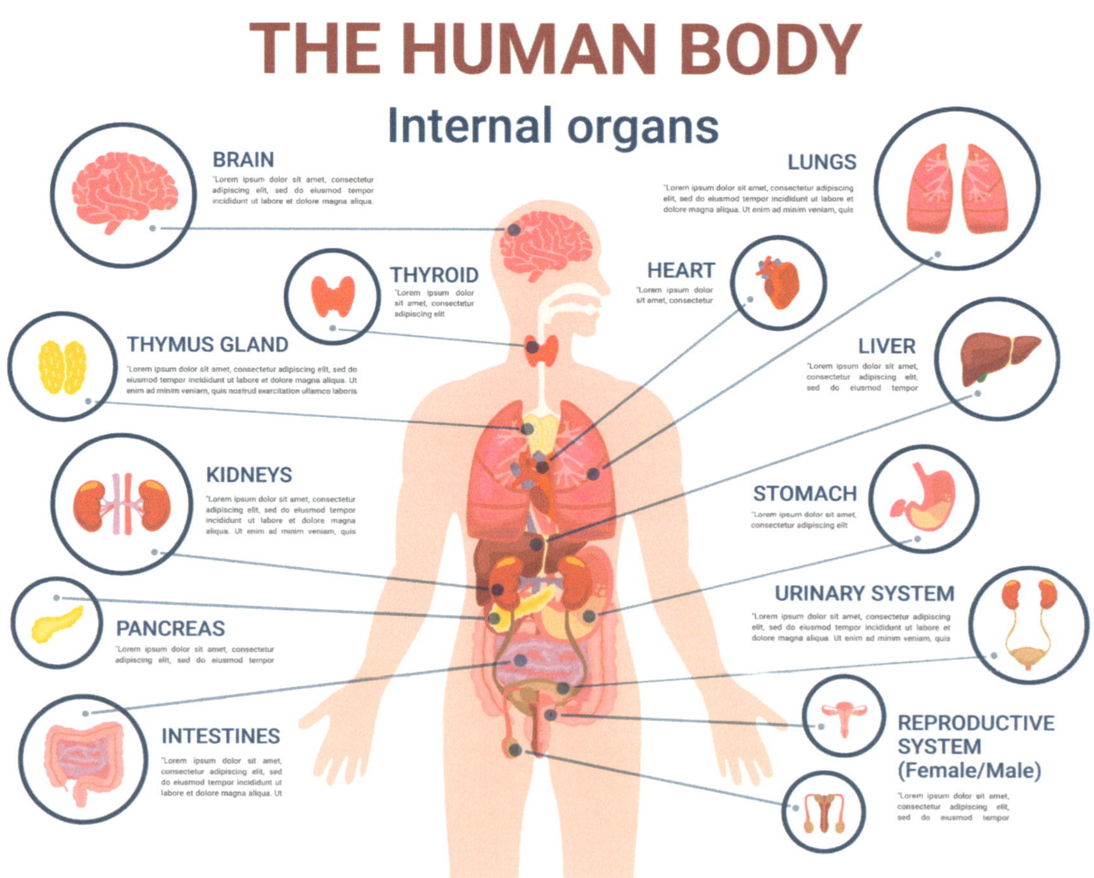

10 Most Essential Health Aspects Everyone Should be targeting (Regardless of Age) for Better Health

Maintaining optimal health requires attention to fundamental aspects that remain crucial throughout life, from childhood to old age. These core elements form the foundation of physical, mental, and emotional well-being, providing the best defense against disease while promoting vitality and longevity.

1. Quality Sleep (7-9 Hours Nightly)

Sleep serves as the body's primary recovery and repair mechanism. During sleep, the brain flushes toxins, consolidates memories, and regulates hormones essential for growth, metabolism, and immune function. Poor sleep disrupts every bodily system, increasing risks of obesity, diabetes, cardiovascular disease, and mental health disorders. Consistent sleep schedules, dark environments, and pre-sleep routines optimize this critical recovery period.

Note: The 7-to-9-hour sleep requirement is questioned by many Hindu Philosophers who state that you need only 4 to 5 hours of sleep time, including the 4 hours 'Delta Sleep'. My respected friend and senior Surya Namaskar practitioner, ***Rev Samuel Nettiyadan*** practiced the 4 to 5 hours sleep pattern since he was about 17 years of age, and now at his 70s, he is physically and mentally well fit. His success story is also related to the strict daily practice of needed light exercises and dietary additions.

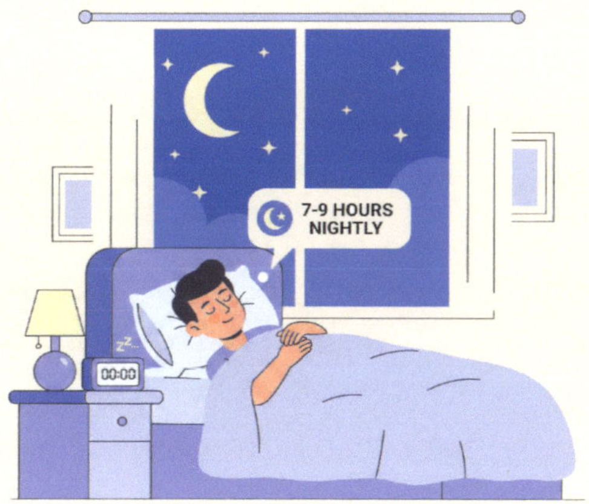

Quality Sleep (7-9 Hours Nightly)

2. Balanced Nutrition and Hydration

Sleep serves as the body's primary recovery and repair mechanism. During sleep, the brain flushes toxins, consolidates memories, and regulates hormones essential for growth, metabolism, and immune function. Poor sleep disrupts every bodily system, increasing risks of obesity, diabetes, cardiovascular disease, and mental health disorders. Consistent sleep schedules, dark environments, and pre-sleep routines optimize this critical recovery period.

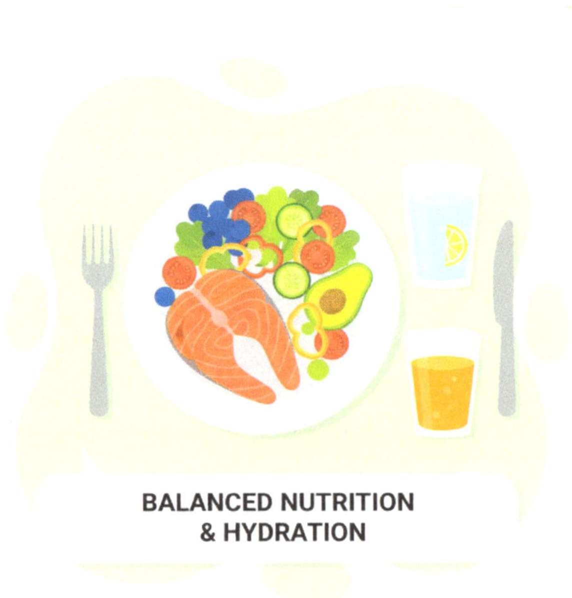

Note: The 7-to-9-hour sleep requirement is questioned by many Hindu Philosophers who state that you need only 4 to 5 hours of sleep time, including the 4 hours 'Delta Sleep'. My respected friend and senior Surya Namaskar practitioner, Rev. Samuel T Thomas practiced the 4

3. Regular Physical Activity

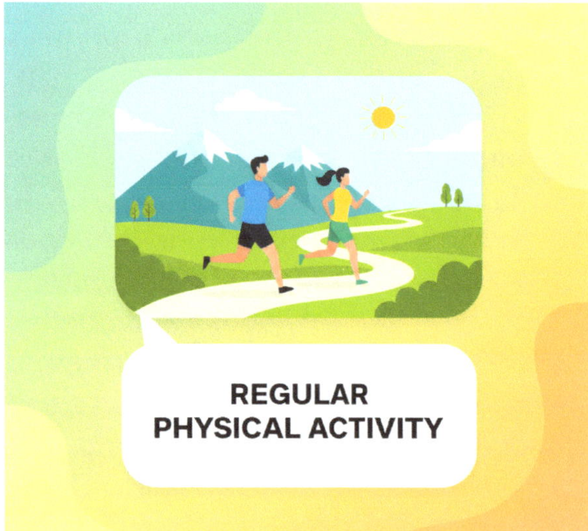

Movement is medicine that benefits every organ system. Regular exercise strengthens muscles and bones, improves cardiovascular health, enhances immune function, and releases mood-boosting endorphins. Whether through walking, swimming, dancing, or structured workouts, consistent physical activity combats obesity, diabetes, depression, and cognitive decline while promoting longevity and quality of life.

4. Stress Management

Chronic stress wreaks havoc on physical and mental health by elevating cortisol levels, suppressing immune function, and contributing to inflammation. Effective stress management through meditation, deep breathing, yoga, or other relaxation techniques protects against anxiety, depression, cardiovascular disease, and digestive disorders. Learning to respond rather than react to stressors builds resilience and emotional stability.

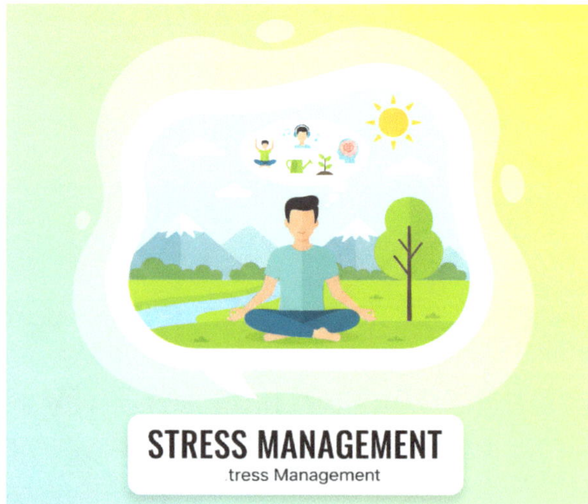

5. Preventive Healthcare and Regular Check-ups

Early detection saves lives and prevents minor issues from becoming major health crises. Regular screenings catch conditions like hypertension, diabetes, and cancer in their most treatable stages. Vaccinations prevent infectious diseases, dental care maintains oral health, and eye exams detect vision problems early. Establi shing relationships with healthcare providers ensures continuity of care and personalized health monitoring.

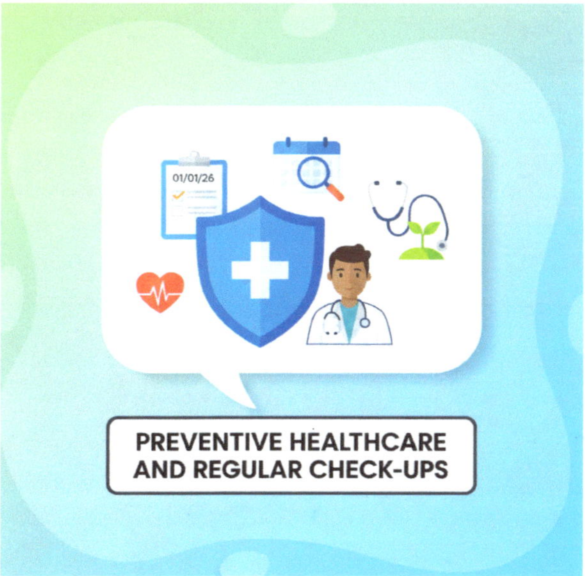

6. Mental Health and Emotional Well-being

Mental health directly impacts physical health through the mind-body connection. Depression and anxiety increase the risk of heart disease, weaken immune function, and accelerate aging. Maintaining emotional well-being through social connections, meaningful activities, professional counseling when needed, and stress reduction protects both mental and physical health throughout life.

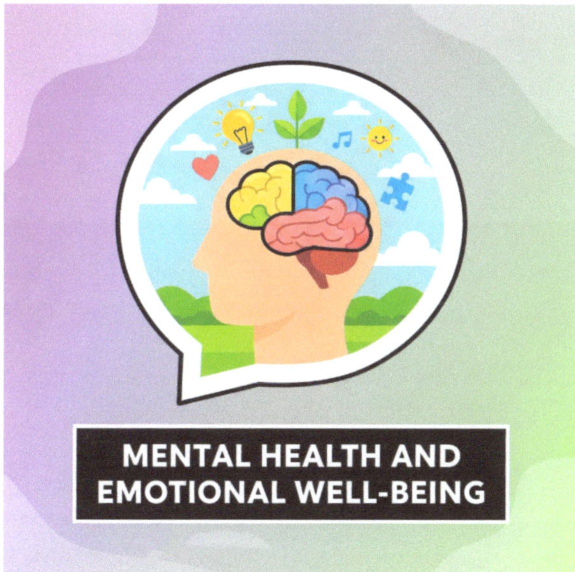

7. Strong Social Connections

Humans are inherently social beings, and meaningful relationships provide profound health benefits. Strong social networks reduce stress, boost immune function, and increase longevity. Loneliness and isolation correlate with increased inflammation, depression, and mortality rates comparable to smoking. Cultivating family bonds, friendships, and community connections supports overall well-being across all life stages.

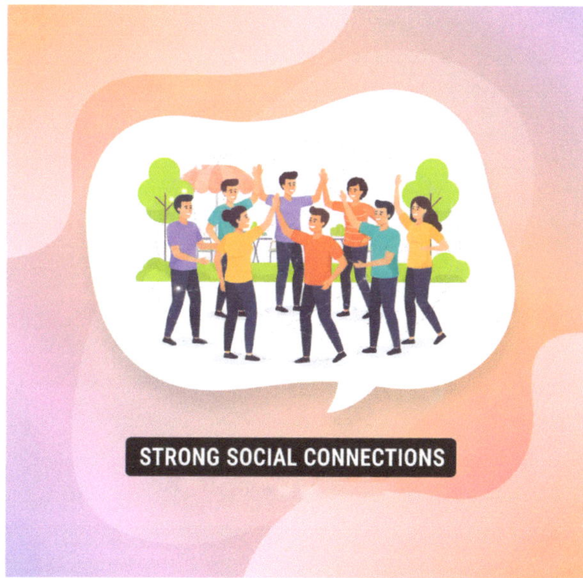

8. Avoiding Harmful Substances

Tobacco use, excessive alcohol consumption, and recreational drugs accelerate aging, increase disease risk, and impair recovery abilities. Smoking alone causes numerous cancers, heart disease, and respiratory disorders. Limiting alcohol intake protects liver function and reduces accident risks. Avoiding harmful substances preserves organ function and maintains the body's natural healing capabilities.

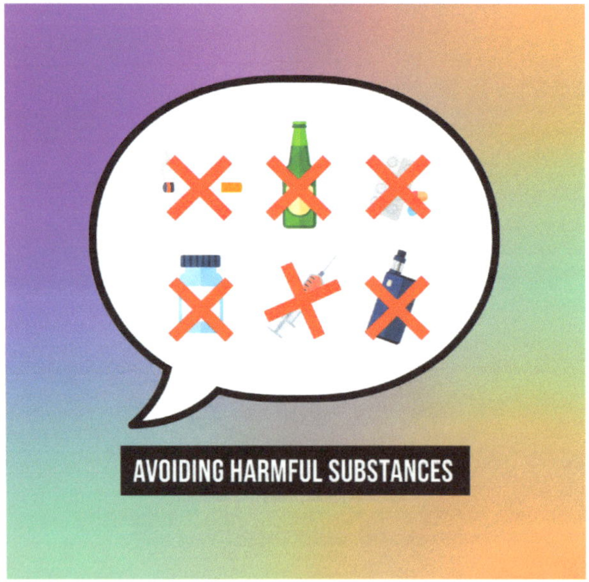

9. Proper Hygiene and Infection Prevention

Basic hygiene practices prevent infectious diseases and maintain health. Regular handwashing, dental care, and personal cleanliness reduce exposure to harmful pathogens. Proper food handling, safe sexual practices, and wound care prevent infections that can become serious health threats. These simple practices form the first line of defense against preventable illnesses.

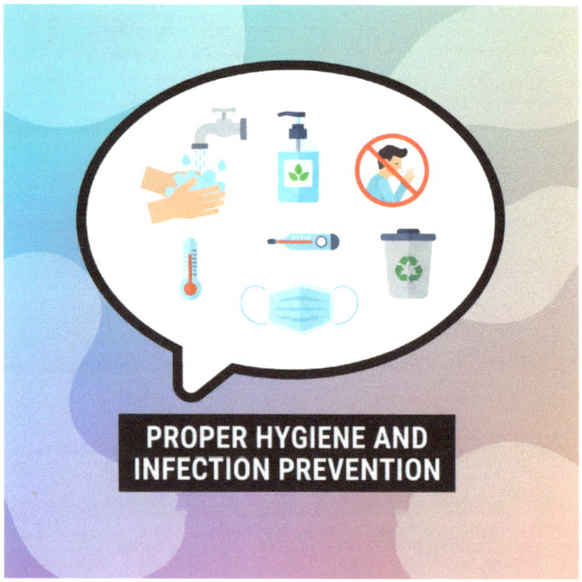

10. Environmental Awareness and Safety

Our surroundings significantly impact health through air quality, chemical exposures, and safety hazards. Using natural cleaning products, ensuring adequate ventilation, practicing safety, and maintaining safe living conditions protect against environmental health risks. Being mindful of pollution exposure, electromagnetic radiation, and toxic substances helps preserve long-term health.

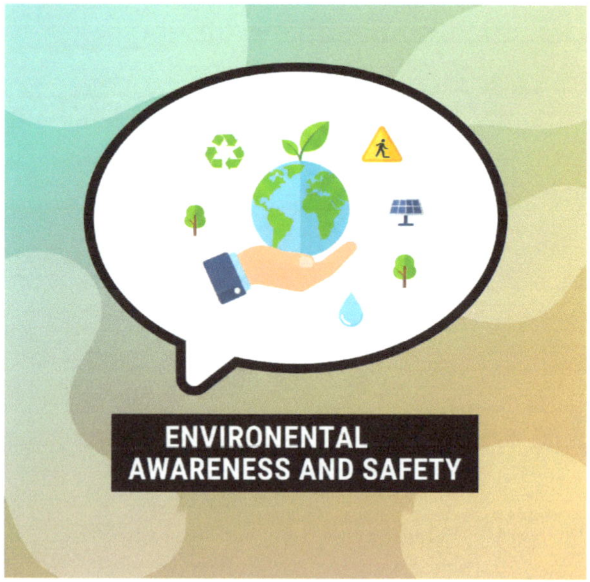

Integration and Balance

These ten aspects work synergistically. Poor sleep affects stress levels, which impacts nutrition choices, which influences energy for exercise. Success comes from viewing health holistically rather than focusing on isolated elements. Small, consistent improvements in each area create compound benefits that dramatically enhance overall well-being.

The beauty of these health fundamentals lies in their accessibility and adaptability. A child needs adequate sleep for growth and learning, while an elderly person needs it for cognitive preservation. Exercise requirements may vary, but movement remains essential throughout life. By prioritizing these ten aspects consistently, regardless of age, individuals create the strongest foundation for lifelong health, vitality, and happiness.

The following Photo was published by Harvard University (Healthy Eating Plate • The Nutrition Source), displaying the proposed proportions of items on your plate.

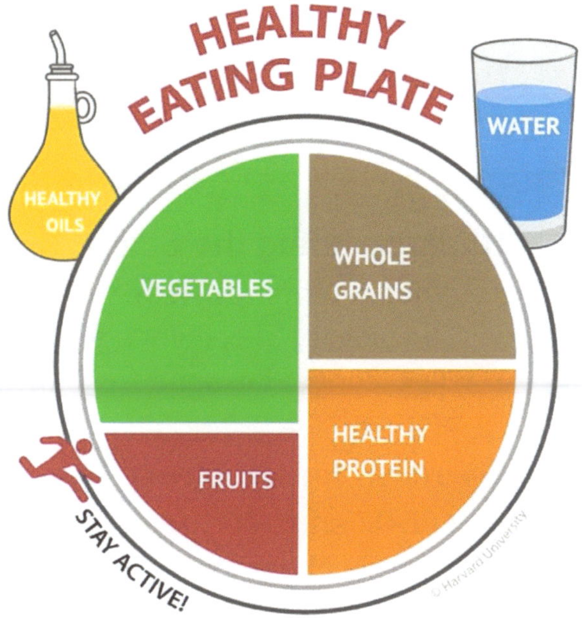

The "7-8-9" Time Management Philosophy

This modern Japanese-influenced approach suggests:

- **7 hours for sleep:** Adequate rest for physical and mental recovery
- **8 hours for work:** The standard professional workday
- **9 hours for personal time:** Everything else, including meals, commute, family, hobbies, and self-care. The 9 hours are divided into 3 sectors of three hours each. First 3 is for your self-care, such as yoga, meditation, exercise, personal hygiene etc. The second 3 is for family time or time spent with close ones. The 3rd sector is for social connections.

The beauty of this framework lies in its recognition that personal time deserves the largest allocation. Those 9 hours encompass morning routines, meals, transportation, exercise, relationships, leisure activities, and evening wind-down time. This acknowledges that life extends far beyond work and sleep.

Most Commonly Accepted Foundations Of Longevity

Part I : Basics

1. **Understanding the Science of Aging**
   - What determines lifespan vs. health span
   - The biology of cellular aging
   - Blue Zones: Lessons from the world's longest-living populations.
2. **Nutrition for Longevity**
   - Anti-inflammatory foods and their benefits
   - The role of antioxidants in preventing disease
   - Optimal macronutrient ratios for different life stages
3. **The Power of Culinary Spices**
   - Healing properties of common spices
   - Incorporating medicinal spices into daily cooking
   - Traditional spice wisdom across cultures
4. **Plant-Based Eating and Longevity**
   - Benefits of increasing plant foods
   - Complete protein sources from plants
   - Practical meal planning strategies
5. **Hydration and Cellular Health**
   - Water's role in aging and disease prevention
   - Herbal teas and functional beverages
   - Signs of chronic dehydration

Part II : Physical Vitality

6. **Movement as Medicine**
   - Exercise recommendations for every age
   - Strength training and bone health
   - Flexibility and balance for fall prevention
7. **Cardiovascular Health Through the Decades**
   - Heart-healthy lifestyle practices
   - Managing blood pressure naturally
   - Understanding cholesterol and heart disease
8. **Maintaining Metabolic Health**
   - Blood sugar regulation and diabetes prevention
   - The impact of intermittent fasting
   - Metabolic syndrome: prevention and reversal
9. **Sleep: The Foundation of Health**
   - Sleep's role in longevity and disease prevention
   - Creating optimal sleep environments
   - Natural strategies for better sleep quality
10. **Brain Health and Cognitive Vitality**
    - Preventing cognitive decline and dementia
    - Neuroplasticity and lifelong learning
    - Memory-boosting activities and nutrition

THE INNATE POWER OF HUMAN SELF - HEALING

Biological Mechanisms and Therapeutic Implications

The human body possesses remarkable self-healing capabilities, orchestrated through complex physiological systems that maintain homeostasis and repair damaged tissues. Understanding these mechanisms provides insight into both natural recovery processes and potential therapeutic interventions.

Immune System Function

The immune system serves as the body's primary defense mechanism, employing innate and adaptive responses to neutralize pathogens and facilitate healing. White blood cells, including macrophages and lymphocytes, identify and eliminate foreign invaders while coordinating tissue repair. The inflammatory response, though often perceived negatively, represents a crucial healing phase that recruits immune cells, increases blood flow, and initiates tissue regeneration.

Cellular Regeneration and Repair

Human tissues exhibit varying regenerative capacities. The liver demonstrates exceptional regenerative ability, restoring functional mass even after significant damage. Bone tissue continuously remodels through osteoblast and osteoclast activity, enabling fracture healing. Skin epithelium regenerates rapidly through stem cell proliferation, closing wounds within days to weeks. However, certain tissues, particularly cardiac and neural tissues, possess limited regenerative capacity, highlighting the variability in self-healing potential across organ systems.

Neuroplasticity and Recovery

The nervous system demonstrates remarkable adaptability through neuroplasticity, allowing neural pathway reorganization following injury. This mechanism underlies recovery from stroke and traumatic brain injury, as surviving neurons form new connections to compensate for damaged areas.

Factors Influencing Self-Healing

Multiple variables affect healing efficiency: adequate nutrition provides essential building blocks for tissue repair; sleep facilitates growth hormone release and cellular restoration; stress management prevents cortisol-mediated immune suppression; and physical activity promotes circulation and metabolic health.

Clinical Implications

Understanding self-healing mechanisms informs medical practice, emphasizing supportive care that optimizes the body's natural recovery processes rather than solely relying on external interventions. This knowledge underpins integrative medicine approaches and rehabilitation protocols that harness innate healing capacity for improved patient outcomes.

Mental Health and Self-Healing

The human mind possesses inherent self-healing capacities that facilitate psychological recovery from trauma, stress, and mental health challenges. Understanding these mechanisms illuminates both natural resilience factors and evidence-based therapeutic approaches that enhance mental wellness.

Neurobiological Foundations

The brain demonstrates neuroplasticity, the ability to form new neural connections and reorganize existing pathways throughout life. This adaptability enables recovery from psychological trauma and supports the development of healthier thought patterns. Research indicates that positive experiences, therapeutic interventions, and mindfulness practices can literally reshape brain structure, strengthening regions associated with emotional regulation while reducing hyperactivity in stress-response centers like the amygdala.

Psychological Resilience

Resilience represents the mind's capacity to adapt to adversity and return to baseline functioning. Key factors include cognitive flexibility, emotional regulation skills, social support networks, and meaning-making abilities. Individuals with strong resilience demonstrate better recovery trajectories following traumatic events, suggesting that psychological self-healing can be cultivated and strengthened.

The Role of Time and Processing

Psychological healing often follows a natural progression through stages of grief, acceptance, and integration. The mind processes difficult experiences during sleep through dream activity and memory consolidation, facilitating emotional resolution. However, this natural healing may be disrupted by avoidance, substance use, or environmental stressors.

Therapeutic Enhancement

While the mind possesses self-healing abilities, professional intervention often accelerates recovery. Cognitive-behavioral therapy helps restructure maladaptive thought patterns, while trauma-focused therapies like EMDR facilitate processing of difficult memories. Medication may support healing by stabilizing neurotransmitter imbalances that impede natural recovery.

Lifestyle Factors

Exercise increases neurotropic factors promoting brain health; adequate sleep consolidates emotional memories; social connection provides validation and support; and creative expression facilitates emotional processing—all enhancing the mind's innate healing capacity.

Conclusion

Mental health self-healing represents a dynamic interplay between biological mechanisms and environmental factors, highlighting both human resilience and the value of supportive interventions.

YOGA AND MEDITATION

A PATH TO MIND-BODY HARMONY

Yoga and meditation represent ancient practices that have transcended cultural boundaries to become essential wellness tools in our modern world. Originating in India over 5,000 years ago, these interconnected disciplines offer profound benefits for physical health, mental clarity, and spiritual well-being.

At its core, yoga means "union" in Sanskrit, referring to the integration of mind, body, and spirit. Traditional yoga encompasses eight limbs, including ethical guidelines, physical postures (asanas), breath control (pranayama), and meditation. The physical practice of yoga posture strengthens muscles, improves flexibility, and enhances balance while promoting proper alignment and body awareness. Regular practice can alleviate chronic pain, reduce inflammation, and boost cardiovascular health.

Meditation, often considered the ultimate goal of yoga, involves training the mind to achieve sustained attention and awareness. Various forms exist, from mindfulness meditation that focuses on present-moment awareness to loving-kindness meditation that cultivates compassion. Concentration practices might involve focusing on the breath, a mantra, or visual imagery, while open awareness techniques allow thoughts and sensations to arise and pass without attachment.

The scientific community has extensively documented the benefits of both practices. Yoga has been shown to lower blood pressure, improve sleep quality, and enhance immune function. Studies indicate that regular yoga practice can reduce symptoms of anxiety, depression, and chronic stress. The combination of physical movement, controlled breathing, and mindful attention creates a powerful therapeutic effect that addresses both psychological and physiological aspects of health.

Meditation research reveals remarkable neuroplasticity benefits. Regular practitioners show increased gray matter density in areas associated with learning, memory, and emotional regulation, while the amygdala, responsible for stress responses, actually shrinks. These changes correlate with improved emotional stability, enhanced focus, and greater resilience to life's challenges.

The relationship between yoga and meditation is synergistic. Physical yoga practices prepare the body for comfortable seated meditation by releasing tension and improving posture. The breath awareness cultivated in yoga naturally leads to deeper meditative states, while meditation enhances the mindful quality of yoga practice. Together, they create a comprehensive system for personal transformation.

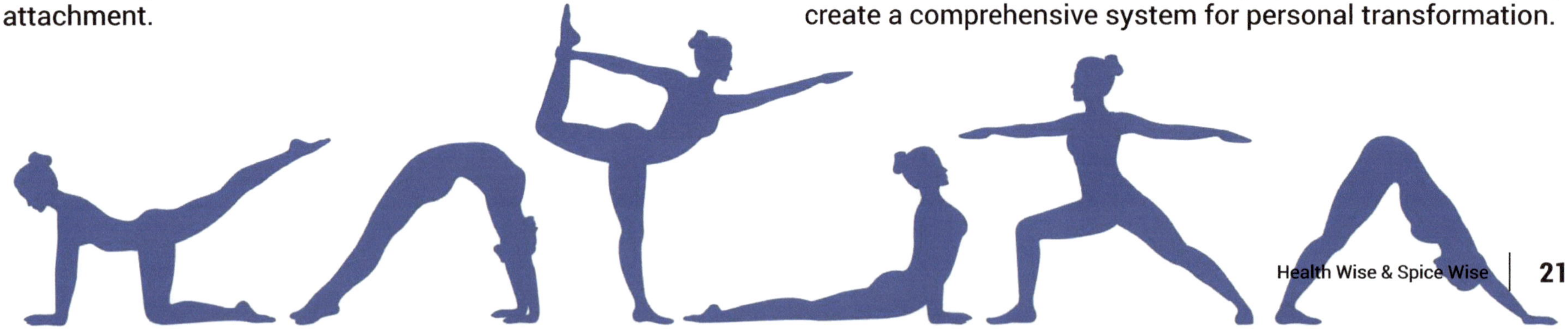

In our fast-paced, digitally dominated world, these practices offer refuge from constant stimulation and stress. The emphasis on present-moment awareness counters our tendency toward multitasking and mental fragmentation. Regular practice develops what practitioners call “witness consciousness” – the ability to observe thoughts and emotions without being overwhelmed by them.

Beginning yoga and meditation requires patience and consistency rather than perfection. Even ten minutes of daily practice can yield significant benefits. Starting with gentle yoga classes or guided meditations provides structure and prevents injury while building confidence and understanding.

The beauty of these practices lies in their accessibility and adaptability. Whether through vigorous vinyasa flow or gentle restorative poses, whether sitting in formal meditation or practicing mindful walking, there are approaches suitable for everybody and every lifestyle.

Ultimately, yoga and meditation offer more than stress relief or physical fitness – they provide tools for cultivating wisdom, compassion, and authentic self-knowledge. In a world that often prioritizes external achievement over inner development, these practices remind us that true well-being emerges from the integration of our physical, mental, and spiritual dimensions.

After migrating to the United States, I have realized the greater value of those traditional practices and routines that have helped in developing a more peaceful and healthier life.

I believe that Yoga, Meditation, and clean-living routines will add to the well-being of any individual and will keep you healthier, no matter what age. As yoga helps breath control and streamlined meditation, it lets you acquire specific bodily postures, all of which in turn help mental tranquility, better health, and strong willpower.

Most Common Yoga Poses:

Since there are many references available on the internet, as well as authored books, I am only going to list the 12 most common poses of Yoga, mostly related to Standing, Balancing, Breathing, Resting, and Bending.

Note: Before you start any exercise or Yoga routines, consult your doctor, as some postures could exacerbate your existing health issues.

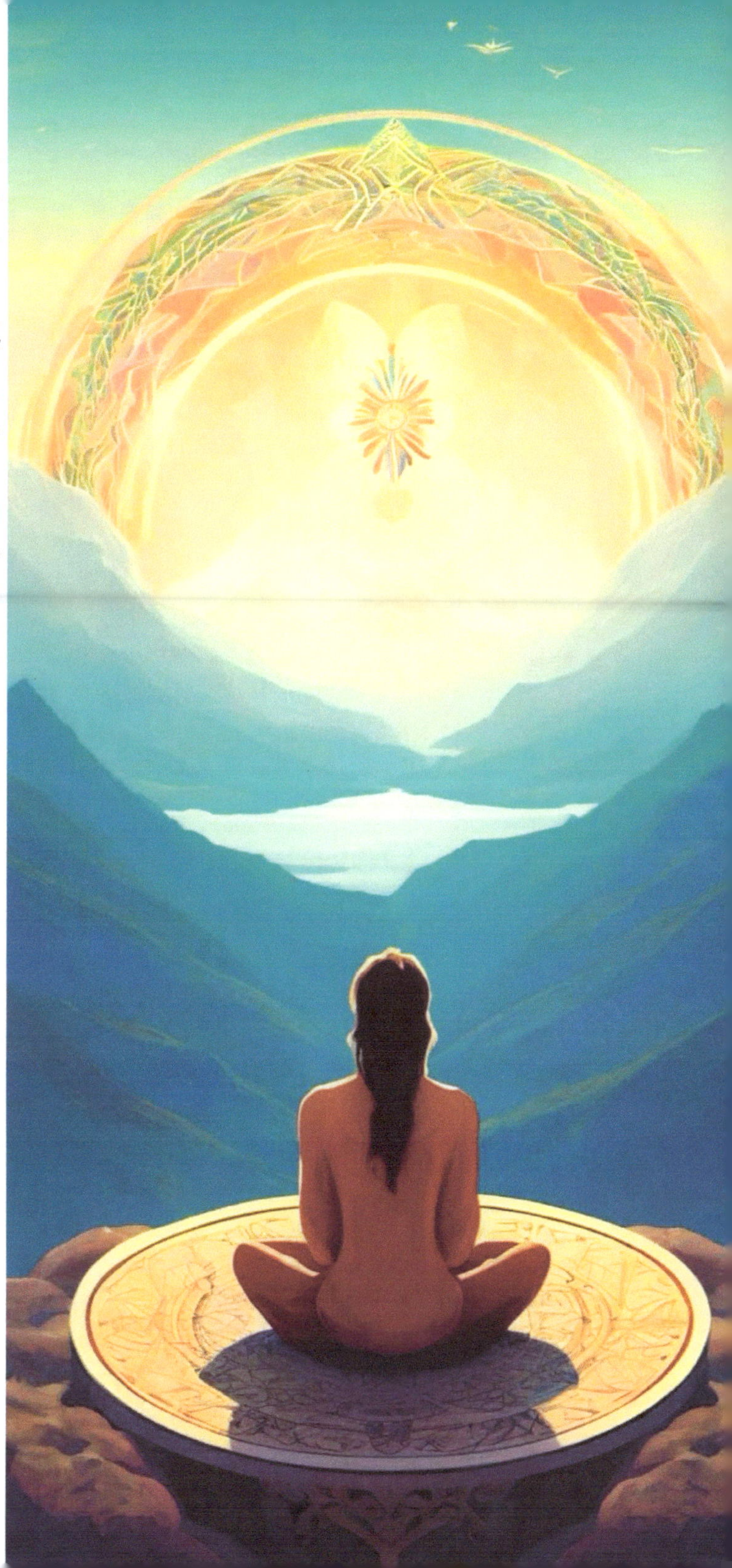

12 Common Postures of Yoga

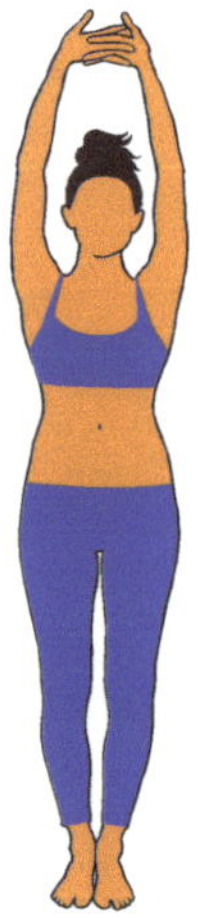

01 Mountain Pose (Tadasana)

Description: The foundation of all standing poses, practiced by standing tall with feet hip-width apart, arms at sides, and weight evenly distributed. Benefits: Improves posture, strengthens legs and core, enhances balance and grounding. Technique: Stand with feet parallel, engage leg muscles, lengthen spine, relax shoulders, and breathe deeply.

02 Downward-Facing Dog (Adho Mukha Svanasana)

Description: An inverted V-shape pose with hands and feet on the ground, hips lifted toward the ceiling. Benefits: Strengthens arms and shoulders, stretches hamstrings and calves, improves circulation, relieves stress. Technique: Start on hands and knees, tuck toes under, lift hips up and back, straighten legs gradually, press hands firmly into mat.

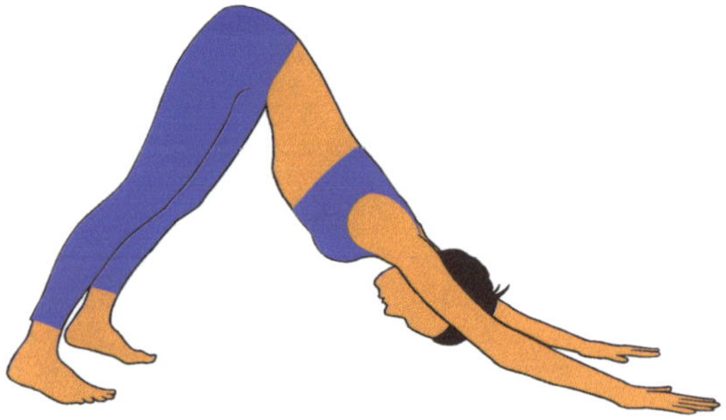

03 Child's Pose (Balasana)

Description: A resting pose where you kneel and sit back on your heels, then fold forward with arms extended or by your sides. Benefits: Calms the nervous system, stretches hips and thighs, relieves stress and fatigue, promotes introspection. Technique: Kneel with big toes touching, sit back on heels, fold forward bringing forehead to mat, extend arms or rest them alongside body.

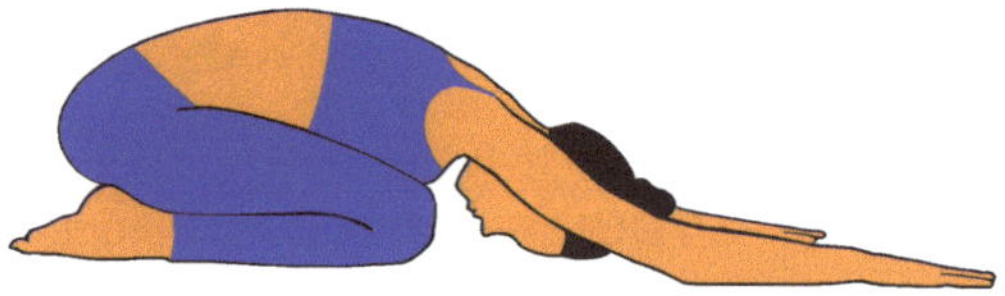

04 Warrior I (Virabhadrasana I)

Description: A powerful standing lunge pose with one foot forward, back leg straight, and arms reaching overhead. Benefits: Strengthens legs and core, opens hips and chest, improves balance and focus, builds confidence. Technique: Step left foot back 3-4 feet, turn left foot out 45 degrees, bend right knee over ankle, square hips forward, raise arms overhead.

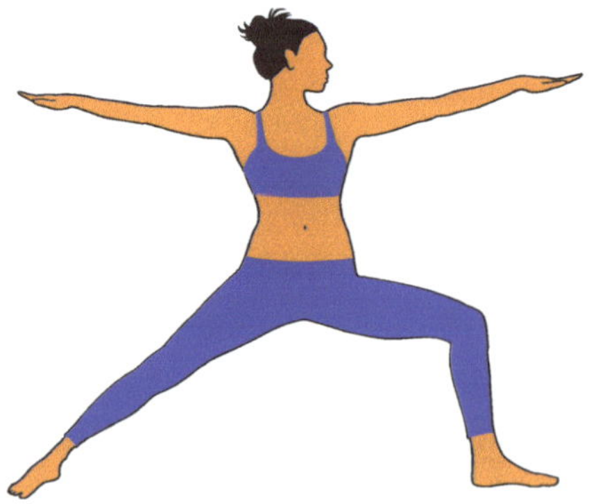

04 Warrior II (Virabhadrasana II)

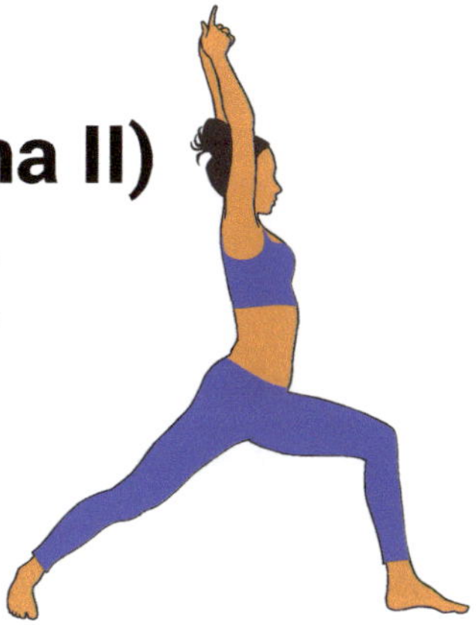

Description: Similar to Warrior I but with arms parallel to the floor and torso facing the side. Benefits: Strengthens legs and core, opens hips and chest, improves stamina and concentration, enhances stability. Technique: From Warrior I, open torso to side, extend arms parallel to floor, gaze over front fingertips, keep front thigh parallel to ground.

05 Tree Pose (Vrikshasana)

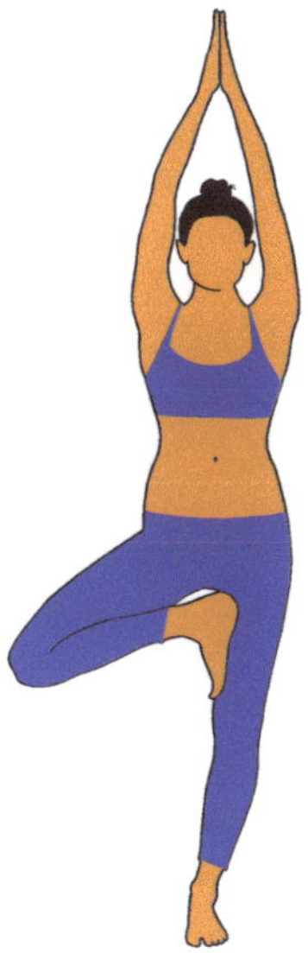

Description: A balancing pose standing on one leg with the other foot placed on the inner thigh or calf. Benefits: Improves balance and concentration, strengthens legs and core, opens hips, enhances focus and mental clarity. Technique: Stand on left leg, place right foot on inner left thigh (avoid knee), press foot into leg and leg into foot, hands in prayer position or overhead.

06 Triangle Pose (Trikonasana)

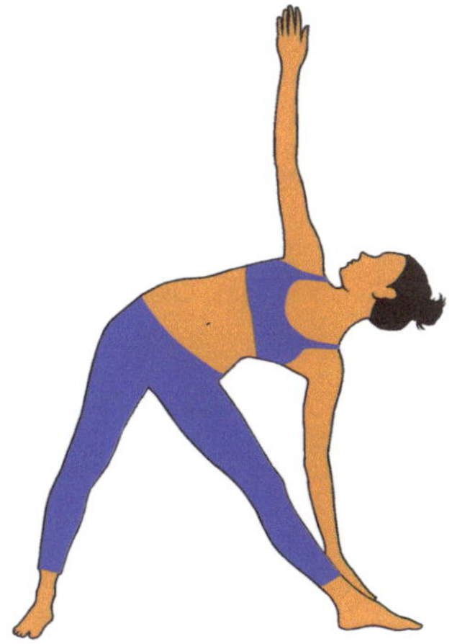

Description: A standing pose forming a triangle shape with legs wide, one hand reaching toward the floor, the other toward the ceiling. Benefits: Strengthens legs, stretches sides of torso, improves balance and digestion, opens chest and shoulders. Technique: Stand with feet 3-4 feet apart, turn right foot out 90 degrees, reach right hand toward floor or shin, extend left arm toward ceiling.

07 Cobra Pose (Bhujangasana)

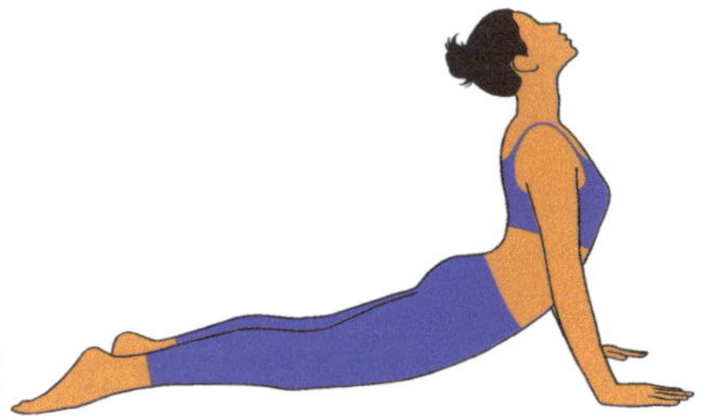

Description: A gentle backbend lying face down, lifting the chest using back muscles and light hand pressure. Benefits: Strengthens back muscles, opens chest and heart, improves spinal flexibility, stimulates abdominal organs. Technique: Lie face down, place palms under shoulders, press pubic bone down, lift chest using back muscles, keep shoulders away from ears.

08 Seated Forward Bend (Paschimottanasana)

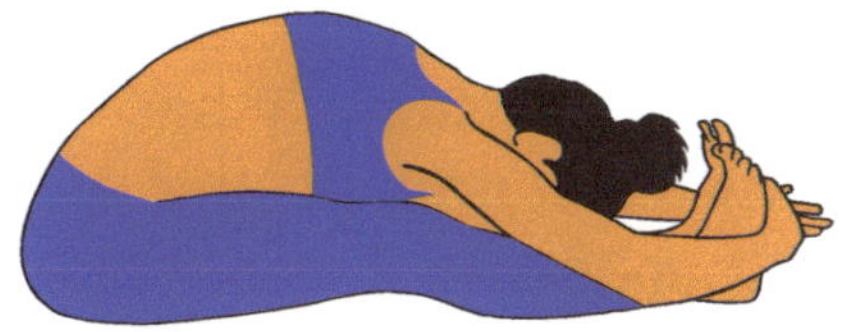

Description: A seated pose folding forward over straight legs, reaching toward feet. Benefits: Stretches hamstrings and spine, calms the nervous system, aids digestion, promotes introspection and patience. Technique: Sit with legs extended, inhale to lengthen spine, exhale to fold forward from hips, keep spine long, reach toward feet or shins.

09 Bridge Pose (Setu Bandhasana)

Description: A gentle backbend lying on your back, lifting hips toward the ceiling while feet and shoulders remain grounded. Benefits: Strengthens back and glutes, opens chest and hip flexors, improves spinal flexibility, energizes the body. Technique: Lie on back with knees bent, feet hip-width apart, press feet down, lift hips, interlace fingers under back or keep arms alongside body.

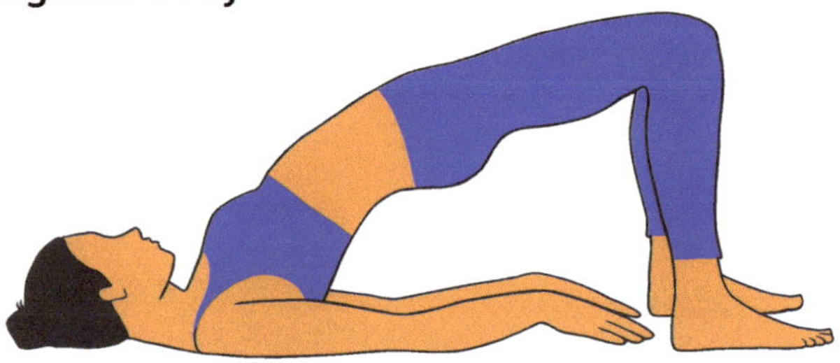

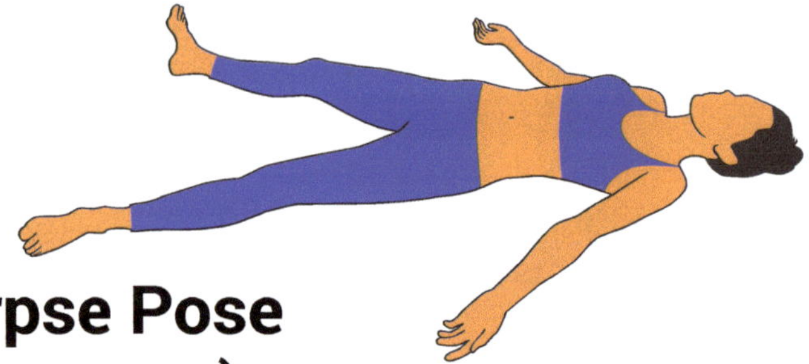

10 Corpse Pose (Savasana)

Description: The final relaxation pose is lying flat on the back with arms and legs comfortably apart, completely relaxed. Benefits: Deep relaxation, stress reduction, integration of practice benefits, calms the nervous system, promotes mindfulness. Technique: Lie on back with legs slightly apart, arms at sides with palms up, close eyes, consciously relax each body part, breathe naturally.

11 Cat-Cow Pose (Marjaryasana-Bitilasana)

Description: A flowing movement between two poses on hands and knees, alternating between arching and rounding the spine. Benefits: Increases spinal flexibility, relieves tension in back and neck, improves posture, warms up the spine. Technique: Start on hands and knees, inhale to arch back (Cow), lift chest and tailbone, exhale to round spine (Cat), tuck chin to chest, repeat fluidly.

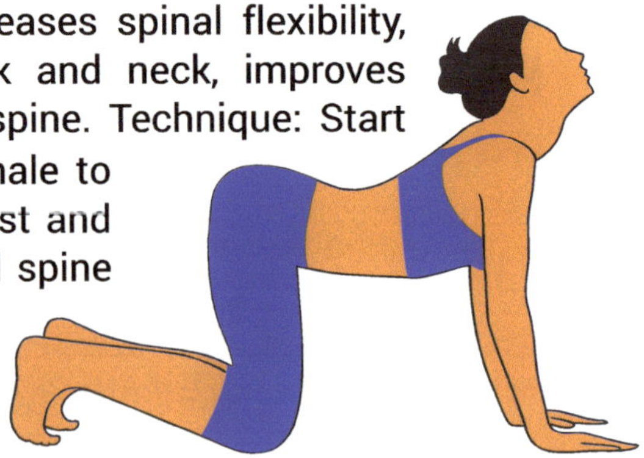

12 Chair Position

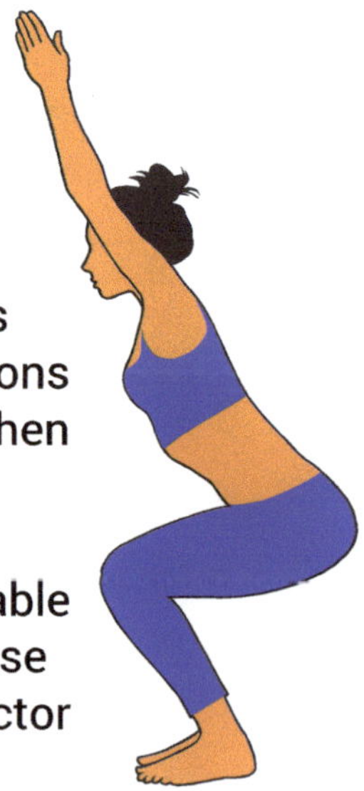

Practice Tips:

- Always warm up before attempting poses
- Listen to your body and never force positions
- Use props (blocks, straps, bolsters) when needed
- Focus on breath throughout practice
- Hold poses for 5-8 breaths or as comfortable
- End practice with relaxation in Corpse Pose
- Consider learning from a qualified instructor for proper alignment.

SURYA NAMASKAR

Surya Namaskar combines most of the above-mentioned beneficial poses and practices of Yoga into one routine with the following steps. I have known friends who practice Surya namaskar daily and are well fit in their physique, avoiding the need for some common adult medications

Surya Namaskar(Sun Salutation) is one of the most complete and powerful yoga practices, often called a "complete body workout" in a single sequence. Here's why it's so important:

Physical Benefits:

Cardiovascular health - When done at a moderate to fast pace, it provides excellent cardio exercise, strengthening the heart and improving circulation throughout the body.

Full-body workout - The sequence engages virtually every major muscle group. You're stretching, strengthening, and toning your arms, shoulders, chest, abs, back, glutes, hamstrings, and calves all in one flow.

Flexibility and strength - The forward folds stretch your hamstrings and spine, while poses like Plank and Chaturanga build arm and core strength. The backward bends open your chest and improve spinal flexibility.

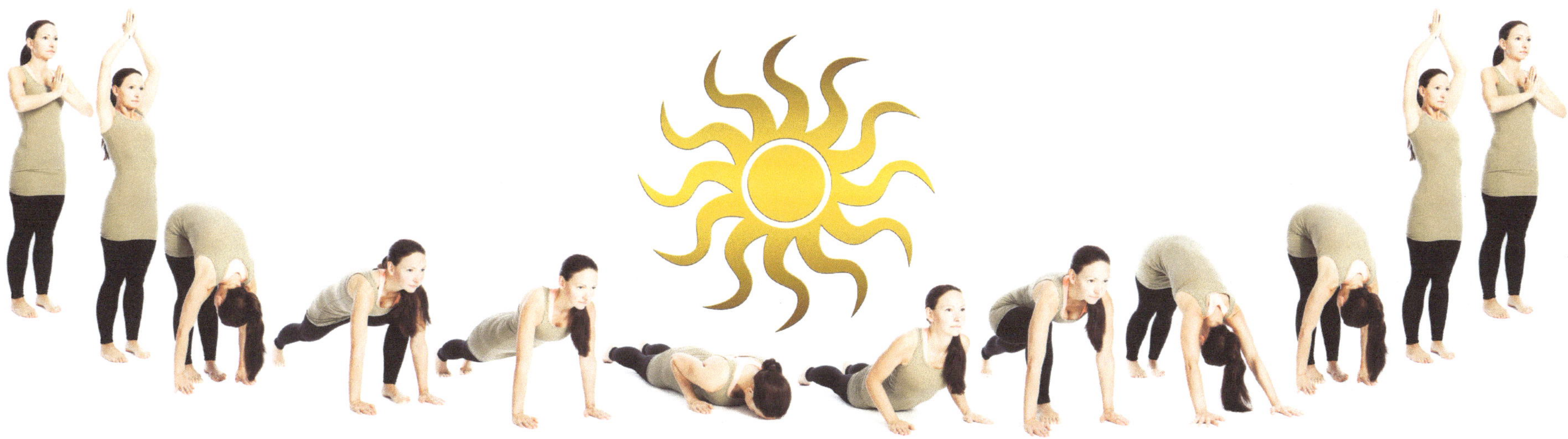

Weight management - A vigorous practice of multiple rounds can burn significant calories and boost metabolism.

Improves posture - The alternating forward and backward bends help correct postural imbalances from sitting and strengthen the muscles that support proper alignment.

Digestive health - The compression and stretching of the abdomen massages internal organs and can improve digestion and elimination.

Mental and Energetic Benefits:

Mind-body connection - Coordinating movement with breath (one pose per inhale or exhale) creates a moving meditation that calms mental chatter and improves focus.

Stress Reduction - The rhythmic breathing and flowing movement activate the parasympathetic nervous system, reducing stress hormones and promoting relaxation.

Energy boost - Despite being calming, it also energizes. Many practitioners do it in the morning to wake up the body and mind.

Breath awareness - It trains proper breathing patterns, increasing lung capacity and oxygen intake.

Spiritual Significance:

Traditional reverence - Historically, it was practiced at sunrise as a way to honor the sun, the source of all life and energy. Each of the 12 positions has a corresponding mantra honoring different aspects of the sun.

Chakra activation - The sequence is believed to activate and balance all seven chakras (energy centers) in the body.

Practical Advantages:

Time-efficient - One complete round takes only 2-3 minutes, making it perfect for busy schedules. Even 5-10 rounds (10-20 minutes) provides substantial benefits.

No equipment needed - Just your body and a small space. It can be done anywhere.

Scalable - Beginners can move slowly with modifications, while advanced practitioners can do 108 rounds for an intense workout!

Foundation for yoga practice - It's often used as a warm-up before other yoga poses because it prepares the entire body.

The Complete Sequence:

The traditional 12-step sequence includes: Prayer Pose →Raised Arms→Forward Fold→Equestrian Pose→Plank→Eight-Limbed Pose→Cobra→Downward Dog→Equestrian Pose→Forward Fold→Raised Arms→Prayer Pose.

This creates a perfect balance of forward bends, backward bends, and inversions.

How many rounds?

Traditional practitioners aim for 12 rounds (representing the 12 sun gods or months), though some do 108 rounds on special occasions. For beginners, even 3-5 rounds daily can make a significant difference in overall health and wellbeing.

Surya Namaskar is truly a complete practice - it's like getting the benefits of multiple yoga poses, cardio exercise, strength training, and meditation all rolled into one beautiful, flowing sequence!

Surya Namaskar (Sun Salutation) Poses of Yoga

Here's a typical 12-pose version of Sun Salutation (Surya Namaskar A)

1. **Mountain Pose** (Tadasana) standing, palms together
2. **Raised Arms Pose** (Urdhva Hastasana) arms reach up
3. **Forward Bend** (Uttanasana) fold forward
4. **Half-Lift** (Ardha Uttanasana) Lift torso midway
5. **Plank Pose** (Dandasana) strong straight body
6. **Four-Limb Staff Pose** (Chaturanga Dandasana) lower halfway
7. **Upward Facing Dog** (Urdhva Mukha Svanasana) back-bend
8. **Downward Facing Dog** (Adho Mukha Svanasana) Hips up
9. **Lunge / Ashwa Sanchalanasana** step foot forward
10. **Forward Bend again** (Uttanasana)
11. **Raised Arms again** (Urdhva Hastasana)
12. **Mountain Pose** (Tadasana) return to standing

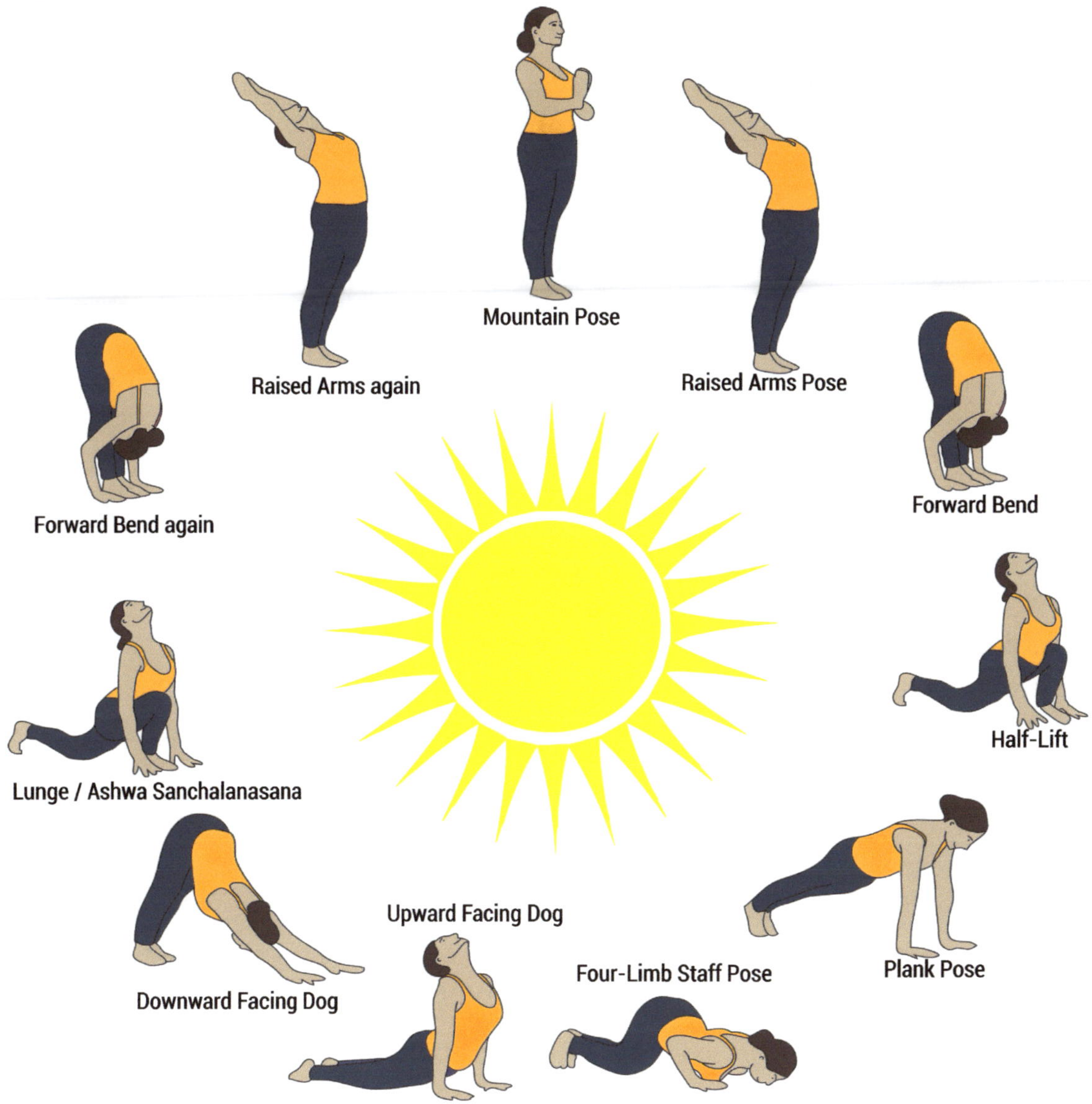

LET THERE BE LIGHT

WHY YOUR BODY AND MIND NEED DAILY SUNLIGHT

A Review of Current Research on Solar Exposure, Neurochemistry, and Emotional Well-Being

Introduction

For most of human history, life unfolded outdoors. Dawn signaled wakefulness, midday brought productive heat, and dusk whispered it was time to rest. The sun was not merely background scenery — it was an active biological regulator, orchestrating hormones, neurotransmitters, and cellular processes across every system of the body. Today, the average adult spends more than 90 percent of waking hours indoors under artificial lighting, a radical departure from our evolutionary heritage that growing evidence links to rising rates of depression, sleep dysfunction, and chronic disease.

Sunlight is not a single, uniform force. It is a complex spectrum of radiation — ultraviolet-A (UVA), ultraviolet-B (UVB), visible light, and infrared — each interacting with the body in distinct and complementary ways. This article examines the science behind those interactions, focusing on what happens in the brain and body when sunlight touches our skin and enters our eyes, and why a daily dose of natural light may be one of the most powerful, cost-free health interventions available.

Sunlight and the Brain: The Serotonin Connection

Among the most well-documented effects of sunlight is its capacity to elevate levels of serotonin, a neurotransmitter often called the "feel-good chemical" because of its central role in mood regulation, appetite control, and sleep.

A landmark study published in The Lancet (Lambert et al., 2002) measured serotonin metabolites in the blood of 101 healthy men and found that the rate of serotonin production by the brain was directly related to the duration of bright sunlight on that day, rising rapidly as luminosity increased and reaching its lowest levels in winter. This neurochemical fluctuation helps explain the well-recognized phenomenon of Seasonal Affective Disorder (SAD), a form of depression that affects an estimated 5 percent of adults in the United States and as much as 10 percent of the population in northern latitudes, where winter daylight can be extremely limited.

A 2024 study lends further clinical weight to these findings, reporting that spending more than one hour in natural daylight during winter months provided meaningful protection against depression symptoms. Serotonin deficiency, meanwhile, is increasingly recognized as a contributor not only to low mood and depression, but also to anxiety disorders, insomnia, and impaired cognitive function — conditions that have become epidemic in modern, predominantly indoor societies.

Dopamine, Endorphins, and the Full Neurochemical Picture

Serotonin is only one piece of the puzzle. Sunlight exposure also stimulates the release of dopamine, a neurotransmitter involved in motivation, reward, and focus, as well as beta-endorphins — the body's natural opioids — which produce feelings of pleasure and reduce pain perception. Additionally, UVA exposure to the skin triggers the production of nitric oxide, a molecule that research has shown can reduce inflammation and oxidative stress, resulting in decreased anxiety and depression. The simultaneous elevation of multiple mood-regulating chemicals helps explain why time spent in sunshine tends to produce a sense of well-being that is difficult to replicate with any single supplement or medication.

Vitamin D: The Sunshine Hormone

Sunlight's most famous gift to the body is vitamin D, often mischaracterized as merely a vitamin but more accurately functioning as a hormone. When UVB rays strike the skin, they convert a cholesterol precursor into vitamin D3 (cholecalciferol), which is then processed by the liver and kidneys into the biologically active form that governs hundreds of physiological processes. More than 90 percent of the body's vitamin D originates from sunlight exposure, not diet — a fact that underscores just how dependent human health is on regular access to the sun.

The mental health implications of vitamin D are substantial and increasingly supported by evidence. Vitamin D receptors have been identified in regions of the brain directly associated with depression and mood regulation. The hormone influences the production of serotonin by activating the genes responsible for its synthesis, and it regulates the Tyrosine Hydroxylase gene, which controls the production of dopamine and norepinephrine. A 2024 prospective cohort study published in the Journal of Psychiatric Research found a statistically significant association between vitamin D deficiency and elevated risk of depression, with sex-specific differences suggesting women may be particularly vulnerable due to hormonal effects on vitamin D metabolism.

Beyond mood, vitamin D deficiency is linked to a striking range of health consequences: weakened bones (rickets in children, osteoporosis in adults), impaired immune response, and — according to a 2024 study of over 269,000 adults — a 19 to 25 percent increased risk of dementia in those with clinically deficient levels. Despite widespread availability of supplements, vitamin D deficiency remains common, particularly in winter months and among those who spend most of their time indoors.

Circadian Rhythms, Sleep, and the Timing of Light

Beyond its neurochemical effects, sunlight serves as the primary time-keeping signal for the body's circadian clock — the internal biological rhythm that governs the sleep-wake cycle, body temperature, hormone secretion, digestion, and even cardiovascular function. The master pacemaker of this system resides in the suprachiasmatic nuclei (SCN) of the hypothalamus, a pair of tiny neural structures that receive light input directly from the retina and use it to synchronize internal biology with the external environment.

Morning sunlight is especially powerful in this regard. A 2025 study published in BMC Public Health involving 1,762 adults found that exposure to natural light before 10 a.m. significantly improved sleep quality and aligned the sleep midpoint — a reliable indicator of circadian health. When morning light enters the eyes, it suppresses melatonin (the sleep-promoting hormone) and activates alerting pathways involving cortisol and dopamine, signaling the body that the day has begun. This cascade improves daytime energy, concentration, and mood, while also ensuring melatonin rises appropriately at night to facilitate deep, restorative sleep.

Practical Guidance: How Much Sunlight Do We Need?

Health experts generally recommend 10 to 30 minutes of direct sunlight on bare skin several times per week as sufficient to maintain healthy vitamin D levels for most lighter-skinned adults — though individuals with darker skin tones, older adults, and those living at higher latitudes may require significantly longer exposure due to differences in UV absorption and skin metabolism. Morning light for circadian entrainment requires as little as 5 to 10 minutes on a clear day, or 15 to 20 minutes on an overcast day, since even diffuse daylight is far brighter than typical indoor artificial lighting.

For those who cannot access sufficient natural sunlight due to geography, season, or health limitations, light therapy boxes that emit bright white light (typically 10,000 lux) for 30 to 60 minutes daily have been shown to replicate many of sunlight's mood and circadian benefits and are a recognized treatment for Seasonal

Affective Disorder. However, light therapy does not deliver UVB radiation and therefore does not stimulate vitamin D synthesis, meaning dietary sources or supplements remain necessary for those with limited sun access.

It is also important to note that sunlight, like most powerful biological agents, requires moderation. Prolonged exposure to UV radiation — particularly during peak hours between 10 a.m. and 2 p.m. in summer — increases the risk of skin cancer. The prudent approach is one of informed balance: seek regular, moderate sunlight exposure with appropriate sun protection for extended periods, rather than avoidance on one extreme or excessive tanning on the other.

Conclusion

The prescription, for most people, is elegantly simple: spend time in natural light every day, especially in the morning. The evidence suggests the return on that investment — in mood, cognition, sleep, and long-term health — may be greater than nearly any pharmaceutical alternative.

References

Lambert, G., Reid, C., Kaye, D., Jennings, G., & Esler, M. (2002). Effect of sunlight and season on serotonin turnover in the brain. The Lancet, 360(9348), 1840–1842. https://doi.org/10.1016/S0140-6736(02)11737-5

Ceolin, G., et al. (2021). Vitamin D and its role in regulating mood and emotional well-being. In: De Oliveira, C., et al. (2018). Cited in: Predicted vitamin D levels and risk of depression in the SUN Project. Journal of Psychiatric Research, 179, 1–7. https://doi.org/10.1016/j.jpsychires.2024.09.028

Chen, H., et al. (2024). Vitamin D supplementation, vitamin D levels, and incidence of dementia: data from 269,229 adults over 14 years. Cited by GrassrootsHealth Nutrient Research Institute. https://www.grassrootshealth.net/blog/improve-brain-power-mood-sunshine-vitamin-d/

Gubin, D. G., Borisenkov, M. F., et al. (2024). Evaluating circadian light hygiene: Methodology and health implications. Russian Open Medical Journal, 13, e0415.

Holick, M. F. (2008). Vitamin D and sunlight: Strategies for cancer prevention and other health benefits. Clinical Journal of the American Society of Nephrology, 3(5), 1548–1554. https://doi.org/10.2215/CJN.01060308

Kent, S. T., McClure, L. A., et al. (2009). Effect of sunlight exposure on cognitive function among depressed and non-depressed participants. Environmental Health, 8, 34. https://doi.org/10.1186/1476-069X-8-34

Mead, M. N. (2008). Benefits of sunlight: A bright spot for human health. Environmental Health Perspectives, 116(4), A160–A167. https://pmc.ncbi.nlm.nih.gov/articles/PMC2290997/

Menon, V., et al. (2020). Vitamin D receptors in brain regions implicated in depression. Cited in SUN Project study above.

Nall, R., & Perkins, S. (2025, August 1). What are the health benefits of sunlight? Healthline. https://www.healthline.com/health/depression/benefits-sunlight

Pereira, M., et al. (2025). The role of sunlight in sleep regulation: Analysis of morning, evening and late exposure. BMC Public Health. https://link.springer.com/article/10.1186/s12889-025-24618-8

Sansone, R. A., & Sansone, L. A. (2013). Sunshine, serotonin, and skin: A partial explanation for seasonal patterns in psychopathology? Innovations in Clinical Neuroscience, 10(7–8), 20–24. https://pmc.ncbi.nlm.nih.gov/articles/PMC3779905/

Shaffer, J. (2025, February 20). The health benefits of sunshine. Cleveland Clinic Health Essentials. https://health.clevelandclinic.org/how-much-sunshine-you-need-daily

Wacker, M., & Holick, M. F. (2013). Sunlight and vitamin D: A global perspective for health. Dermato-Endocrinology, 5(1), 51–108.

BREATHING EXERCISES

Breathing exercises are incredibly valuable and significant in physical, mental, and emotional well-being. Here's why:

Physical Benefits

Improved Oxygen Flow: They help deliver more oxygen to your body and organs, boosting overall function.

Better Lung Capacity: Breathing exercises strengthen the lungs, which is especially helpful for people with asthma or other respiratory conditions.

Stress Reduction: Deep breathing activates the parasympathetic nervous system, which calms the body and reduces stress-related tension.

Mental and Emotional Benefits

Stress and Anxiety Relief: Controlled breathing techniques are proven to reduce cortisol (stress hormone) levels.

Enhanced Focus and Clarity: Mindful breathing helps clear mental clutter and improves concentration.

Emotional Regulation: Breathing exercises can stabilize mood and bring a sense of balance during difficult times.

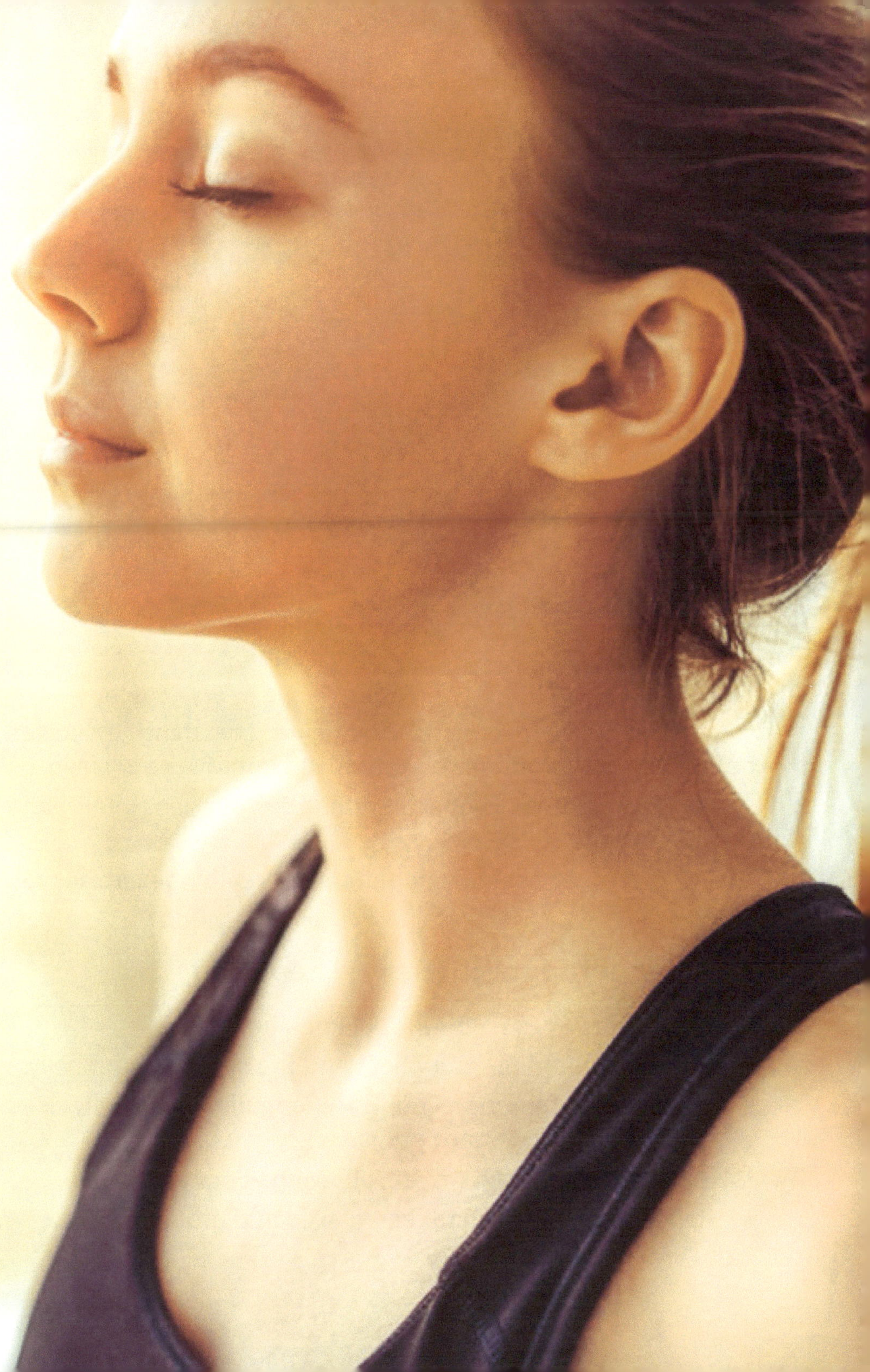

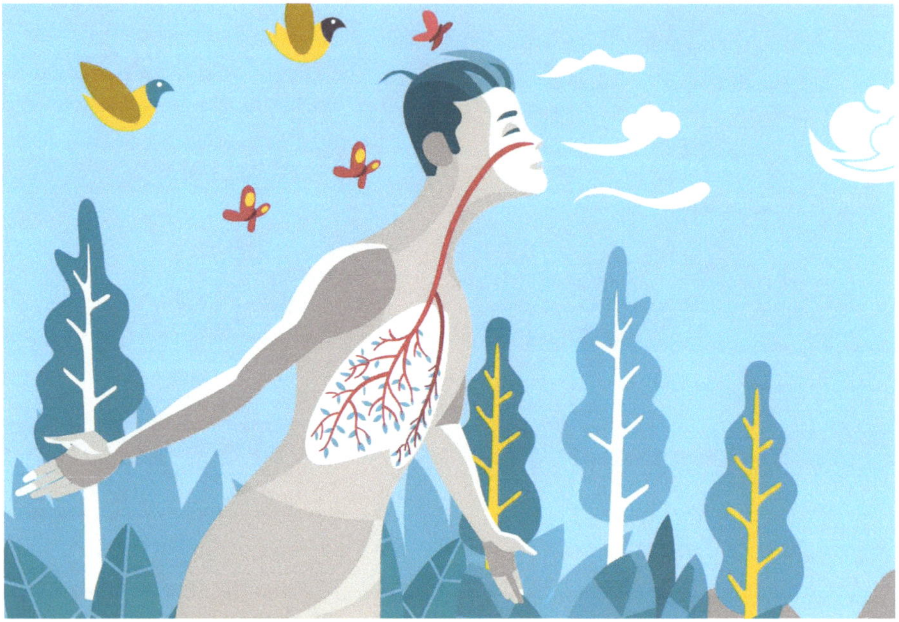

Overall Wellness

Sleep Improvement: Practicing breathing exercises before bed can promote relaxation and improve your sleep.

Energy Boost: Proper breathing can increase vitality and combat fatigue.

Here are a few simple and effective breathing exercises you can try:

1. Diaphragmatic (Belly) Breathing

- Sit or lie down in a comfortable position.
- Place one hand on your chest and the other on your belly.
- Inhale deeply through your nose, ensuring your belly rises (your chest should stay still).
- Exhale through your mouth, allowing your belly to fall.
- Repeat 5-10 minutes to feel relaxed and grounded.

2. Box Breathing:

- Inhale through your nose for a count of 4.
- Hold your breath for a count of 4.
- Exhale slowly through your mouth for a count of 4.
- Hold your breath again for a count of 4 before repeating the cycle.
- Continue for a few minutes to calm your mind.

3. Alternate Nostril Breathing (Nadi Shodhana)

- Sit comfortably and use your thumb to close your right nostril.
- Inhale deeply through your left nostril.
- Close your left nostril with your ring finger and release your thumb from the right nostril.
- Exhale through the right nostril.
- Inhale through the right nostril, then switch and exhale through the left nostril.
- Repeat for 5–10 cycles to feel balanced.

4. 4-7-8 Breathing:

- Inhale through your nose for a count of 4.
- Hold your breath for a count of 7.
- Exhale completely through your mouth for a count of 8.
- Repeat for 4–5 cycles; this technique is great for relaxation and sleep.

THE IMPORTANCE & BENEFITS OF MEDITATION & Life Longevity

An Evidence-Based Review of Scientific Research, Clinical Findings, and Ancient Wisdom

INTRODUCTION

Ancient Practice in a Modern Age

For more than 5,000 years, meditation has been woven into the spiritual and healing traditions of civilizations from India to China, Japan to the Middle East. Practiced by Buddhist monks, Vedic sages, Christian contemplatives, and Sufi mystics alike, it has long been valued as a path to inner stillness and transcendent wisdom. What distinguishes our era is that, for the first time in human history, we possess the scientific tools — neuroimaging, molecular biology, epidemiology, and randomized controlled trials — to investigate what these ancient practitioners claimed: that meditation does not merely calm the mind. It changes the body at the deepest levels, and may, in doing so, extend healthy human life.

The scope of research has expanded enormously in recent decades. Institutions including Harvard Medical School, Johns Hopkins University, the Max Planck Institute, and the University of Massachusetts Medical School have produced hundreds of peer-reviewed studies on the physiological, neurological, and psychological effects of meditation. Their collective findings converge on a remarkable picture: consistent meditation practice is associated with measurable improvements in cellular aging, cardiovascular health, brain structure, immune function, stress regulation, and psychological resilience — each of which is directly relevant to longevity.

This article reviews the principal mechanisms through which meditation influences the ageing process and lifespan, examines the strongest available evidence, considers the different types of practice and their effects, and offers practical guidance for beginning a sustained practice. It draws on findings from mindfulness-based stress reduction (MBSR), transcendental meditation (TM), loving-kindness meditation (LKM), Zen practice, and yoga-based meditation, and synthesis results from meta-analyses, randomized controlled trials, neuroimaging studies, and longitudinal cohort investigations.

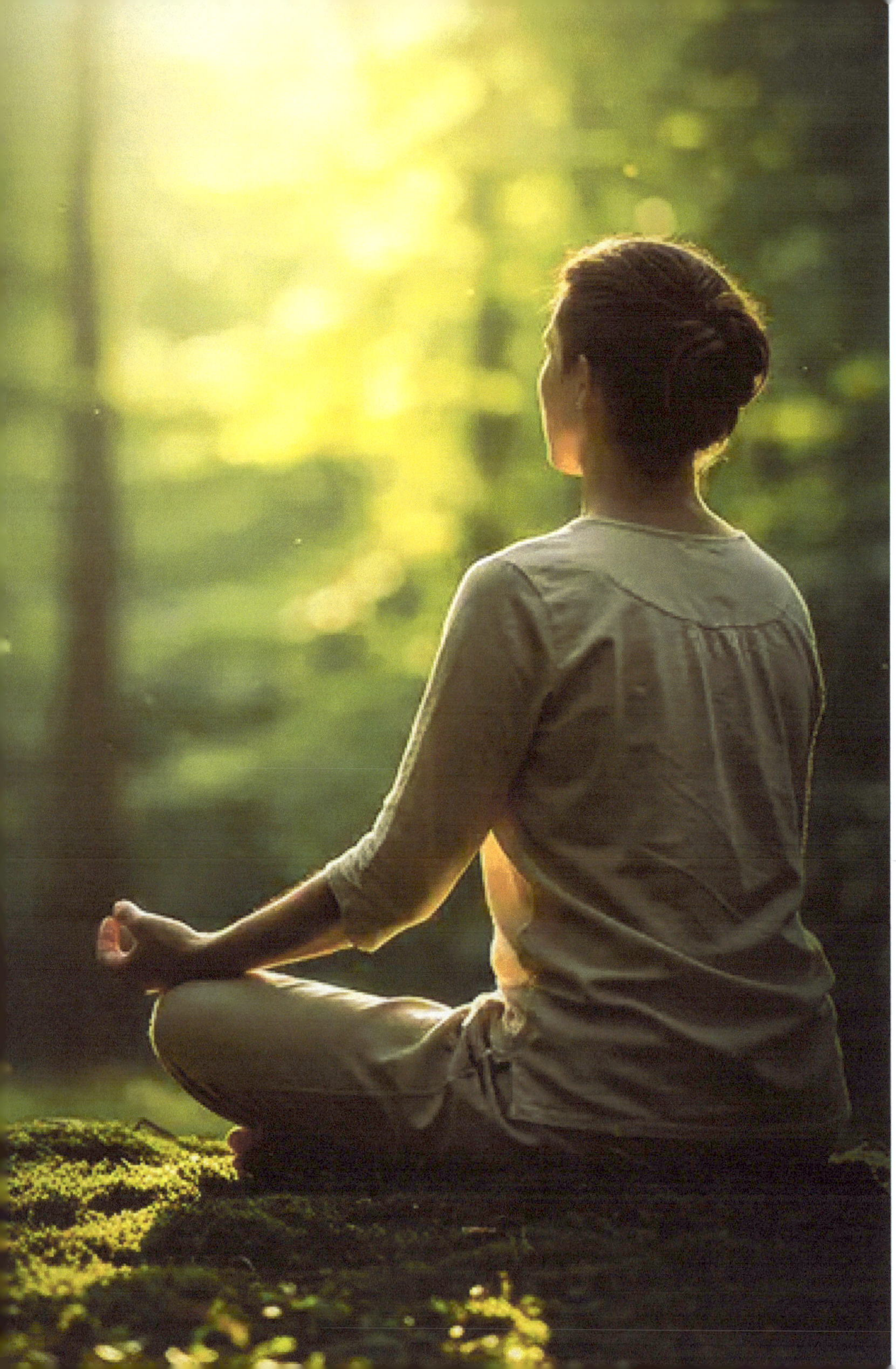

Telomeres, Telomerase, and the Biology of Cellular Ageing

At the heart of the modern science of longevity lies the telomere — the protective cap at the end of each chromosome, functionally analogous to the plastic tip on a shoelace. With each cell division, telomeres shorten. When they become critically short, the cell either enters a state of senescence (permanently halting division) or undergoes programmed death (apoptosis). Telomere length is therefore a direct measure of cellular age and a predictive biomarker for a range of age-related diseases including cardiovascular disease, Alzheimer's, cancer, and diabetes.

The enzyme telomerase partially counteracts this shortening by adding telomeric sequences back to chromosome ends. Research now demonstrates that psychological stress accelerates telomere attrition — by increasing oxidative stress and cortisol-mediated damage to DNA — while practices that reduce stress appear to preserve or even restore telomere integrity. This is the central biological pathway linking meditation to longevity.

Evidence from Meta-Analyses and Clinical Trials

The research based on meditation and telomere biology is substantial and growing. A 2020 meta-analysis published in PubMed, consolidating results from 11 studies and 12 comparisons, found that meditating individuals had significantly longer telomeres than those in control conditions, with an overall weighted effect size of g = 0.40 (Schutte & Malouff, 2020). While trimming for outliers reduced this to g = 0.16, the directional consistency was clear: more hours of meditation practice was associated with proportionally larger protective effects.

A 2023 comprehensive systematic review and meta-analysis published in Mindfulness (Bossert et al., 2023) the most thorough synthesis to date — incorporated 25 studies involving 2,099 participants. The review found that mindfulness-based interventions produced small-to-medium positive effects on both telomere length (g = 0.23; 95% CI [0.07, 0.39]; p = 0.006) and telomerase activity (g = 0.37 [0.01, 0.73]; p = 0.046). The study found that greater meditation does more hours practiced — was the strongest moderator of effect size across both outcomes.

A case-control study from the University of Colombo, Sri Lanka (Dasanayaka et al., 2023), recruited 30 long-term meditators matched with 30 non-meditating controls. Long-term meditators demonstrated not only longer relative telomere lengths and higher telomerase enzyme levels, but also elevated expression of the hTERT and hTR genes — the genetic machinery directly responsible for telomerase activity. Critically, the meditators showed lower levels of nitric oxide and higher antioxidant capacity, suggesting that meditation reduces the oxidative stress environment that damages telomeres. Notably, in this cohort, age showed no significant association with telomere length among meditators — a finding that starkly contrasts with the normal age-telomere relationship seen in non-meditators.

An influential earlier study (Hoge et al., 2013) found that women who practiced loving-kindness meditation had significantly longer telomeres than age, gender, education, and trauma-matched controls — raising the intriguing possibility that compassion-based meditative practices may carry specific benefits for cellular longevity beyond stress-reduction effects alone.

> To understand the importance of meditation is to understand the biology of ageing itself — for the two are more deeply connected than most people realize.
>
> — **Dr. Elizabeth Blackburn,** Nobel Laureate in Physiology (2009)

Meditation and Cellular Longevity: Key Findings

- Long-term meditators show longer telomere length across multiple independent studies and meta-analyses.
- Meditation is associated with higher telomerase activity — the enzyme that rebuilds protective chromosome caps.
- Long-term meditators show elevated expression of hTERT and hTR genes, the molecular machinery of telomere maintenance.
- Age showed no significant association with telomere length in one cohort of experienced meditators — compared to the expected negative correlation in non-meditators.
- Meditation reduces oxidative stress and cortisol — both established accelerants of telomere attrition.
- Higher meditation dose (total hours practiced) is the strongest predictor of telomere-protective effect across studies.

The theoretical framework linking meditation to telomere maintenance was most elegantly described by Epel, Daubenmier, Blackburn, and colleagues (2009) in their foundational paper published in the Annals of the New York Academy of Sciences. They proposed that mindfulness meditation preserves telomere length via two complementary pathways: (1) by reducing threat-based stress cognitions and attenuating HPA-axis stress arousal, thereby lowering cortisol and oxidative stress; and (2) by directly increasing positive psychological states and hormonal factors that upregulate telomerase activity. Aspects of this model have since been confirmed in multiple independent studies.

NEUROSCIENCE

The Meditating Brain: Neuroplasticity and Cognitive Ageing

The brain was long assumed to be a fixed structure in adulthood — a hardwired organ incapable of meaningful structural change after the critical developmental periods of childhood and adolescence. Decades of neuroimaging research have conclusively overturned this view, establishing that the brain retains significant structural plasticity throughout life. Among the most striking demonstrations of adult neuroplasticity is the finding that meditation literally reshapes the brain's grey matter — and in doing so, counteracts some of the most defining structural changes of normal biological ageing.

Grey Matter, Cortical Thickness, and Ageing

Dr. Sara Lazar and her team at Harvard Medical School and Massachusetts General Hospital produced some of the most impactful findings in this area. In their landmark 2005 study published in NeuroReport, brain scans of 20 long-term meditators were compared with 15 age-matched non-meditators. The meditators showed significantly greater cortical thickness in the prefrontal cortex — the region governing working memory, decision-making, and fluid intelligence — and in the insula, which underlies interoceptive awareness and emotional integration. Most strikingly, while cortical thickness in the prefrontal cortex typically declines with age, 50-year-old meditators in Lazar's study had the same amount of grey matter there as adults half their age (Lazar et al., 2005). The increases in grey matter thickness were proportional to total lifetime hours of meditation practice.

In a critical follow-up longitudinal study (Hölzel et al., 2011), 16 healthy, meditation-naive individuals underwent brain imaging before and after completing an eight-week MBSR program. After just eight weeks of practice averaging 27 minutes daily, significant increases in grey matter concentration were documented in the left hippocampus (critical for learning, memory, and emotional regulation), the temporo-parietal junction (associated with empathy and perspective-taking), and the pons (a brainstem structure involved in regulatory neurotransmitter production). Simultaneously, grey matter

> Meditation may have a bit of an anti-aging effect on the brain. It may protect our brains from the normal effects of aging.
> — **Dr. Sara Lazar**, Harvard Medical School / Massachusetts General Hospital

density in the amygdala — the brain's primary threat-detection and stress-response hub — decreased significantly, correlating directly with participants' self-reported reductions in stress. These structural changes occurred in just eight weeks: a timeframe with profound implications for the accessibility of meditation's benefits.

Implications for Age-Related Cognitive Decline

The prefrontal cortex and hippocampus are precisely the regions that atrophy most significantly in normal ageing and neurodegenerative disease. A systematic review of meditation's effects on age-related cognitive decline (Gard, Hölzel & Lazar, 2014) concluded that meditation practice may slow age-related cognitive decline through its effects on these vulnerable regions, and through its enhancement of neuroplasticity more broadly. The review also highlighted meditation's role in increasing Brain-Derived Neurotrophic Factor (BDNF) — a molecular growth hormone that supports neurogenesis, synaptic plasticity, and neuronal survival — levels of which are typically reduced in Alzheimer's disease and age-related cognitive impairment.

These structural brain changes translate into measurable cognitive performance advantages. Long-term meditators consistently demonstrate superior performance on tests of sustained attention, working memory, fluid intelligence, and cognitive flexibility compared to non-meditating controls, including individuals decades their junior. The evidence suggests that meditation does not merely slow cognitive decline — it actively builds a neurological reserve that confers protection against the onset of dementia-spectrum conditions.

CARDIOVASCULAR HEALTH

Cardiovascular Health and Mortality Risk

Cardiovascular disease (CVD) remains the leading cause of death globally, accounting for an estimated 17.9 million deaths annually (WHO, 2021). The cardiovascular effects of meditation have attracted substantial research attention, culminating in a 2017 Scientific Statement from the American Heart Association (Levine et al., 2017) — the most authoritative review to date — which systematically evaluated dozens of studies and concluded that meditation may be considered as an adjunct to guideline-directed cardiovascular risk reduction, given its low cost and favourable risk profile.

Studies across multiple meditation modalities have found consistent improvements in hypertension — one of the primary modifiable risk factors for stroke and heart disease. A 2024 systematic review and meta-analysis (Wu et al., 2024) published in BMC Cardiovascular Disorders, pooling data from studies published to May 2023, confirmed that mindfulness-based interventions produce significant reductions in both systolic and diastolic blood pressure, with greater effects observed in participants with higher pre-intervention blood pressure. The clinical significance is substantial: even a modest 5 mmHg reduction in systolic blood pressure reduces cardiovascular mortality by 9% and stroke mortality by 14%.

Perhaps the most striking cardiovascular findings come from long-term Transcendental Meditation (TM) studies. A post-hoc analysis of two randomized controlled trials in patients with established coronary artery disease found that TM practitioners showed a 23% reduction in all-cause mortality, a 30% reduction in cardiovascular mortality, and a non-statistically significant 51% reduction in cancer mortality compared to controls — findings that, if replicated in larger studies, would place meditation among the most effective lifestyle interventions for primary cardiovascular prevention (Levine et al., 2017).

A large-scale analysis of more than 61,000 participants in the National Health Interview Survey found that meditators had substantially lower rates of hypertension (76% as likely), high cholesterol (65% as likely), diabetes (70% as likely), stroke, and coronary artery disease — with meditators being only 51% as likely as non-meditators to have coronary artery disease (Krittanawong et al., 2020). The effect persisted after controlling for multiple confounding variables, though the authors appropriately noted the observational limitations of the design.

The physiological mechanisms are multifaceted. Meditation activates the parasympathetic nervous system — reducing heart rate, lowering cortisol, decreasing circulating catecholamines, and reducing vascular resistance. It consistently improves heart rate variability (HRV), a marker of autonomic cardiac regulation strongly associated with cardiovascular health and longevity. It also reduces C-reactive protein (CRP) and other inflammatory cytokines — the chronic low-grade inflammation that underlies much of cardiovascular ageing.

Mechanisms by Which Meditation Supports Longevity

- Telomere preservation and elevated telomerase activity — slowing cellular ageing at the chromosomal level.
- Structural brain changes preserving cortical thickness and hippocampal volume against age-related atrophy.
- HPA-axis down-regulation reducing chronic cortisol and its multi-system ageing effects.
- Reduction of systemic inflammation (CRP, IL-6, TNF-α) — the driver of most age-related chronic diseases.
- Improved heart rate variability and cardiovascular risk factor profiles.
- Enhanced immune function and greater resistance to infection and stress-induced immunosuppression.
- Increased BDNF — the brain's neuroplasticity and neuroprotection factor.
- Improved sleep architecture, which is critical for cellular repair and immune homeostasis.
- Reduced psychological stress, anxiety, and depression — all independently associated with shorter lifespan.

STRESS & IMMUNITY

Stress Biology, Cortisol, and Immune Resilience

Chronic psychological stress is one of the most potent accelerants of biological ageing known to medicine. Via sustained activation of the hypothalamic-pituitary-adrenal (HPA) axis, chronic stress produces chronically elevated cortisol, which impairs immune function, disrupts sleep architecture, promotes visceral adiposity, suppresses hippocampal neurogenesis, and accelerates telomere attrition. In short, chronic stress ages the body from the inside out. Meditation's capacity to down-regulate the HPA axis is therefore among the most longevity-relevant mechanisms in its pharmacological profile.

A meta-analysis of 45 randomized controlled trials (Sanada et al., 2016, cited in Nassif et al., 2022) identified strong evidence that mindfulness meditation produces consistent reductions in serum cortisol, with effect sizes that increase with longer intervention duration. Programs exceeding 20 total hours of meditation appear to be particularly effective. A comprehensive meta-analysis (Grasmann et al., 2020) found that meditation interventions efficiently reduce cortisol levels in at-risk samples — those under elevated psychological or physiological stress — with preliminary evidence that benefits are sustained over the long term, not merely transient stress-relief effects.

The immune system benefits of meditation extend beyond cortisol modulation. A 3-month intensive yoga and meditation retreat study (Bhasin et al., 2017) found significantly increased BDNF levels alongside alterations in cytokine profiles consistent with enhanced immune readiness and resilience. Mindfulness-based interventions have been shown to reduce pro-inflammatory markers including IL-6, TNF-alpha, and CRP — the same inflammatory signatures implicated in accelerated ageing, cancer progression, cardiovascular disease, and neurodegenerative conditions.

The practical implication is significant: by consistently deactivating the stress response and allowing the parasympathetic nervous system to predominate, regular meditators create a physiological milieu that is less hospitable to the inflammation-driven processes that shorten healthy lifespan. Harvard research has documented that participants in relaxation programs — including meditation — used 43% fewer medical services than they did the previous year, suggesting that these biological effects translate into tangible clinical and economic outcomes (Stahl et al., 2015).

PSYCHOLOGY & WELLBEING

Purpose, Presence, and Psychological Longevity

The relationship between psychological wellbeing and longevity is one of the most robustly supported findings in epidemiology. Individuals who experience higher levels of purpose, positive affect, social connection, and life satisfaction live measurably longer, healthier lives — and show slower rates of biological ageing — than those who do not. Meditation addresses each of these factors simultaneously.

Regular meditation practice is among the most effective non-pharmacological interventions for anxiety and depression — two conditions independently associated with shorter telomere length, accelerated cardiovascular ageing, and elevated all-cause mortality. A seminal meta-analysis of 209 studies (Goyal et al., 2014) published in JAMA Internal Medicine found that mindfulness meditation programs produced moderate evidence of improvement in anxiety, depression, and pain, with effect sizes comparable to those of antidepressant medications but without side-effect burden.

The Monastic Evidence

A natural experiment on the relationship between contemplative practice and longevity exists in the well-documented longevity of cloistered religious communities. Research consistently demonstrates that monks and nuns in contemplative orders have significantly lower mortality risk than the general population — a finding that holds across Catholic, Buddhist, and other contemplative traditions (Luy, 2003; cited in Bossert et al., 2023). While confounding factors such as abstinence from alcohol, tobacco, and a regulated diet contribute, the shared practice of daily meditation and prayer, the strong community bonds, and the sense of meaning and purpose inherent in contemplative life are widely regarded as major contributing factors.

The ancient Vedic and Buddhist traditions that gave rise to modern meditation practices always understood longevity consequently — not a goal — of right living and deep practice. What modern science is now confirming, pathway by pathway, is that these traditions were physiologically correct: the practice of attending fully and compassionately to the present moment, over years and decades, appears to alter the very machinery by which cells age, hearts beat, brains think, and immune systems defend. Meditation does not promise immortality. It offers something more useful: a life that is not only longer in years, but richer in the qualities that make those years worth living.

TYPES OF PRACTICE

Types of Meditation and Their Relative Benefits

Meditation encompasses a wide family of practices, and the research evidence — while largely convergent on shared mechanisms — does identify certain differences in emphasis and effect.

Mindfulness-Based Stress Reduction (MBSR), developed by Jon Kabat-Zinn at the University of Massachusetts in 1979, is the most extensively studied secular meditation intervention. Its structured 8-week curriculum has been tested in hundreds of RCTs and consistently demonstrates benefits across stress reduction, depression and anxiety, blood pressure, immune markers, grey matter density, and pain management. MBSR is the gold standard for clinical research and serves as the intervention framework for many of the neuroimaging and telomere studies reviewed in this article.

Transcendental Meditation (TM) has the strongest evidence base for cardiovascular outcomes, with multiple long-term RCTs showing reductions in blood pressure, hypertension, and — most remarkably — in cardiovascular mortality itself. TM's unique twice-daily 20-minute structure, focusing on a personally assigned mantra, may produce particularly robust parasympathetic activation.

Loving-Kindness Meditation (LKM) has been specifically linked to longer telomere length in women (Hoge et al., 2013) and to measurable increases in positive affect, compassion, and social connection — the psychological pillars associated with longevity in epidemiological research. The Dasanayaka et al. (2023) study found positive telomere effects across mindfulness, loving-kindness, and Zen meditation, suggesting that the specific technique may matter less than the consistency and depth of practice.

Mantra-based practices — including Vedic meditation and Om chanting — activate the vagus nerve via extended exhalation and sustained vocalization, producing parasympathetic effects on blood pressure, heart rate, and cortisol that complement and overlap with breath-focused mindfulness practices.

> It is not that long-term meditators live forever. It is that they age more slowly, suffer less from chronic disease, and maintain their cognitive and emotional capacities far longer into old age.
>
> — Synthesis of current meditation research

Yoga-based meditation integrates physical posture (asana), breath regulation (pranayama), and meditative concentration. Research by Lazar's group at MGH found that long-term yoga practitioners and meditation practitioners showed virtually identical cortical preservation patterns — suggesting that the meditative component of yoga carries comparable brain-protective effects to dedicated silent meditation practice.

PRACTICAL GUIDANCE

Beginning a Longevity-Oriented Meditation Practice

The scientific evidence is clear that the benefits of meditation are dose-dependent: more consistent, longer-duration practice produces greater effects on telomere biology, cortical thickness, cardiovascular markers, and psychological wellbeing. However, the threshold for benefit is lower than many people assume. Hölzel et al.'s 2011 study demonstrated measurable brain changes after just eight weeks of practice averaging 27 minutes daily. Even five minutes per day, practiced consistently, has been shown to produce measurable improvements in perceived stress and mood regulation within four weeks.

For longevity-oriented benefits, the research suggests: starting with a structured eight-week program (MBSR courses are widely available online and in person, and have the strongest clinical evidence base); progressing to 20–30 minutes of daily practice over time; integrating both focused-attention practice (breath or mantra) and open-monitoring practice (observing thoughts and sensations without attachment); and, where possible, engaging in group or community practice, which adds the social connection dimension that independently supports longevity.

As Lazar herself notes, the benefits are cumulative and progressive — proportional to total lifetime hours of practice. Beginning at any age appears to yield significant benefits; the brain's neuroplasticity and the telomere-protective effects of stress reduction are accessible across the full adult lifespan. The most important meditation practice, in every tradition that has considered the question, is the one you actually do.

CONCLUSION

A Practice for the Long Game

The evidence reviewed in this article points toward a consistent and scientifically grounded conclusion: meditation is not merely a stress-management technique or a spiritual exercise. It is a physiologically active practice that engages with the biology of ageing at multiple levels simultaneously — preserving telomere length, protecting cortical grey matter, reducing systemic inflammation, down-regulating the HPA stress axis, improving cardiovascular function, and cultivating the psychological conditions that epidemiology consistently associates with longer, healthier lives.

None of these benefits require advanced practice or monastic dedication. They emerge from the simple, repeatable act of sitting still, attending to the breath or a chosen anchor of awareness, and returning — again and again — when the mind wanders. In this return, in this daily recommitment to the present moment, something biological is happening at the level of chromosomes, neurons, and heart cells. Something that the body, with its own deep intelligence, appears to regard as profoundly protective.

The ancient traditions were, it turns out, pointing at something real. We now have the tools to see it. What we need, individually and collectively, is the practice to act on what the evidence so clearly suggests.

REFERENCES

1. Bossert, M., Kleindienst, N., Klimke, A., Bosch, J., & Kleindienst, N. (2023). The effects of mindfulness-based interventions on telomere length and telomerase activity: A systematic review and meta-analysis. Mindfulness. https://doi.org/10.1007/s12671-023-02075-x

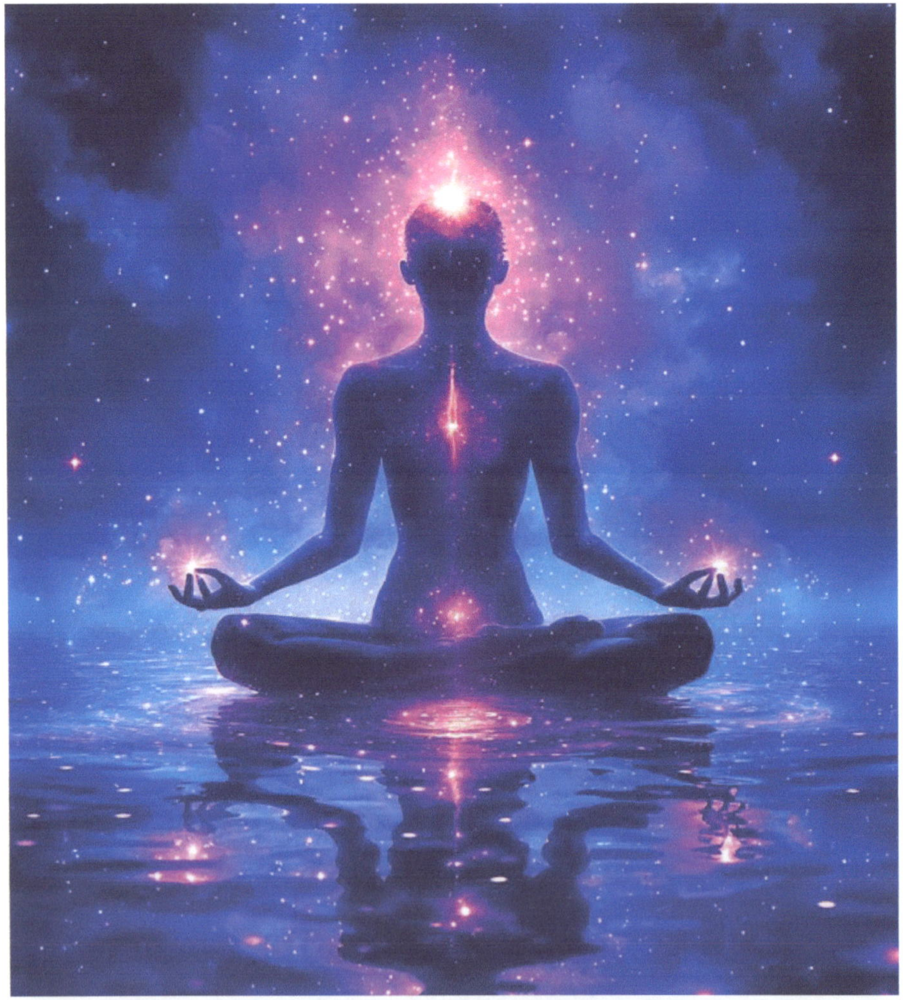

2. Dasanayaka, N.N., Sirisena, N.D., & Samaranayake, N. (2023). Associations of meditation with telomere dynamics: A case-control study in healthy adults. Frontiers in Psychology. https://doi.org/10.3389/fpsyg.2023.1222863
3. Epel, E., Daubenmier, J., Moskowitz, J.T., Folkman, S., & Blackburn, E. (2009). Can meditation slow rate of cellular aging? Cognitive stress, mindfulness, and telomeres. Annals of the New York Academy of Sciences, 1172, 34–53. https://doi.org/10.1111/j.1749-6632.2009.04414.x
4. Gard, T., Hölzel, B.K., & Lazar, S.W. (2014). The potential effects of meditation on age-related cognitive decline: A systematic review. Annals of the New York Academy of Sciences, 1307(1), 89–103. https://doi.org/10.1111/nyas.12348
5. Goyal, M., Singh, S., Sibinga, E.M., et al. (2014). Meditation programs for psychological stress and well-being: A systematic review and meta-analysis. JAMA Internal Medicine, 174(3), 357–368. https://doi.org/10.1001/jamainternmed.2013.13018
6. Grasmann, D., Schroeder, A., Faessler, L., &Glombiewski, J.A. (2020). Meditation interventions efficiently reduce cortisol levels of at-risk samples: A meta-analysis. Health Psychology Review. https://doi.org/10.1080/17437199.2020.1760727
7. Hoge, E.A., Chen, M.M., Orr, E., et al. (2013). Loving-Kindness Meditation practice associated with longer telomeres in women. Brain, Behavior, and Immunity, 32, 159–163. https://doi.org/10.1016/j.bbi.2013.04.005
8. Hölzel, B.K., Carmody, J., Vangel, M., et al. (2011). Mindfulness practice leads to increases in regional brain gray matter density. Psychiatry Research:

Neuroimaging, 191(1), 36–43. https://doi.org/10.1016/j.pscychresns.2010.08.006 [PMC3004979]

9. Krittanawong, C., et al. (2020). Meditation and cardiovascular health in the United States. American Journal of Cardiology, 131, 23–26. https://doi.org/10.1016/j.amjcard.2020.06.043

10. Lazar, S.W., Kerr, C.E., Wasserman, R.H., et al. (2005). Meditation experience is associated with increased cortical thickness. NeuroReport, 16(17), 1893–1897. https://doi.org/10.1097/01.wnr.0000186598.66243.19

11. Levine, G.N., Lange, R.A., Bairey-Merz, C.N., et al. (2017). Meditation and cardiovascular risk reduction: A Scientific Statement from the American Heart Association. Journal of the American Heart Association, 6(10), e002218. https://doi.org/10.1161/JAHA.117.002218

12. Mendioroz, M., Puebla-Guedea, M., Montero-Marín, J., et al. (2020). Telomere length correlates with subtelomeric DNA methylation in long-term mindfulness practitioners. Scientific Reports, 10, 4564. https://doi.org/10.1038/s41598-020-61241-6

13. Schutte, N.S., & Malouff, J.M. (2020). Meditation and telomere length: A meta-analysis. PubMed. https://pubmed.ncbi.nlm.nih.gov/31903785/

14. Tolahunase, M., Sagar, R., & Dada, R. (2017). Impact of yoga and meditation on cellular aging in apparently healthy individuals: A prospective, open-label single-arm exploratory study. Oxidative Medicine and Cellular Longevity. https://doi.org/10.1155/2017/7928981

15. Wu, J., et al. (2024). Effect of mindfulness-based interventions on people with prehypertension or hypertension: A systematic review and meta-analysis. BMC Cardiovascular Disorders. https://doi.org/10.1186/s12872-024-03746-w

16. Bhasin, M.K., Denninger, J.W., Huffman, J.C., et al. (2017). Yoga, meditation and mind-body health: Increased BDNF, cortisol awakening response, and altered inflammatory marker expression after a 3-month yoga and meditation retreat. Frontiers in Human Neuroscience. https://doi.org/10.3389/fnhum.2017.00315

17. Kabat-Zinn, J. (2003). Mindfulness-Based Stress Reduction (MBSR). Constructivism in the Human Sciences, 8(2), 73–107.

18. Brand, S., Holsboer-Trachsler, E., Naranjo, J.R., & Schmidt, S. (2012). Influence of mindfulness practice on cortisol and sleep in long-term and short-term meditators. Neuropsychobiology. https://doi.org/10.1159/000336559

19. Stahl, J.E., Dossett, M.L., LaJoie, A.S., et al. (2015). Relaxation response and resiliency training and its effect on healthcare resource utilization. PLoS ONE. https://doi.org/10.1371/journal.pone.0140212

20. World Health Organization. (2021). Cardiovascular diseases (CVDs) — Fact Sheet. https://www.who.int/news-room/fact-sheets/detail/cardiovascular-diseases-(cvds)

This article is intended for informational and educational purposes only. It does not constitute medical advice. Consult a qualified healthcare professional before making changes to your health regimen.

Word to Remember

As you are probably aware, **M-E-N-T-A-L** (mental) is a great way to remember the six aspects that should be integrated into our life routines to achieve a quality life, with each letter representing a necessary activity.

M Meditate daily, at least for a few minutes, in a quiet and serene surrounding within or outside your home. Focus on your breath. Breath awareness is important in meditation

E Exercise daily. Any kind of exercise that you can do, based on your age, general health, and physique, will largely help you.

N No: Learn to say NO to anything that will not help to move towards your general life goals.

T Talk: Make sure to talk to your loved ones, your close friends, other family members, co-workers, your neighbors, and anyone who directly or indirectly impacts your daily life.

A Accept what comes along in life, especially things that are not under your direct control. Do not keep dwelling on negative aspects that you fight to accept, which did not originate from your actions. Such negative thinking can increase your blood pressure, anxiety, and even cause depression

L Laughter. Do things and watch things that will let you laugh and unwind. Join family and friends in sharing funny incidents or jokes that do not hurt anyone's feelings.

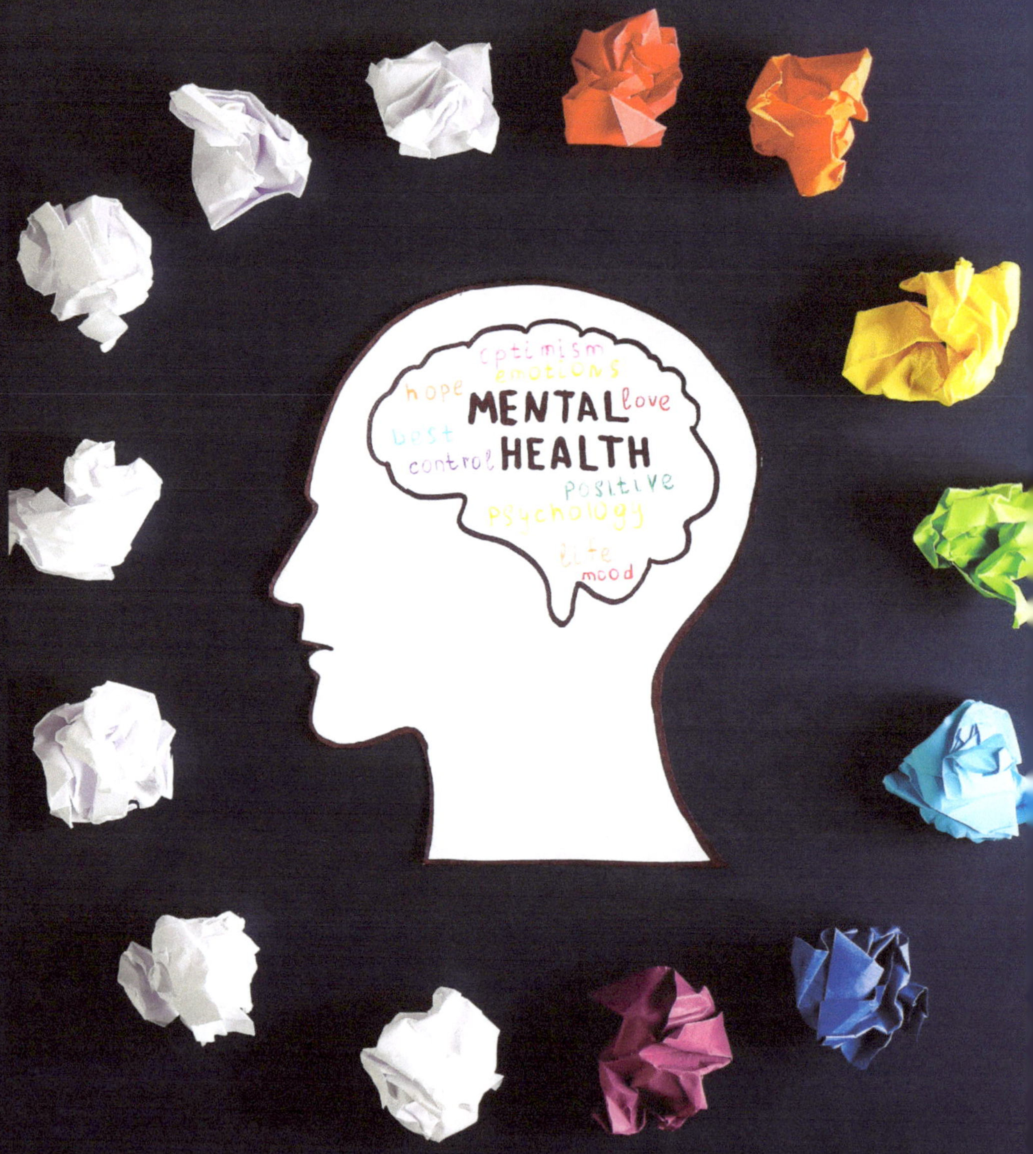

Barefoot Simple Slow Walking

Recent Studies on Barefoot Walking and General Health Due to Earth's Electromagnetic Fields.

Recent research on "grounding" or "earthing" - the practice of direct physical contact with the Earth's surface through barefoot walking - has revealed intriguing health benefits that may be linked to the planet's electromagnetic fields. Here's what the latest studies show:

What is Grounding / Earthing?

Earthing (or grounding) refers to the discovery of benefits-including better sleep and reduced pain-from walking barefoot outside or sitting, working, or sleeping indoors connected to conductive systems that transfer the Earth's electrons from the ground into the body. The theory suggests that bodily contact with the Earth's natural electric charge stabilizes the physiology at the deepest levels, reduces inflammation, pain, and stress, improves blood flow, energy, and sleep, and generates greater well-being

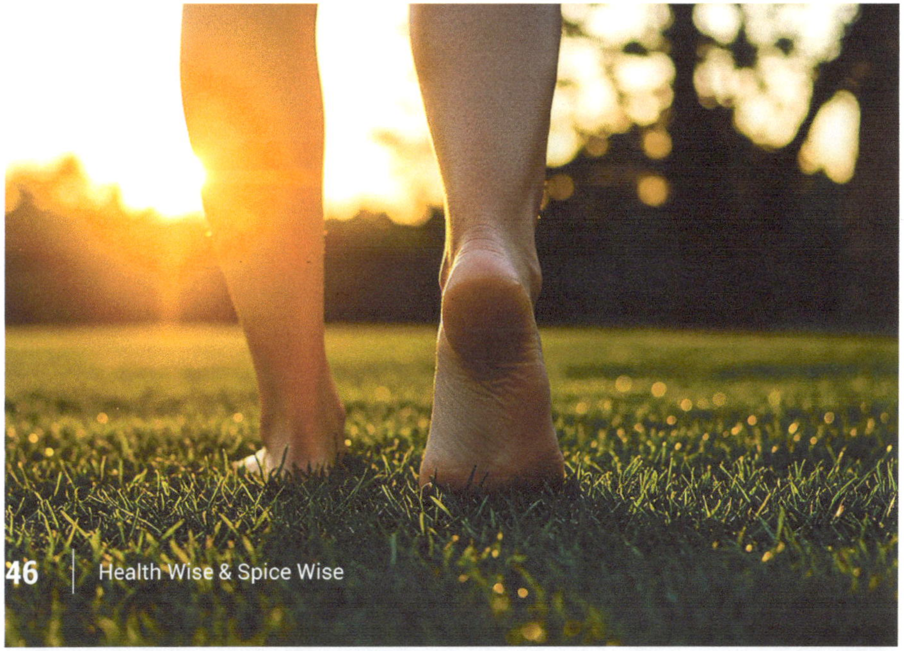

Recent Research Findings
Anti-Inflammatory Effects

Studies show that earthing lowers inflammatory markers like C-reactive protein (CRP) and cytokines, which are associated with chronic diseases such as arthritis and cardiovascular conditions. The research indicates that in the Earthing studies, as well as global feedback from thousands of individuals who have grounded themselves, we have consistent evidence of people whose pain has been reduced. Such reduction of pain is evidence (but not proof) that inflammation is reduced.

Cardiovascular Benefits

Emerging research is revealing that direct physical contact of the human body with the surface of the earth (grounding or earthing) has intriguing effects on human physiology and health, including beneficial effects on various cardiovascular risk factors. In one study published in a peer-reviewed journal, researchers observed that grounding can decrease blood viscosity, a marker linked to inflammation and cardiovascular risk.

Improved Blood Flow and Circulation

In another small study of adults, one two-hour session of grounding reduced inflammation and improved blood flow. This suggests that even short-term exposure to grounding can produce measurable physiological changes.

Immune System Enhancement

There's a growing body of evidence that earthing may enhance the body's immune response, though more research is needed to fully understand these mechanisms.

The Scientific Theory

An ever-expanding body of research over the past several decades suggests that directly touching the earth, a practice known as grounding, puts the body into a healing state. The natural universe conducts an energy current known as a direct current (DC). The hypothesis is that when we don't have contact with the ground, our bodies "pick up a positive charge relative to the Earth", causing illness. But connection to the ground, like being barefoot, equalizes this potential difference.

Study Limitations and Considerations

While the research shows promise, it's important to note that the science is shaky at best, according to some medical experts. Studies tend to be small and are done indoors using wires that connectparticipants to grounding systems rather than actual outdoor barefoot walking.

Practical Applications

Earthing is as simple as routinely walking barefoot outdoors and/or using inexpensive grounding systems indoors while sleeping or sitting, practices that restore a lost and needed electric connection with the Earth Activities that are commonly promoted by earthing practitioners include: Walking barefoot: Whether on grass, sand, or even mud, walking without shoes or socks allows the skin to touch the natural ground, which can provide grounding energy.

Recent Clinical Evidence

Based on the above hypothesis, some research has explored grounding as a therapeutic option for inflammation, cardiovascular disease, muscle damage, chronic pain, and mood. In an older study from 2018, 16 massage therapists participated in a controlled trial examining grounding effects, and proven to be true.

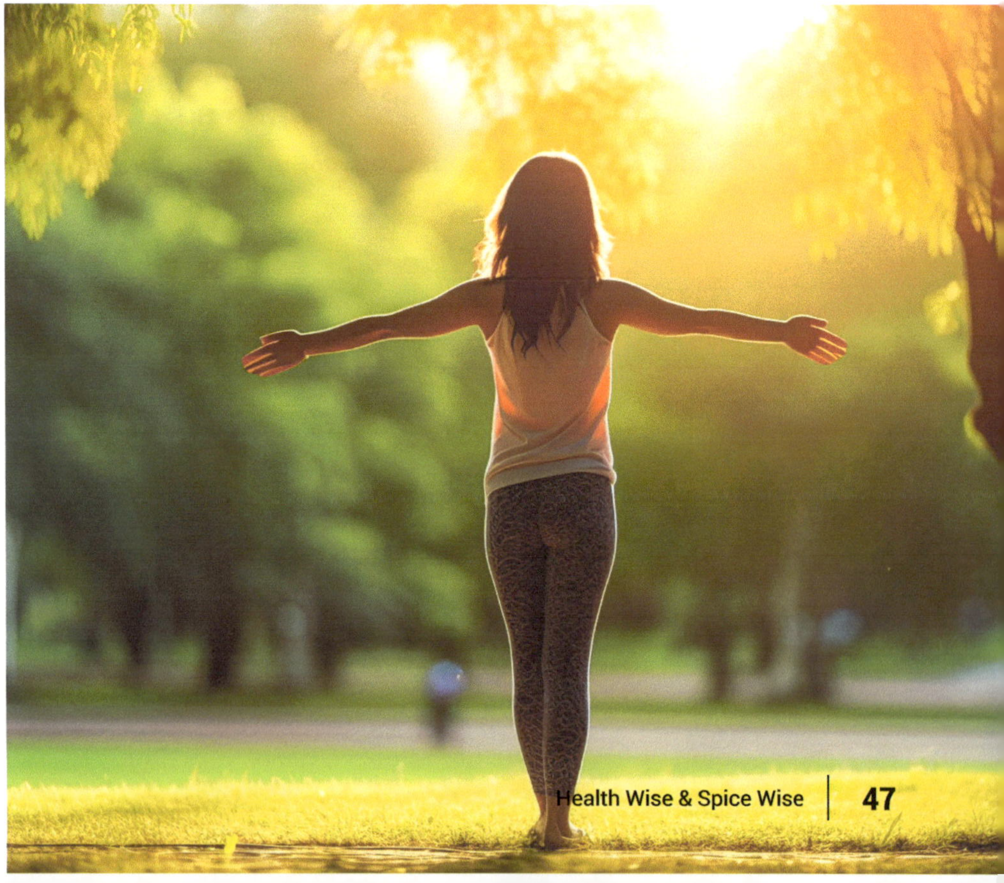

THE IMPORTANCE OF INTERMITTENT FASTING & Better Health

A Review of the Science, Methods, and Evidence-Based Benefits

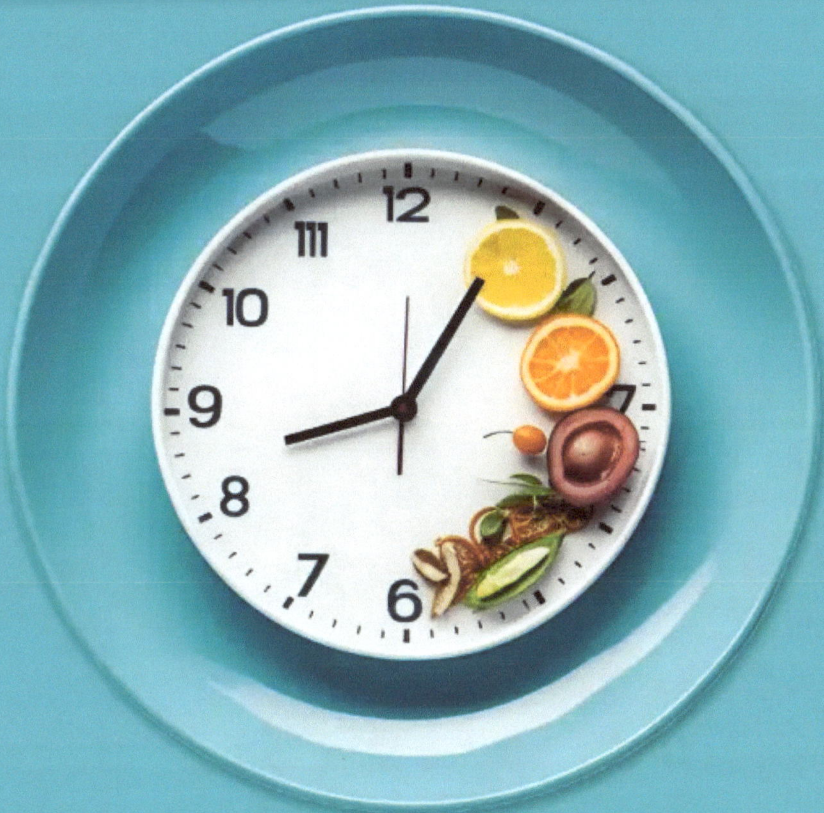

Introduction

Intermittent fasting (IF) — an eating pattern that cycles between periods of fasting and unrestricted eating — has emerged as one of the most studied dietary interventions of the 21st century. Unlike calorie-restricted diets that require daily food reduction, IF restructures when we eat rather than simply what we eat. This simple shift in timing triggers a cascade of metabolic, cellular, and neurological changes that peer-reviewed research now links to significant improvements in weight management, metabolic health, brain function, cardiovascular markers, and longevity.

A landmark 2019 review published in the New England Journal of Medicine by Mattson et al. noted that eating within a 6-hour window and fasting for 18 hours can trigger a metabolic switch from glucose-based to ketone-based energy — with associated increases in stress resistance, longevity, and a decreased incidence of diseases including cancer and obesity (Mattson et al., 2019).

What Is Intermittent Fasting?

Intermittent fasting is not a diet in the conventional sense; it is a structured eating pattern. The most widely practiced protocols include:

- 16:8 Method — 16 hours of fasting with an 8-hour eating window (e.g., eating between 12pm–8 pm).
- 5:2 Diet — Normal eating for five days per week, with caloric restriction (under 500 kcal) on two non-consecutive days.
- Alternate Day Fasting (ADF) Alternating days of normal eating with fasting or severe caloric restriction.
- Extended Fasting — Fasting periods of 24–72 hours, typically practised monthly or less frequently.

Weight Management and Metabolic Health

The most extensively documented benefit of IF is its effect on body composition and metabolic markers. A 2025 systematic review and meta-analysis of 15 randomized controlled trials involving 758 overweight or obese adults (Wang et al., 2025) confirmed that IF significantly improves total cholesterol, LDL cholesterol, fasting plasma glucose, and body weight compared to control diets.

A comprehensive 2024 umbrella review published in eClinicalMedicine (The Lancet) synthesized data from RCTs across six health outcome categories — anthropometric measures, lipid profiles, glycemic markers, circulatory function, appetite, and others — and found consistent beneficial effects of IF across most metabolic parameters (Liu et al., 2024).

Crucially, IF improves insulin sensitivity. A pivotal early study by Sutton et al. (2018) demonstrated that early time-restricted feeding improved insulin sensitivity, blood pressure, and oxidative stress in men with prediabetes — even without weight loss — underscoring that the benefits of IF extend beyond simple caloric reduction.

Autophagy and Cellular Regeneration

One of the most significant — and least discussed — mechanisms by which IF promotes health is through the activation of autophagy: the body's intrinsic cellular housekeeping process. When fasting reduces glucose availability, the body suppresses the mTOR signalling pathway and upregulates autophagy — a process by which cells break down and recycle damaged proteins, dysfunctional organelles, and metabolic waste.

This cellular self-repair mechanism is associated with protection against neurodegeneration, cancer, and accelerated ageing. Yoshinori Ohsumi was awarded the 2016 Nobel Prize in Physiology or Medicine specifically for his foundational work uncovering the mechanisms of autophagy — lending

Key Metabolic Benefits at a Glance

- Reduces body weight and visceral fat, primarily from fat tissue rather than lean mass.
- Lowers fasting blood glucose and improves insulin sensitivity.
- Improves lipid profiles reduces LDL, total cholesterol, and triglycerides.
- Reduces C-reactive protein (CRP) and other inflammatory markers.
- Activates AMPK and suppresses mTOR — pathways linked to cellular longevity.

significant scientific weight to the fasting practices that trigger it.

Brain Health and Cognitive Function

Research by Dr. Mark Mattson of Johns Hopkins University has established that IF can enhance neurotrophic factor signaling — particularly Brain-Derived Neurotrophic Factor (BDNF) — a protein critical for cognition, synaptic plasticity, neurogenesis, and mood regulation (Mattson, 2019).

A 2021 PMC review (Gudden et al., 2021) confirmed that ketones produced during fasting periods serve as an alternative, efficient brain fuel. Lower glucose levels during fasting also suppress mTOR — increasing autophagy in neural tissue — while upregulating BDNF and promoting mitochondrial biogenesis. These effects support cognitive resilience, memory, and protection against neurodegenerative disease.

A 2025 review in Frontiers in Nutrition further demonstrated that IF improves brain health through the gut–brain axis: by improving gut microbiota diversity, raising short-chain fatty acids, and lowering systemic inflammation, IF supports neuroinflammation reduction, synaptic plasticity, and cognitive resilience (Chen et al., 2025).

Clinical evidence also shows benefits for epilepsy, Alzheimer's disease, and multiple sclerosis in terms of disease symptoms and progression, though human research in these areas is still maturing and further large-scale trials are needed.

Cardiovascular and Inflammatory Markers

Intermittent fasting has been linked to improvements in several cardiovascular risk factors, including blood pressure, resting heart rate, LDL cholesterol, triglycerides, and inflammatory markers such as CRP and IL-6 (Kim et al., 2023). The beneficial effects are partly direct — through metabolic switching and reduced oxidative stress — and partly indirect through weight loss.

It is important to note, however, that a preliminary observational analysis presented at the 2024 American Heart Association conference (Zhong et al., 2024) suggested an association between 8-hour TRE and increased cardiovascular mortality risk in individuals with pre-existing heart conditions, highlighting that IF protocols should

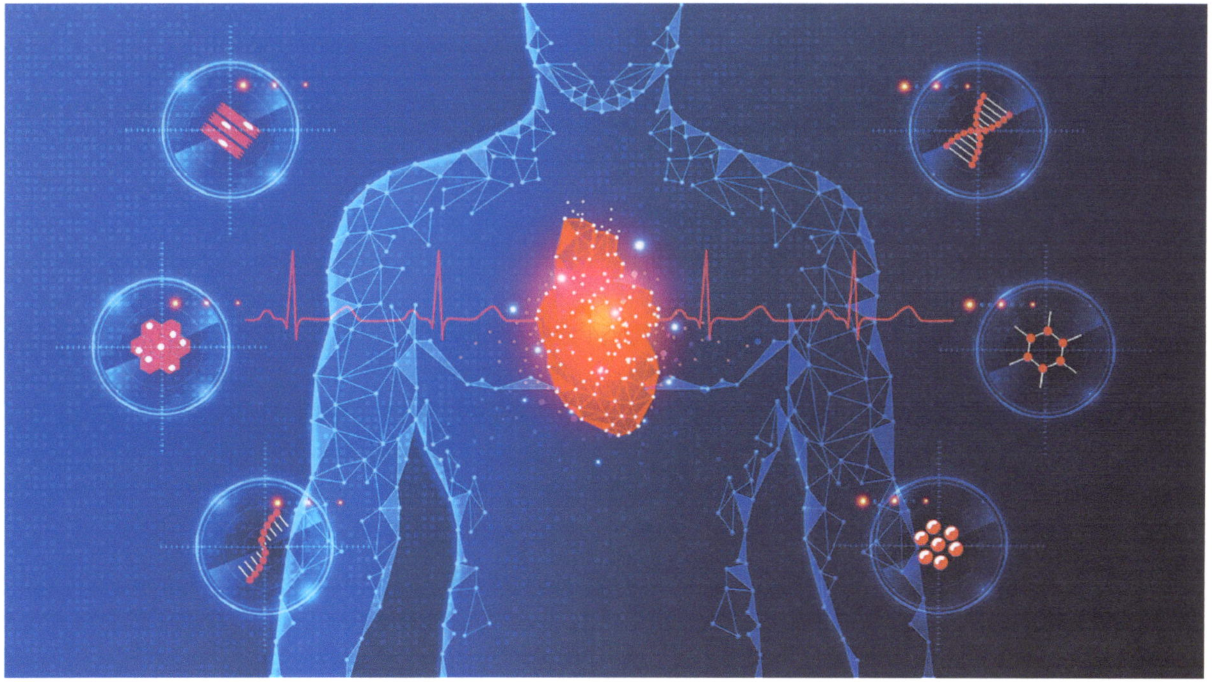

be tailored — particularly for high-risk populations — and undertaken with appropriate medical guidance.

Longevity, Circadian Rhythm, and Ageing

IF aligns eating patterns with the body's circadian biology. Aligning food intake with daylight hours — as early time-restricted eating does — synchronizes insulin secretion, cortisol, and digestive enzyme activity with their natural peaks, producing superior metabolic outcomes compared to late-night eating. Longo & Panda (2016) was established in a landmark Cell Metabolismpaper that time-restricted feeding in healthy subjects improves metabolic health and appears to support healthy lifespan through circadian entrainment.

At the molecular level, IF activates AMPK (an energy-sensing enzyme), deactivates mTOR, and upregulates FOXO transcription factors and sirtuins (SIRT1 in particular) a set of longevity-associated pathways also activated by caloric restriction in model organisms, where they consistently extend lifespan (Longo & Panda, 2016).

Who Should Consider IF and Who Should Avoid It

While evidence for IF is strong in healthy adults with overweight or metabolic dysfunction, it is not universally appropriate. Individuals who should seek medical guidance before beginning IF include those with type 1 or 2 diabetes, pregnant or breastfeeding women, children and adolescents, those with a history of eating disorders, and individuals with cardiovascular disease. Clinicians should be involved in protocol selection, particularly for longer fasting windows.

For the general healthy adult population, the 16:8 method has the strongest evidence base for adherence and safety, while the 5:2 method has demonstrated efficacy comparable to continuous caloric restriction in multiple meta-analyses. A 2025 comparative study confirmed that both 5:2 and 16:8 show similar effectiveness for weight loss in overweight individuals (Wang et al., 2025).

Conclusion

Intermittent fasting represents a scientifically validated, accessible, and flexible approach to improving metabolic health, body composition, brain function, and cellular longevity. Backed by decades of basic research, a rapidly growing body of randomized controlled trials, and multiple systematic meta-analyses, IF has moved firmly from fringe practice to mainstream evidence-based nutrition.

The most compelling insight from science is that IF does not merely reduce calories — it activates ancient biological pathways of resilience, repair, and renewal that are inherent to human physiology. As the field matures, personalized IF protocols — guided by metabolic biomarkers, lifestyle, and individual health context — promise to make this ancient practice increasingly precise and powerful.

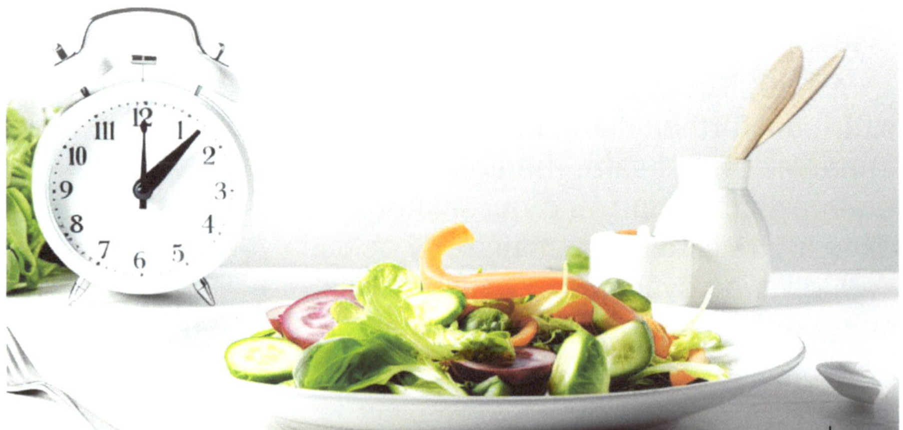

REFERENCES

1. Mattson, M.P., Longo, V.D., & Harvie, M. (2019). Effects of intermittent fasting on health, aging, and disease. New England Journal of Medicine, 381(26), 2541–2551. https://doi.org/10.1056/NEJMra1905136
2. Liu, M.-S., Wu, Y., Gao, T.-T., & Wen, Q.-J. (2024). Intermittent fasting and health outcomes: An umbrella review of systematic reviews and meta-analyses of randomised controlled trials. eClinicalMedicine (The Lancet). https://doi.org/10.1016/S2589-5370(24)00098-1
3. Wang, B., & Wang, C. (2025). The impact of intermittent fasting on body composition and cardiometabolic outcomes in overweight and obese adults: A systematic review and meta-analysis of randomized controlled trials. Nutrition Journal. https://doi.org/10.1186/s12937-025-01178-6
4. Sutton, E.F., Beyl, R., Early, K.S., Cefalu, W.T., Ravussin, E., & Peterson, C.M. (2018). Early time-restricted feeding improves insulin sensitivity, blood pressure, and oxidative stress even without weight loss in men with prediabetes. Cell Metabolism, 27(6), 1212–1221. https://doi.org/10.1016/j.cmet.2018.04.010
5. Gudden, J., Arias Vasquez, A., & Bloemendaal, M. (2021). The effects of intermittent fasting on brain and cognitive function. Nutrients, 13(9), 3166. https://doi.org/10.3390/nu13093166
6. Chen, X., et al. (2025). Effects of intermittent fasting on brain health via the gut–brain axis. Frontiers in Nutrition. https://doi.org/10.3389/fnut.2025.1696733
7. Yılmaz, E., & Özcan, M. (2024). Intermittent fasting and its potential effects on health. Cyprus Journal of Medical Sciences. https://doi.org/10.4274/cjms.2024.2023-109
8. Longo, V.D., & Panda, S. (2016). Fasting, circadian rhythms, and time-restricted feeding in healthy lifespan. Cell Metabolism, 23(6), 1048–1059. https://doi.org/10.1016/j.cmet.2016.06.001
9. Kim, Y., et al. (2023). Beneficial effects of intermittent fasting: A narrative review. Clinical Nutrition Research, PMC9946909. https://pmc.ncbi.nlm.nih.gov/articles/PMC9946909/
10. Zhong, V.W., et al. (2024). Cardiovascular mortality associated with 8-hour time-restricted eating. Preliminary analysis presented at American Heart Association Scientific Sessions 2024.
11. Longo, V.D., et al. (2025). Critical assessment of fasting to promote metabolic health and longevity. Endocrine Reviews. https://doi.org/10.1210/endrev/bnaf007
12. de Cabo, R., & Mattson, M.P. (2019). Effects of intermittent fasting on health, aging, and disease [extended references]. New England Journal of Medicine, 381, 2541–2551.
13. Ohsumi, Y. (2016). Nobel Lecture: Autophagy — an intracellular recycling system. Nobel Prize in Physiology or Medicine. Karolinska Institutet, Stockholm.

Note: This article is intended for informational purposes only. Consult a qualified healthcare professional before beginning any fasting regimen.

CHANTING FOR BETTER HEALTH

THE ANCIENT ART OF CHANTING

How the sustained practice of vocal resonance quiets the nervous system, restores the mind, and heals the body from within.

For thousands of years, across every major civilization on earth — from the Vedic forests of ancient India to the monastic cloisters of medieval Europe, from Tibetan high-altitude temples to the sweat lodges of the Americas — humans have turned to rhythmic, repetitive vocalization as a portal to inner stillness. Modern neuroscience is now confirming what the ancients understood intuitively: chanting is not merely a spiritual ceremony. It is a precise, physiologically active practice that measurably transforms both the body and the brain.

"The universe began with a sound. To chant is to remember that origin — and to reconnect the nervous system with its own deepest frequency."

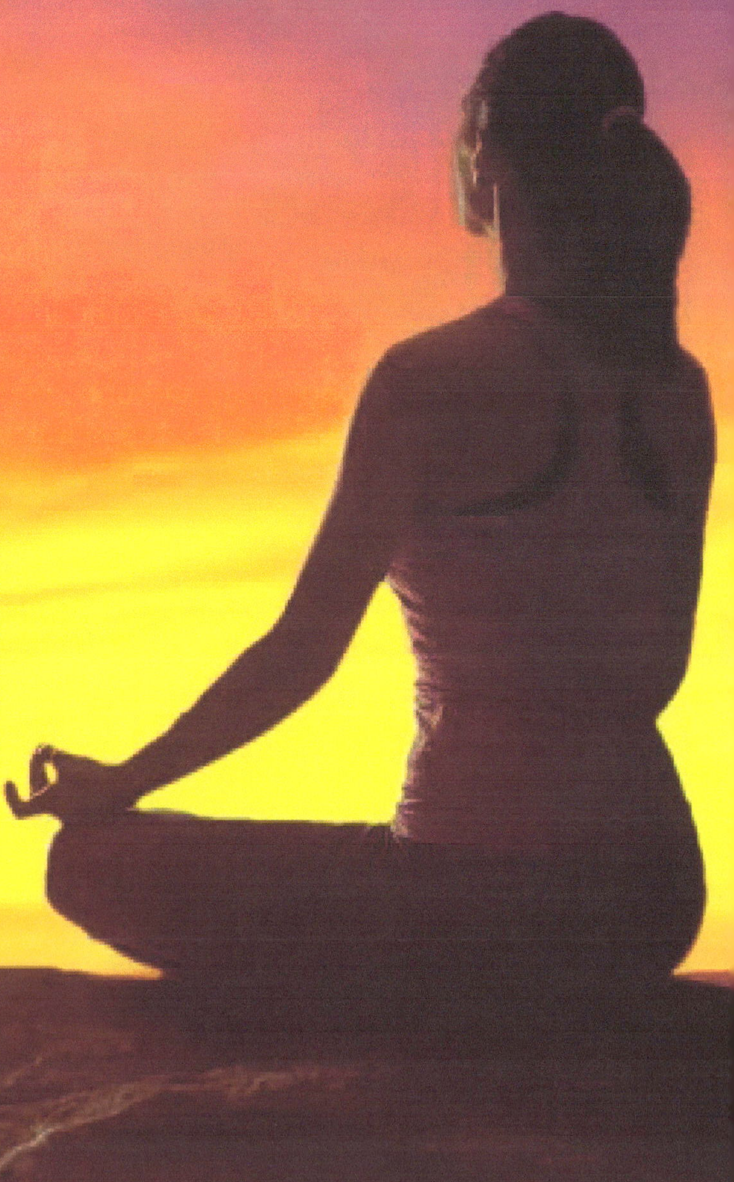

Ancient Vedic Teachi Foundation

What Is Chanting?

Chanting is the sustained, melodic or rhythmic repetition of words, syllables, or sounds — most often performed with breath as the governing force. Unlike ordinary speech, chanting synchronizes breath, voice, and attention into a single unified flow. This synchronization is precisely what gives it its remarkable power.

Across traditions, chanting takes many forms. The common thread is intentionally prolonged vocalization — the elongation of sound that forces the practitioner to inhabit the present moment, breath by breath.

Mantra Chanting

Sanskrit syllables like Om, So Hum, or the Maha Mrityunjaya mantra, repeated to create internal resonance.

Gregorian Chant

Monophonic liturgical song from the Western Catholic tradition, characterized by modal melodies and sacred Latin text.

Tibetan Overtone

Deep harmonic chanting that produces multiple tones simultaneously, used in Buddhist practice for meditative absorption.

Kirtan & Bhajan

Devotional call-and-response singing from the Hindu tradition, often involving community, melody, and percussion.

Physiology

Chanting and the nervous system

The most immediate and measurable effect of chanting is on the autonomic nervous system — the body's internal regulator of stress and recovery. When we chant, we naturally extend the exhale. This extended exhalation directly stimulates the vagus nerve, the long cranial nerve that connects the brain to the heart, lungs, and digestive system.

Vagal stimulation triggers what scientists call the parasympathetic response — commonly known as "rest and digest." Heart rate slows. Blood pressure drops. Cortisol levels decline. The body shifts from a state of alert reactivity into one of calm, restorative presence.

The Vagal Tone Connection

Research published in peer-reviewed journals has shown that regular chanting increases vagal tone — essentially, the baseline strength and responsiveness of the parasympathetic nervous system. Higher vagal tone is associated with greater emotional resilience, reduced anxiety, better cardiovascular health, and stronger immune function. In this sense, chanting is not merely relaxing in the moment; it trains the nervous system to be calmer over time.

What Happens Inside the Brain

Neuroimaging studies using fMRI and EEG have offered extraordinary windows into the chanting brain. The findings are consistent across cultures and chanting styles: sustained vocalization shifts brain activity in profound and measurable ways.

Brainwave Shifts

In ordinary waking life, the brain predominantly operates in the beta frequency (14–30 Hz) – the frequency of active thinking, problem-solving, and alertness. Chanting gradually decelerates brainwave activity toward alpha (8–13 Hz) and, in deeper practice, toward theta (4–7 Hz). Alpha is associated with calm, relaxed awareness – the state we enter just before sleep or in light meditation. Theta is the twilight zone between waking and dreaming, linked to deep creativity, emotional processing, and spiritual insight.

The Default Mode Network

The Default Mode Network (DMN), the brain's "chattering mind," responsible for rumination, self-referential thought, and worry, shows markedly reduced activity during chanting. This is the neurological equivalent of giving the inner critic a rest. Simultaneously, activity increases in the prefrontal cortex (associated with focused attention) and the insula (linked to interoception and body awareness), creating a state of alert, embodied calm.

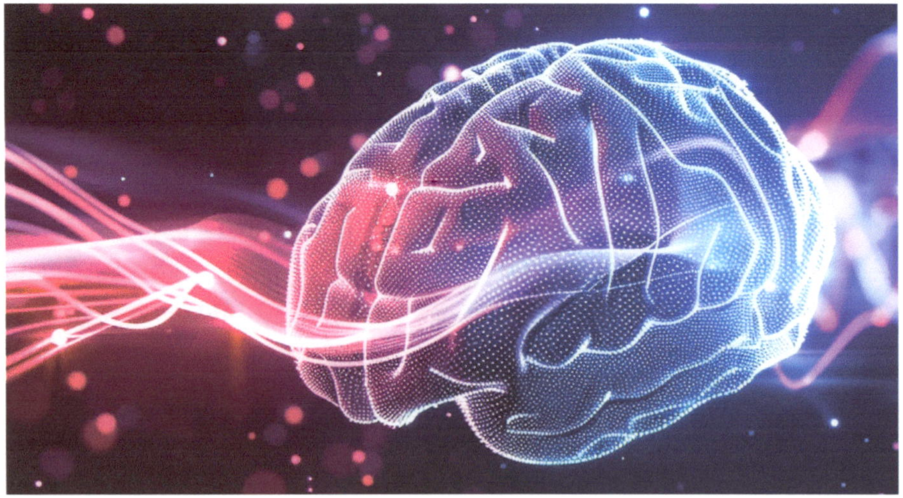

Key Neurological Effects Of Chanting

- Increased alpha and theta brainwave activity – promoting deep relaxation without drowsiness
- Reduced activation of the amygdala – the brain's fear and stress response center
- Elevated serotonin and dopamine production – neurotransmitters of mood and wellbeing
- Reduced activity in the Default Mode Network – quieting repetitive thought loops
- Enhanced synchrony between the left and right hemispheres – supporting whole-brain integration
- Stimulation of the pineal and pituitary glands via physical vibration in the skull cavity

BREATH

The Breath at the Centre

All chanting is, at its core, a breathwork practice. To sustain a chant – whether a single syllable like Om or a long Gregorian phrase – the practitioner must breathe with intention. The typical chanting breath involves a moderately deep inhalation followed by a long, controlled exhalation that carries the sound. This pattern naturally produces six to eight breath cycles per minute, a rate, researchers have identified as optimal for heart rate variability (HRV) a key marker of cardiovascular and nervous system health.

This slow, resonant breathing is essentially identical to the pranayama practices of yoga and the coherent breathing practices prescribed in clinical stress-reduction programs. Chanting achieves the same physiological state through the vehicle of sound and devotion, making it a practice that is simultaneously deeply spiritual and rigorously physiological.

The breath is the bridge between the conscious and the unconscious. Chanting makes that bridge luminous.

INTEGRAL YOGA TRADITION

PSYCHOLOGY

The Psychological Dimension

Beyond the neurological, chanting exerts a profound influence on psychological well-being. Clinical researchers at institutions including Harvard Medical School and the National Institute of Mental Health have studied chanting-based interventions for anxiety, depression, PTSD, and addiction recovery — with results that are consistently encouraging.

Anxiety and Rumination

The rhythmic, repetitive nature of chanting occupies the analytical mind sufficiently to interrupt the cycle of anxious rumination. Unlike watching television or scrolling — which numb but do not resolve — chanting processes, the nervous system's backlog of stress while simultaneously building capacity for stillness. Participants in structured chanting programs report significant reductions in trait anxiety within as little as eight weeks of regular practice.

Emotional Regulation

Chanting activates the anterior cingulate cortex, a brain region central to emotional regulation and empathy. Regular practitioners show greater capacity to tolerate difficult emotions without being overwhelmed — what psychologists call "distress tolerance." This is partly physiological (stronger

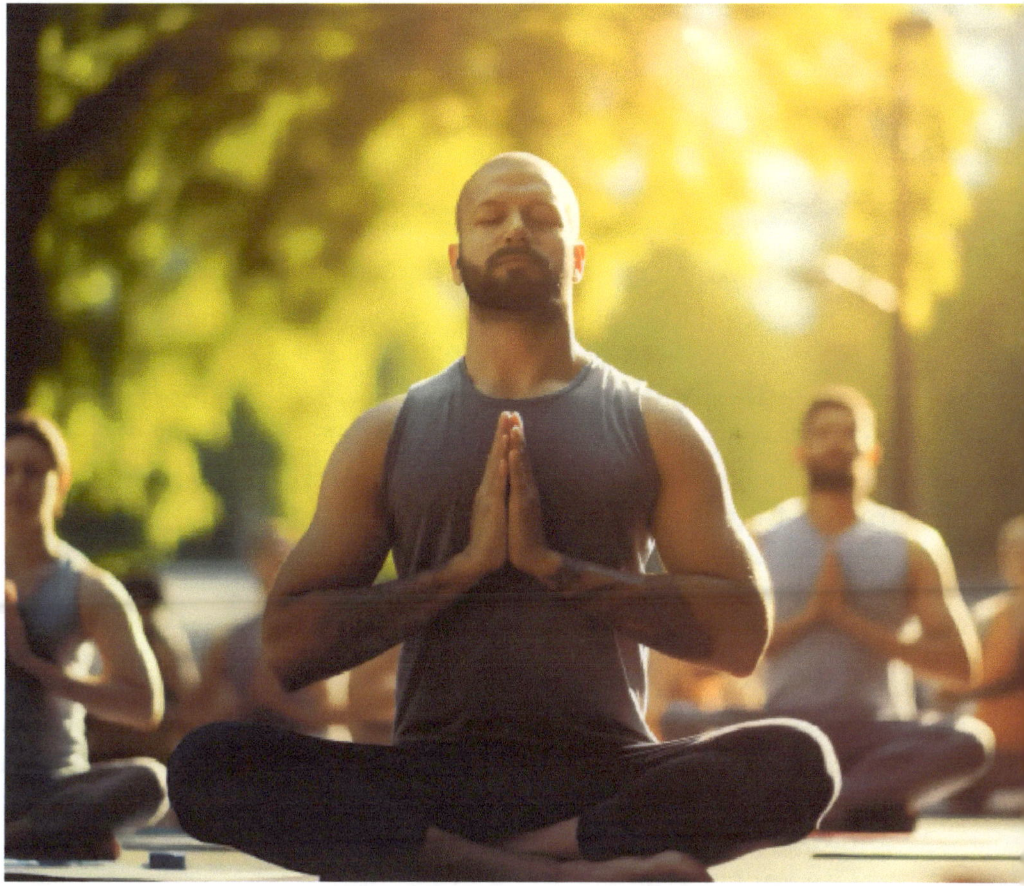

vagal tone) and partly cognitive: the discipline of returning attention to the chant trains is the same "return" skill that is central to all meditative practice.

The Community Factor

Group chanting adds a powerful social dimension. Research on group synchrony — where multiple people breathe, move, or vocalize in unison — shows measurable increases in oxytocin (the bonding hormone), elevated pain thresholds, and a felt sense of connection and belonging. In an age of endemic loneliness, the communal quality of kirtan, choir, or group mantra practice may be among its most therapeutically significant features.

VIBRATION

The Physics of Sacred Sound

Sound is vibration. When we chant, we are not merely producing sound waves in the air — we are vibrating our own bodies from the inside out. The chest, sinuses, skull cavity, and even individual cells participate in the resonance of sustained vocalization. This internal vibration has direct physical effects.

The sound Om (or Aum), arguably the most studied chant in scientific literature, produces a vibration of approximately 136.1 Hz when intoned at its natural pitch — a frequency that interestingly corresponds to the resonant frequency of the Earth's orbital period. More practically, research using functional MRI has shown that Om chanting deactivates the limbic system — including the amygdala, hippocampus, and orbitofrontal cortex — far more effectively than a comparable non-chanting vocalization, suggesting that the specific vibrational quality of Om carries unique neurological properties.

Nitric Oxide and the Sinuses

Studies by Swedish researchers discovered that humming and certain chanting patterns dramatically increase nitric oxide production in the paranasal sinuses by as much as 1500% compared to quiet breathing. Nitric oxide is a critical signaling molecule involved in cardiovascular health, immune function, and the regulation of inflammation. This mundane physiological pathway may be one of the reasons why chanting practitioners across traditions reports improved respiratory health and a general sense of physical vitality.

PRACTICE

Beginning Your Own Practice

The remarkable thing about chanting as a relaxation and healing modality is its accessibility. No special equipment is needed — only the willingness to use the instrument you already carry. A simple starting practice might look like this:

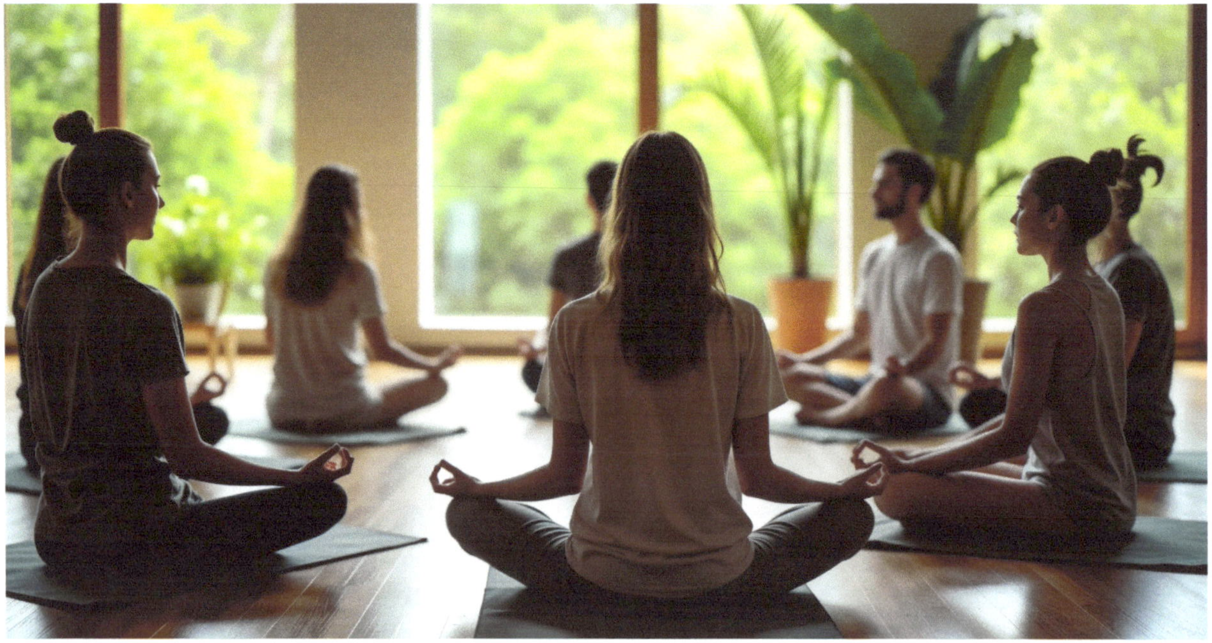

A SIMPLE CHANTING PRACTICE

- Sit comfortably with the spine upright, either cross-legged on the floor or in a chair with feet flat
- Take three slow, deep breaths through the nose to settle the body and arrive fully present
- On the next exhale, allow the sound Om to emerge — beginning with the "Aah" sound, transitioning to "Oh," and sealing with a long humming "Mmm"
- Feel the vibration in the chest, throat, and skull. Let the exhale be as long and complete as is comfortable
- Inhale gently and repeat. Continue for 5–20 minutes, allowing the mind to rest on the sound

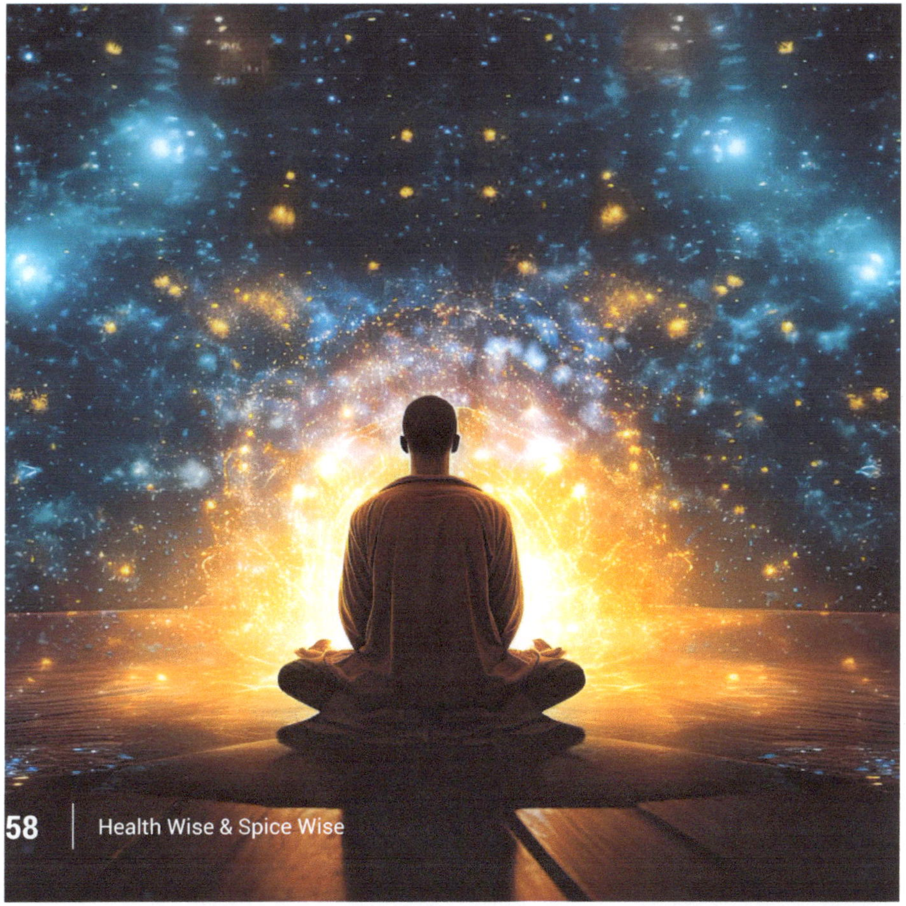

- When finished, sit in silence for 2–3 minutes before returning to activity — honoring the stillness that chanting cultivates

Even five minutes of daily chanting — practiced with consistency over several weeks — is enough to begin reshaping the nervous system's default tone. Longer and deeper practices yield proportionally richer results. The tradition has always held that chanting is not something you do occasionally as a remedy; it is something you become, over time, through repetition and devotion.

You do not need to believe in anything for chanting to work. You only need to do it. The body will understand before the mind does.

CONTEMPORARY MEDITATION TEACHING CLOSING

An Ancient Medicine Rediscovered

What is striking about the modern science of chanting is not that it reveals something new — it is that it confirms, in the precise and dispassionate language of neuroscience and physiology, what contemplative practitioners have always known. The human voice, used with intention and sustained attention, is a remarkably powerful healing instrument. It slows the heart, steadies the breath, quiets the storm of thought, bathes the brain in restorative neurochemistry, and connects the individual to something larger than themselves.

In a culture saturated with noise, distraction, and chronic stress, chanting offers a counterweight that is at once ancient and urgently relevant. It asks nothing more of us than our voice, our breath, and a few minutes of willingness to be still.

The sound is always waiting. We need only open our mouths.

REFERENCES

Physiology & the Nervous System

1. Kalyani, B.G., Venkatasubramanian, G., Arasappa, R., et al. (2011). Neurohemodynamic correlates of 'OM' chanting: A pilot functional magnetic resonance imaging study. International Journal of Yoga, 4(1), 3–6. doi:10.4103/0973-6131.78171The foundational fMRI study demonstrating that Om chanting produces significant deactivation of the amygdala, hippocampus, insula, orbitofrontal cortex, and thalamus — comparable to effects of clinical vagus nerve stimulation.
2. Rao, N.P., Deshpande, G., Gangadhar, K.B., et al. (2018). Directional brain networks underlying OM chanting. Asian Journal of Psychiatry, 37, 20–25. doi:10.1016/j.ajp.2018.07.025Follow-up fMRI connectivity study showing reduced output from insula, anterior cingulate, and orbitofrontal cortices to the amygdala during Om chanting, with implications for depression treatment.
3. Bernardi, L., Sleight, P., Bandinelli, G., et al. (2001). Effect of rosary prayer and yoga mantras on autonomic cardiovascular rhythms: Comparative study. BMJ, 323(7327), 1446–1449. doi:10.1136/bmj.323.7327.1446Landmark study in 23 healthy adults showing that both Ave Maria recitation and yoga mantra chanting spontaneously slow breathing to approximately 6 breaths per minute, significantly enhancing heart rate variability and baroreflex sensitivity.
4. Inbaraj, G., Rao, R.M., Ram, A., et al. (2022). Immediate effects of OM chanting on heart rate variability measures compared between experienced and inexperienced yoga practitioners. International Journal of Yoga, 15(1), 52–58. doi:10.4103/ijoy.ijoy_141_21Demonstrates enhanced parasympathetic activity (measured via HRV) following brief Om chanting sessions.
5. Porges, S.W. (2017). The Pocket Guide to Polyvagal Theory: The Transformative Power of Feeling Safe. W.W. Norton & Company. Theoretical framework explaining how the voice, social engagement, and vocalization are directly linked to vagal regulation of safety and autonomic tone.

Nitric Oxide & Respiratory Physiology

6. Weitzberg, E. & Lundberg, J.O. (2002). Humming greatly increases nasal nitric oxide. American Journal of Respiratory and Critical Care Medicine, 166(2), 144–145. doi:10.1164/rccm.200202-138BCDemonstrated a 15-fold increase in nasal nitric oxide during humming compared with quiet exhalation, mediated by oscillating airflow increasing sinus ventilation — with implications for respiratory health and immune function.
7. Maniscalco, M., Weitzberg, E., Sundberg, J., Sofia, M., & Lundberg, J.O. (2003). Assessment of nasal and sinus nitric oxide output using single-breath humming exhalations. European Respiratory Journal, 22(2), 323–329. doi:10.1183/09031936.03.00017903

Brainwaves & Neural Correlates

8. Harne, B.P., Bobade, Y., Dhekekar, R.S., &Hiwale, A. (2019). SVM classification of EEG signal to analyze the effect of Om Mantra chanting on the brain. IEEE Xplore Conference Proceedings.Demonstrated significant increases in alpha and theta brainwave activity during mantra chanting.
9. Thanneeru, S.K., Kushwah, A., & Agrawal, A. (2023). "Om" chanting and its impact on selected neurological functions. Manipal Journal of Medical Sciences. Available via Manipal University PressSystematic review of fMRI and EEG studies of Om chanting documenting consistent reductions in limbic activity, alpha/theta shifts, and improvements in anxiety and stress.

Cortisol, Anxiety & Psychological Effects

10. Niva, W.J., Sekar, L., Manikandan, A., Maheshkumar, K., & Ganesan, T. (2021). Mahamantra chanting as an effective intervention for stress reduction among nursing professionals — A randomized controlled study. Complementary Therapies in Clinical Practice. doi:10.1016/j.ctcp.2020.101278Randomized controlled trial finding significant reductions in serum cortisol and salivary amylase in nursing professionals who chanted the Hare Krishna Mahamantra for 20 minutes daily over 45 days.
11. Koh, E., &Calear, A. (2023). Exploring the physiological and psychological effects of group chanting in Australia: Reduced stress, cortisol and enhanced social connection. Journal of Religion and Health. doi:10.1007/s10943-023-01967-5Thirty-four-participant study showing that 12 minutes of group Om chanting reduced cortisol and anxiety and increased feelings of social connection.
12. Bormann, J.E., et al. (2014). Mantram repetition for veterans with PTSD. Journal of Clinical Psychology — referenced in Koh &Calear (2023) above. A randomized controlled trial of 146 veterans showing that 6 weeks of silent mantra repetition reduced PTSD symptoms and increased mindful attention.

Group Synchrony & Oxytocin

13. Wiltermuth, S.S. & Heath, C. (2009). Synchrony and cooperation. Psychological Science, 20(1), 1–5. Foundational research showing that behavioural synchrony (including vocal synchrony) increases cooperation, prosocial behaviour, and feelings of connection — mediated in part by oxytocin and elevated pain thresholds.

General Reviews

14. Lim, D., & Mak, M. (2022). Scientific evidence of health benefits by practicing mantra meditation: Narrative review. JMIR Serious Games / PMC. PMC9623891Comprehensive narrative review covering the evidence base for mantra meditation across stress, anxiety, hypertension, and immunity, including the Bernardi et al. respiratory findings.
15. DeFrancesco, M., Johnson, L., Cruz, G., & Stryker, M. (2025). The vagus nerve and voice. NCVS Insights. ncvs.orgReview of vocalization, the vagus nerve, and autonomic regulation, including research on chanting and humming as non-invasive vagal stimulation techniques.

MUSIC THERAPY

Healing Through Sound and Rhythm

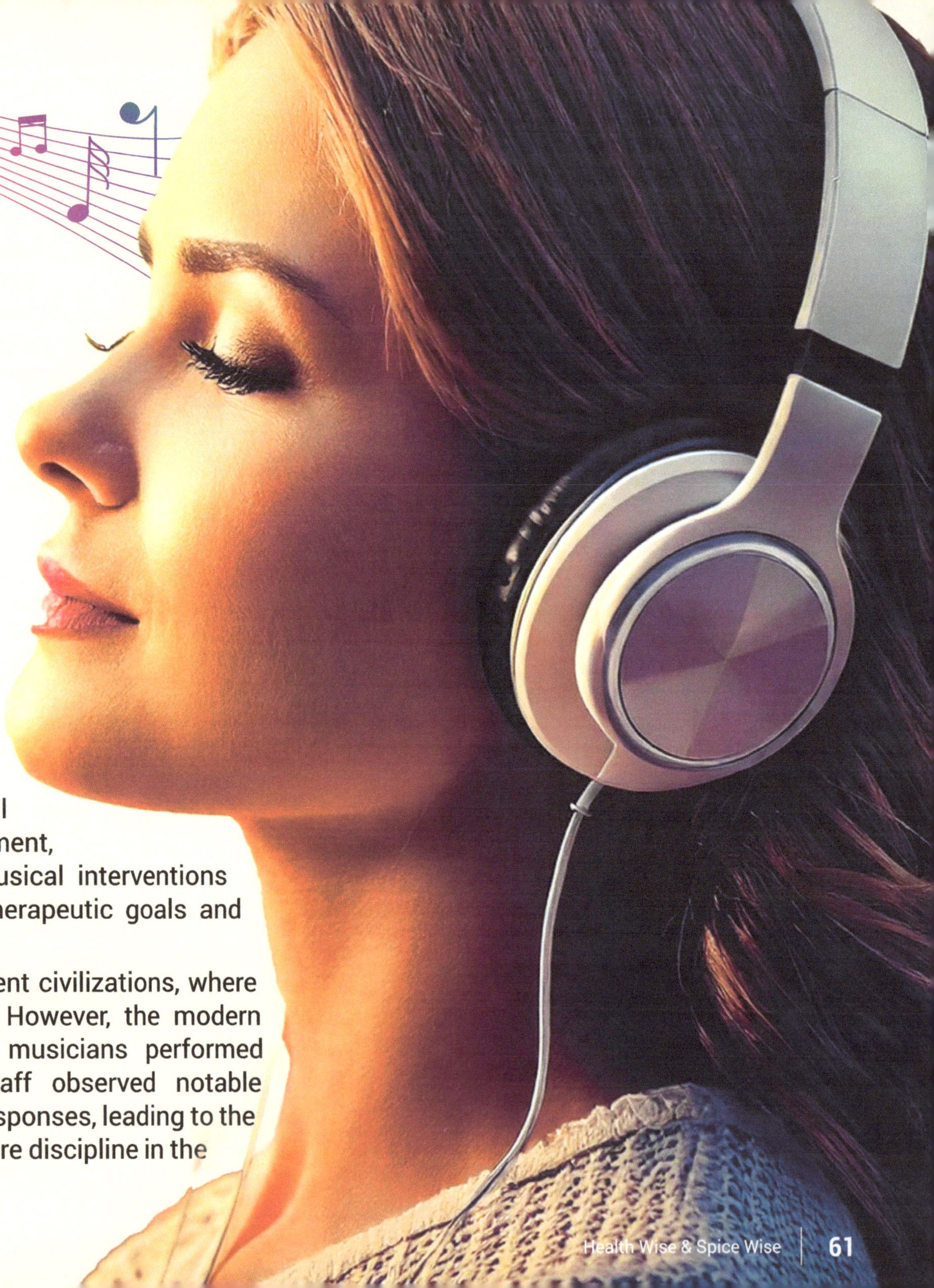

Music therapy is a clinical and evidence-based healthcare profession that harnesses the inherent power of music to address the physical, emotional, cognitive, and social needs of individuals across all age groups. Far beyond casual listening or entertainment, music therapy involves the systematic use of musical interventions by trained professionals to accomplish specific therapeutic goals and improve quality of life.

The roots of music therapy stretch back to ancient civilizations, where music was recognized for its healing properties. However, the modern profession emerged during World War II when musicians performed for wounded veterans in hospitals. Medical staff observed notable improvements in patients' physical and emotional responses, leading to the formal establishment of music therapy as a healthcare discipline in the

1940s.

Board-certified music therapists complete rigorous academic and clinical training, studying music, psychology, anatomy, research methods, and therapeutic techniques. They assess clients' needs and develop individualized treatment plans incorporating various musical elements: rhythm, melody, harmony, and lyrics. Interventions might include active music-making, songwriting, improvisation, music listening, or movement to music, each tailored to specific therapeutic objectives.

The neurological basis for music therapy's effectiveness lies in music's unique ability to activate multiple brain regions simultaneously. Music processing involves areas responsible for motor control, emotion, memory, and language, creating rich neural networks that can be leveraged for rehabilitation. This widespread brain activation explains why music therapy succeeds where traditional therapies sometimes fall short.

Research demonstrates music therapy's effectiveness across numerous conditions. For stroke patients, rhythmic auditory stimulation can improve gait patterns and motor coordination. Individuals with Alzheimer's disease often retain musical memories long after other cognitive functions decline, making music a powerful tool for accessing communication and reducing agitation. Children with autism spectrum disorders benefit from structured musical interactions that enhance social skills and communication abilities.

In mental health treatment, music therapy provides emotional expression outlets for those struggling to verbalize feelings. Songwriting allows clients to process trauma, while group drumming circles foster social connection and reduces isolation. For individuals battling addiction, music therapy offers healthy coping mechanisms and supports recovery through creative expression and community building.

Pediatric settings showcase music therapy's versatility. Hospitalized children experience reduced anxiety and pain through musical interventions, while premature infants in NICUs show improved vital signs and feeding responses when exposed to therapeutic music. Music therapy also supports children with developmental delays, using musical play to enhance motor skills, language development, and social interaction.

The profession continues expanding into diverse settings: psychiatric facilities, rehabilitation hospitals, schools, nursing homes, hospice care, and private practice. Music therapists work within interdisciplinary teams, collaborating with physicians, psychologists, physical therapists, and social workers to provide comprehensive care.

Technology is revolutionizing music therapy delivery through apps, virtual reality experiences, and biofeedback-integrated musical devices. These innovations expand access to therapeutic music interventions while maintaining the essential human connection between therapist and client.

Perhaps most remarkably, music therapy recognizes that musical ability or training is unnecessary for therapeutic benefit. The intervention focuses on the client's response to music rather than musical performance quality, making it universally accessible.

As healthcare increasingly embraces holistic approaches, music therapy stands as a testament to music's profound healing capacity. By addressing the whole person rather than isolated symptoms, music therapy offers hope, healing, and human connection through the universal language of music, proving that sometimes the most powerful medicine comes not from a pharmacy, but from the heart of human creativity.

ANGER CONTROL

Mastering Your Emotional Responses

Anger is a natural human emotion that serves as a warning signal when we perceive threats, injustices, or frustrations. While anger itself isn't inherently problematic, uncontrolled anger can damage relationships, impair decision-making, and negatively impact both mental and physical health. Learning effective anger control techniques is essential for maintaining emotional well-being and fostering healthy interactions with others.

Understanding anger's physiological mechanisms is the first step toward control. When triggered, the body's fight-or-flight response activates, releasing stress hormones like adrenaline and cortisol,heart rate increases, muscles tense, and breathing becomes shallow. This biological response, evolved for survival, can overwhelm rational thinking and lead to impulsive reactions that we later regret.

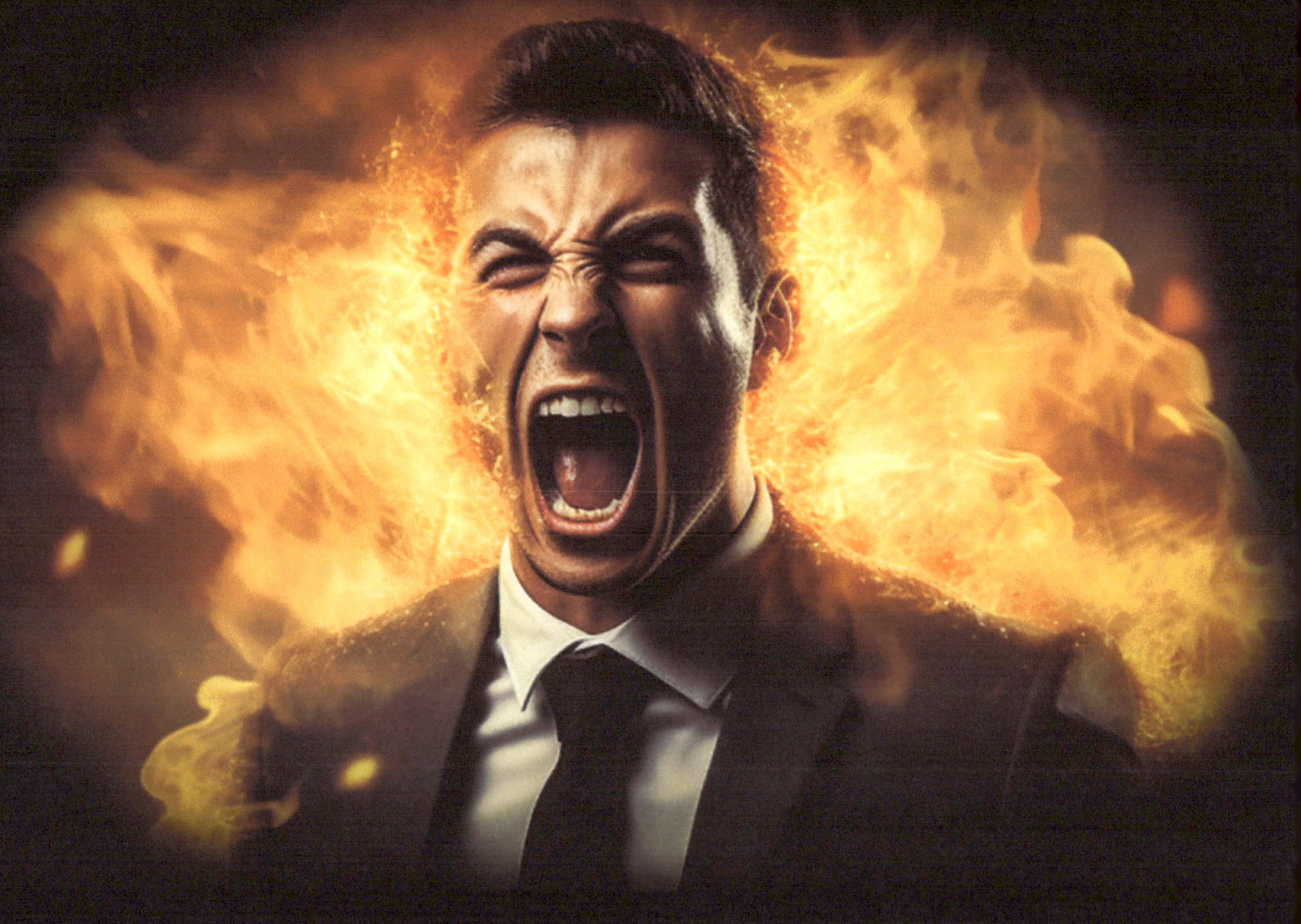

The cognitive component of anger often involves distorted thinking patterns. Common triggers include perceived unfairness, feeling disrespected, experiencing frustration when goals are blocked, or interpreting neutral situations as personal attacks. Recognizing these thought patterns helps interrupt the anger cycle before it escalates.

Early warning signs of anger include physical sensations like tension headaches, clenched jaw, rapid heartbeat, or feeling hot. Emotional indicators might include irritability, resentment, or feeling overwhelmed. Behavioral changes such as speaking louder, pacing, or withdrawing from others also signal mounting anger. Developing awareness of these personal warning signs enables proactive intervention.

Deep breathing techniques form the cornerstone of immediate anger management. The 4-7-8 technique involves inhaling for four counts, holding for seven, and exhaling for eight. This activates the parasympathetic nervous system, naturally calming the body's stress response. Progressive muscle relaxation, systematically tensing and releasing muscle groups, also helps discharge physical tension associated with anger.

Cognitive restructuring challenges angry thoughts by examining their accuracy and helpfulness. Instead of thinking "This always happens to me," try "This is frustrating, but it's a temporary situation I can handle." Reframing situations from different perspectives reduces anger intensity and opens possibilities for constructive solutions.

The timeout strategy involves removing yourself from anger-provoking situations when you notice escalation beginning. This isn't avoidance but rather a strategic pause to regain emotional equilibrium before addressing the issue constructively. During timeouts, engage in calming activities like walking, listening to music, or practicing mindfulness.

Physical exercise provides an excellent outlet for anger's energy. Regular cardiovascular activity reduces overall stress levels and provides healthy emotional release. Activities like boxing, running, or even vigorous housework can help discharge angry energy constructively.

Communication skills play a crucial role in anger management. Using "I" statements instead of "you" accusations reduce defensiveness in others. For example, say "I feel frustrated when meetings start late" rather than "You never start on time." This approach expresses feelings without attacking others, making productive dialogue more likely.

Long-term anger management involves addressing underlying causes. Chronic anger often stems from deeper issues like unresolved trauma, depression, anxiety, or learned behavioral patterns. Professional counseling can help identify and address these root causes through techniques like cognitive-behavioral therapy or anger management courses.

Lifestyle factors significantly impact anger control. Adequate sleep, regular exercise, balanced nutrition, and stress reduction practices create a foundation for emotional stability. Limiting alcohol and caffeine consumption also helps maintain emotional equilibrium.

Remember that anger control is a skill requiring practice and patience. Setbacks are normal parts of the learning process. The goal isn't eliminating anger entirely but developing healthy ways to express and manage it. With consistent effort and appropriate strategies, anyone can learn to harness anger's energy constructively while maintaining important relationships and personal well-being.

COMMON HEADACHES

Causes, Symptom Treatments & Daily Routine Relationships

A Comprehensive Health Reference • April 2026

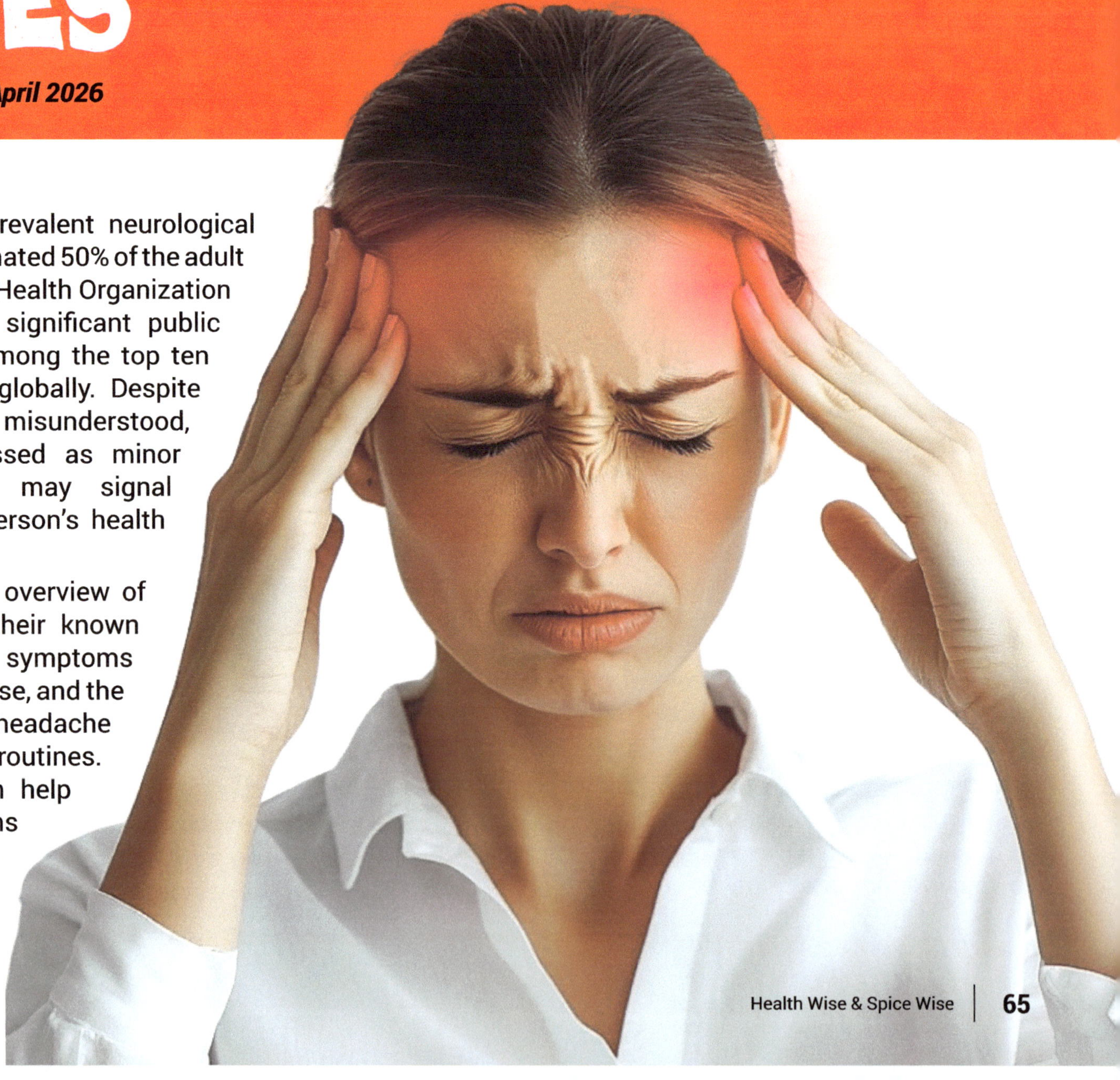

INTRODUCTION

Headaches are among the most prevalent neurological complaints worldwide, affecting an estimated 50% of the adult population in any given year. The World Health Organization recognizes headache disorders as a significant public health concern, noting that they are among the top ten causes of years lived with disability globally. Despite their ubiquity, headaches are frequently misunderstood, inappropriately self-treated, or dismissed as minor inconveniences, even though they may signal meaningful underlying patterns in a person's health and lifestyle.

This article provides an accessible overview of the most common headache types, their known causes, approaches to managing symptoms without necessarily treating the root cause, and the often-overlooked relationship between headache frequency and daily habits and routines. Understanding these connections can help individuals make informed decisions about their own well-being and when to seek professional medical advice.

PART I: TYPES & KNOWN CAUSES OF COMMON HEADACHES

1.1 Tension-Type Headaches

Tension-type headaches (TTH) are the most common headache disorder, affecting up to 78% of the general population at some point in their lives. They are characterized by a dull, pressing, or tightening pain — often described as a "band" or "vice" around the head — typically bilateral in nature and of mild to moderate intensity. Unlike migraines, they are not usually worsened by routine physical activity.

Known causes and triggers include:

- Prolonged muscle contraction in the head, neck, and shoulder regions, often from poor posture
- Psychological stress and anxiety, which increase muscle tension around the cranium
- Sleep disturbances, including both insufficient and excessive sleep
- Eye strain from extended screen use or uncorrected vision
- Dehydration and irregular meal patterns
- Caffeine dependence and withdrawal

1.2 Migraine

Migraines are a complex neurological disorder affecting approximately 15% of the global population, with a notably higher prevalence in women (roughly 3:1 female-to-male ratio). A migraine episode typically involves throbbing, moderate-to-severe head pain — most often unilateral — accompanied by nausea, vomiting, and heightened sensitivity to light (photophobia) and sound (phonophobia). Episodes can last between 4 and 72 hours and are frequently debilitating.

Approximately one-third of migraine sufferers experience an "aura," transient neurological symptoms such as visual disturbances (flashing lights, zigzag lines), tingling in the limbs, or speech difficulties that precede or accompany the headache phase.

Established causes and common triggers include:

- Genetic predisposition: migraines have a strong hereditary component, with first-degree relatives of migraine sufferers at significantly elevated risk
- Hormonal fluctuations, particularly changes in estrogen levels around menstruation, pregnancy, and menopause
- Dietary triggers: aged cheeses, processed meats, alcohol (especially red wine), MSG, and aspartame
- Sensory stimuli: bright or flickering lights, strong odors, and loud sounds
- Barometric pressure changes and weather shifts
- Stress and post-stress relaxation (the so-called "weekend migraine" phenomenon)
- Disrupted sleep patterns and jet lag

1.3 Cluster Headaches

Cluster headaches are the least common of the primary headache disorders discussed here, yet they are often regarded as among the most severe pain conditions known to medicine. They occur in cyclical patterns or "clusters," typically one to eight attacks per day lasting 15 to 180 minutes each, followed by remission periods that can last months or years. They are significantly more prevalent in men and typically manifest between the ages of 20 and 50.

The pain is typically described as excruciating, burning, or piercing, localized around or behind one eye. Distinctive autonomic features include a red or watering eye, drooping eyelid, nasal congestion, and facial sweating on the affected side.

Known causes and triggers include:

- Hypothalamic dysfunction — abnormal activity in the region of the brain that regulates circadian rhythms is strongly implicated
- Alcohol consumption, which is a reliable trigger during active cluster periods
- Strong smells such as solvents, paint, or petrol
- Changes in sleep-wake cycles, including seasonal shifts and altitude changes
- Cigarette smoking (found in a disproportionate number of cluster headache patients)

1.4 Secondary Headaches

Secondary headaches are attributable to an underlying condition rather than representing a primary disorder themselves. Common causes include sinusitis and upper respiratory infections, cervicogenic (neck-related) dysfunction, hypertension, medication overuse ("rebound headache"), caffeine withdrawal, sleep apnea, andrarer conditions requiring urgent medical attention, such as meningitis, intracranial bleeding, or brain tumors. Any headache described as a sudden, severe "thunderclap" onset, or accompanied by fever, stiff neck, confusion, or vision loss, warrants immediate medical evaluation.

> ***Clinical Note:*** *Medication Overuse Headache (MOH) affects an estimated 1–2% of the general population and is one of the most underdiagnosed causes of chronic daily headache. If you are taking pain relief more than 2–3 times per week, consult a healthcare professional.*

PART II: SYMPTOM TREATMENT APPROACHES

Symptom management — as distinct from addressing the root cause — focuses on reducing pain intensity, shortening episode duration, and improving quality of life during a headache. The following strategies span pharmacological, physical, and behavioral domains.

2.1 Over-the-Counter Analgesics

For tension-type headaches and mild-to-moderate migraines, non-prescription analgesics represent the first line of symptomatic relief for most adults. These include:

- Paracetamol (acetaminophen): effective for tension-type headaches; generally well tolerated and considered safe for most adults when used as directed
- NSAIDs (Non-Steroidal Anti-Inflammatory Drugs): ibuprofen, naproxen sodium, and aspirin reduce both pain and associated inflammation; ibuprofen has substantial evidence for migraine symptom relief
- Combination analgesics: products containing paracetamol, aspirin, and caffeine (e.g. Excedrin Migraine) can be more effective for migraine than single-ingredient options

Important caution: Frequent use of analgesics — more than 10 to 15 days per month — can paradoxically lead to medication overuse headache (MOH), a form of chronic daily headache that is itself difficult to treat. Adherence to recommended frequencies is essential.

2.2 Prescription Triptans for Migraine

Triptans (e.g., sumatriptan, rizatriptan, Ele triptan) are serotonin receptor agonists specifically developed for acute migraine treatment. They work by constricting blood vessels and inhibiting the release of inflammatory neuropeptides. Available in oral, nasal spray, and injectable forms, triptans are highly effective when taken early in a migraine episode. They are not suitable for individuals with cardiovascular disease, and a healthcare provider should be consulted before use.

2.3 Physical and Non-Pharmacological Approaches

Cold and Heat Therapy

Applying a cold pack or ice wrapped in cloth to the forehead or back of the neck can reduce the throbbing sensation associated with migraines by constricting blood vessels. Conversely, heat application to the neck and shoulders is often more effective for tension-type headaches, where muscle tightness is a primary contributor.

Hydration

Dehydration is one of the most overlooked headache triggers. Drinking 400–500 ml of water at headache onset — and maintaining adequate daily hydration of approximately 2–2.5 liters — can prevent a significant proportion of dehydration-related episodes and shorten their duration.

Rest and Environmental Control

Migraine sufferers in particular benefit substantially from resting in a quiet, dark room during an acute episode. Reducing sensory input — turning off screens, dimming lights, and using earplugs — directly addresses the photophobia and phonophobia that amplify pain perception during attacks.

> ***Key Principle:*** *Symptom treatments are most effective when applied early. Waiting until pain is severe significantly reduces the efficacy of most interventions, both pharmacological and non-pharmacological.*

Caffeine (Targeted Use)

Caffeine in moderate amounts can enhance the effectiveness of analgesics and, when consumed at headache onset, may abort mild attacks. However, habitual caffeine consumption creates dependency, and withdrawal itself becomes a headache trigger. Strategic use — not daily reliance — is the relevant approach here.

Pressure Point and Massage Techniques

Gentle massage of the temples, suboccipital muscles (at the base of the skull), and the LI-4 acupressure point (the web between thumb and index finger) has demonstrated modest symptomatic benefit in some studies. These approaches are particularly appropriate as adjunctive measures for tension-type headaches.

Biofeedback and Relaxation Training

Biofeedback — a technique in which individuals learn to control physiological responses (such as muscle tension and skin temperature) through real-time monitoring — has robust evidence as a non-pharmacological treatment for both tension-type and migraine headaches. Progressive muscle relaxation and guided breathing techniques offer accessible alternatives with comparable benefits when practiced consistently.

2.4 Oxygen Therapy for Cluster Headaches

High-flow inhaled oxygen (100% O_2 at 7–15 liters per minute via a non-rebreather mask for 15–20 minutes) is one of the most effective acute treatments for cluster headache, producing relief in up to 70% of cases. Portable oxygen setups can be prescribed for home use during active cluster periods. Sumatriptan injection or nasal spray is also used acutely.

PART III: HEADACHES & DAILY ROUTINES

Perhaps the most actionable insight in headache research over the past two decades is how strongly everyday habits and routines influence both headache frequency and severity. The concept of "lifestyle medicine," using modifiable behavioral factors as therapeutic tools, is directly applicable to headache management.

3.1 Sleep: The Foundation

There is a bidirectional relationship between sleep and headaches. Poor sleep quality or insufficient duration (below 7 hours for most adults) significantly increases headache risk the following day. Conversely, migraines and cluster headaches frequently disrupt sleep, creating a reinforcing cycle. Equally problematic is excessive sleep: oversleeping on weekends is a well-recognized trigger for "weekend migraines" linked to schedule disruption and delayed caffeine intake.

Practical recommendations for sleep-headache management include:

- Maintaining a consistent sleep and wake time, including weekends and holidays
- Targeting 7–9 hours of sleep per night for most adults
- Limiting screen exposure to 60 minutes before bedtime
- Keeping the sleep environment cool, dark, and quiet — conditions that also reduce migraine vulnerability
- Addressing sleep apnea through medical consultation if morning headaches are frequent

3.2 Hydration and Nutrition Patterns

As noted previously, dehydration is among the most common — and most preventable — headache triggers. Many individuals find that distributing water intake evenly throughout the day, rather than drinking large volumes infrequently, is most effective. Caffeinated beverages do not substitute for water and contribute to the overall dehydration cycle.

Meal regularity is equally significant. Skipping meals leads to hypoglycemia (low blood sugar), a well-documented headache trigger. For individuals prone to migraines, maintaining stable blood glucose through regular meals — including a small protein source — can meaningfully reduce attack frequency. For those tracking dietary migraine triggers, a food diary maintained over 4–6 weeks is the most reliable method for identifying personal sensitivities.

3.3 Physical Activity and Posture

Regular, moderate aerobic exercise is associated with reduced headache frequency. A landmark study published in Cephalalgia demonstrated that three sessions per week of cycling or brisk walking were as effective as preventive migraine medication (topiramate) in reducing monthly migraine frequency, with fewer side effects. The mechanism likely involves the release of endorphins, improved cardiovascular function, and normalization of the stress response.

However, high-intensity exercise can trigger migraines in susceptible individuals (exertional headache), and gradual escalation of intensity is recommended for those new to exercise as a preventive strategy.

Posture and ergonomics represent an underappreciated driver of tension-type and cervicogenic headaches. Sustained forward head posture — prevalent in remote workers and those spending extended periods at computers — places considerable mechanical load on the cervical spine and suboccipital musculature. Workstation adjustments (monitor at eye level, chair support for lumbar and thoracic spine, keyboard at elbow height) and regular movement breaks (every 30–45 minutes) are evidence-supported interventions.

3.4 Stress Management and Psychological Routines

Psychological stress is the single most frequently cited headache trigger in population surveys. The mechanisms are both direct (stress hormones such as cortisol and adrenaline promote vascular changes and muscle tension) and indirect (stress disrupts sleep, increases caffeine consumption, and promotes irregular eating). Importantly, the "let-down" phase following a period of intense stress — such as the end of the working week or a demanding project — is also a common migraine window.

Evidence-based stress management approaches that have demonstrated headache reduction include:

- Mindfulness-Based Stress Reduction (MBSR): structured 8-week programs with strong evidence for chronic pain reduction
- Cognitive Behavioral Therapy (CBT): particularly effective for chronic daily headache and headache-associated anxiety
- Regular mindfulness meditation: even 10–15 minutes daily, with apps such as Headspace or Calm offering accessible entry points
- Journaling: tracking stressors, mood, and headache occurrence helps identify patterns and gives a sense of agency
- Social connection and adequate leisure time: consistently associated with lower chronic pain levels in epidemiological research

When to Seek Medical Advice: *Consult a doctor if headaches occur more than 15 days per month, are progressively worsening, begin after age 50, are accompanied by neurological symptoms (weakness, vision changes, confusion), follow a head injury, or are described as the "worst headache of your life." These features require professional evaluation.*

3.5 Screen Use and Digital Habits

In the contemporary working and social environment, extended screen exposure has emerged as a significant contributor to headache burden. Blue light exposure, reduced blink rate (causing eye strain and dry eye), and the posture associated with device use all contribute. Practical mitigations include the 20-20-20 rule (every 20 minutes, look at something 20 feet away for 20 seconds), blue light filtering glasses or screen settings, and ensuring adequate ambient lighting to reduce screen contrast.

3.6 Building a "Headache Routine" Putting It Together

For individuals experiencing frequent or recurring headaches, a structured daily routine incorporating the elements discussed represents the most sustainable preventive strategy. The following framework consolidates the evidence:

- Morning: consistent wake time; immediate hydration (400–500 ml water upon waking); balanced breakfast including protein
- Work/day: ergonomic workspace; 30-minute movement breaks; regular water intake; screen management with 20-20-20 rule
- Exercise: 3–5 sessions per week of moderate aerobic activity, 30–45 minutes
- Evening: wind-down routine including stress-reduction practice; limiting caffeine after midday; screen dimming
- Sleep: consistent bedtime; 7–9 hours; cool, dark, quiet environment
- Monitoring: maintain a headache diary noting triggers, duration, severity, medications taken, and potential lifestyle factors.

REFERENCES

The following sources informed the content of this article. Readers are encouraged to consult peer-reviewed literature and qualified healthcare providers for personalised guidance.

1. Stovner, L.J., et al. (2022). Global, regional, and national burden of headache disorders, 1990–2016: A systematic analysis for the Global Burden of Disease Study 2016. The Lancet Neurology, 17(11), 954–976.
2. World Health Organization. (2016). Headache disorders. WHO Fact Sheet No. 277. Geneva: WHO. https://www.who.int/news-room/fact-sheets/detail/headache-disorders
3. Headache Classification Committee of the International Headache Society (IHS). (2018). The International Classification of Headache Disorders, 3rd edition. Cephalalgia, 38(1), 1–211.
4. Smitherman, T.A., Burch, R., Sheikh, H., & Loder, E. (2013). The prevalence, impact, and treatment of migraine and severe headaches in the United States: A review of statistics from national surveillance studies. Headache, 53(3), 427–436.
5. Linde, M., et al. (2012). Aerobic exercise and topiramate as preventive therapies for migraine: A randomised controlled trial. Cephalalgia, 32(14), 1055–1065.
6. Diener, H.C., et al. (2012). Medication-overuse headache: A worldwide problem. The Lancet Neurology, 11(5), 457–470.
7. Bigal, M.E., & Lipton, R.B. (2011). Obesity is a risk factor for transformed migraine but not chronic tension-type headache. Neurology, 67(2), 252–257.
8. Hindiyeh, N.A., et al. (2020). The role of diet and nutrition in migraine triggers and treatment: A systematic literature review. Headache, 60(7), 1300–1316.
9. Rains, J.C. (2018). Sleep disorders and headache. Headache, 58(7), 1074–1091.
10. Nestoriuc, Y., & Martin, A. (2007). Efficacy of biofeedback for migraine: A meta-analysis. Pain, 128(1–2), 111–127.
11. Garza, I., & Swanson, J.W. (2006). Prophylaxis of migraine. Neuropsychiatric Disease and Treatment, 2(3), 281–291.
12. Silberstein, S.D., et al. (2012). Evidence-based guideline update: Pharmacologic treatment for episodic migraine prevention in adults. Neurology, 78(17), 1337–1345.
13. Sutherland, H.G., & Griffiths, L.R. (2017). Genetics of migraine: Insights into the molecular basis of migraine disorders. Headache, 57(4), 537–569.
14. National Institute for Health and Care Excellence (NICE). (2021). Headaches in over 12s: Diagnosis and management. NICE guideline NG218. London: NICE.
15. Robbins, M.S., & Lipton, R.B. (2010). The epidemiology of primary headache disorders. Seminars in Neurology, 30(2), 107–119.

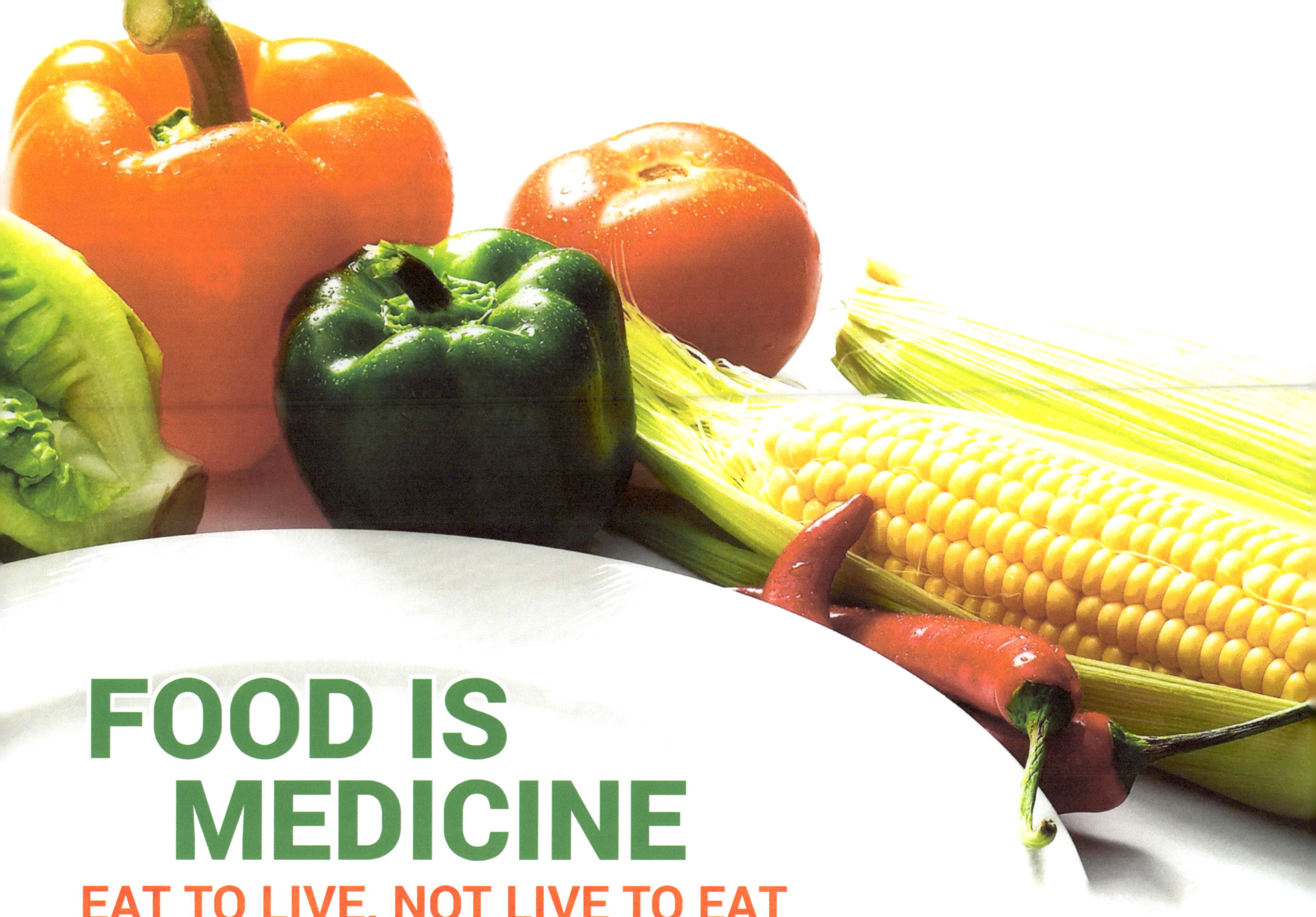

FOOD IS MEDICINE

EAT TO LIVE, NOT LIVE TO EAT

The ancient wisdom "eat to live, not live to eat" has never been more relevant than in our modern world of processed foods and convenience eating. This profound principle, attributed to philosophers like Socrates, reminds us that food should serve as fuel for our bodies and minds rather than becoming the primary focus of our existence. Understanding food as medicine transforms our relationship with nutrition from pleasure-seeking to health-building.

Throughout history, civilizations have recognized food's therapeutic properties. Traditional Chinese Medicine categorizes foods by their energetic qualities and healing properties, while Ayurveda emphasizes eating according to individual constitution and seasonal needs. Hippocrates, the father of modern medicine, proclaimed "Let food be thy medicine and medicine be thy food," establishing a foundational principle that modern science continues to validate.

Contemporary research overwhelmingly supports food's medicinal qualities. Chronic diseases like diabetes, heart disease, and certain cancers are directly linked to dietary choices. Anti-inflammatory foods such as leafy greens, berries, fatty fish, and nuts can reduce disease risk and promote healing. Conversely, processed foods high in sugar, unhealthy fats, and artificial additives contribute to inflammation and disease progression.

The "eat to live" philosophy emphasizes mindful consumption focused on nutritional value rather than sensory pleasure alone. This doesn't mean eliminating enjoyment from eating but rather finding satisfaction in foods that nourish and energize. When we prioritize nutrient density over calorie density, we naturally gravitate toward whole foods that support optimal health.

Functional foods demonstrate a food's medicinal potential. Turmeric's curcumin compounds fight inflammation, while garlic's sulfur compounds support cardiovascular health. Probiotics in fermented foods promote gut health, which influences immune function, mood, and cognitive performance. These examples illustrate how strategic food choices can address specific health concerns naturally.

The opposite approach - living to eat - often leads to emotional eating, overconsumption, and food addiction. When food becomes entertainment or emotional comfort rather than sustenance, we lose connection with hunger and satiety cues. This disconnection contributes to obesity, digestive issues, and metabolic dysfunction that plague modern society.

Adopting an "eat to live" mindset requires practical strategies. Meal planning based on nutritional needs rather than cravings helps establish healthy patterns. Reading ingredient labels and choosing whole, unprocessed foods becomes second nature. Portion control aligns with body's actual energy requirements rather than external influences like restaurant serving sizes.

Mindful eating practices support this philosophy. Eating slowly, chewing thoroughly, and paying attention to hunger and fullness cues help distinguish between physical and emotional hunger. This awareness prevents overeating and increases satisfaction with smaller portions of nutritious foods.

The timing of eating also matters. Eating regular meals prevents energy crashes that lead to poor food choices. Starting the day with protein and healthy fats stabilizes blood sugar and supports sustained energy. Avoiding late-night eating allows digestive systems to rest and repair.

Cultural and social aspects of food need not be abandoned when embracing food as medicine. Sharing meals with others and celebrating with food can coexist with healthy choices. The key lies in balance and intentionality—making most daily food choices based on nutritional value while allowing occasional indulgences without guilt.

This paradigm shift from eating for pleasure to eating for health creates profound changes in energy levels, mental clarity, and overall well-being. When we truly understand that every meal is an opportunity to either fight disease or feed it, our food choices become acts of self-care and preventive medicine, transforming our relationship with food from destructive to healing.

Natural foods are much more nutritious and healthier than factory mass-produced products. Remember that your food needs are also based on the calories you burn daily. In other words, a person practicing and playing a heavy sport has different intake needs than an office worker. It's better to keep starchy vegetables to a minimum (potatoes, corn, peas, etc.), and add leafy vegetables, which are rich in many minerals and vitamins. You need your protein to build and maintain muscles, provide energy sources, and help nervous system development.

Children should be directed by adults in their food choices. Avoid any shelf food with too much or too many additives. Studies prove that eating smaller portions at different intervals is beneficial than eating one large meal at one sitting.

Avoiding drinks that are highly caffeinated, alcoholic, or with too much sugar content will certainly help you in the long run.

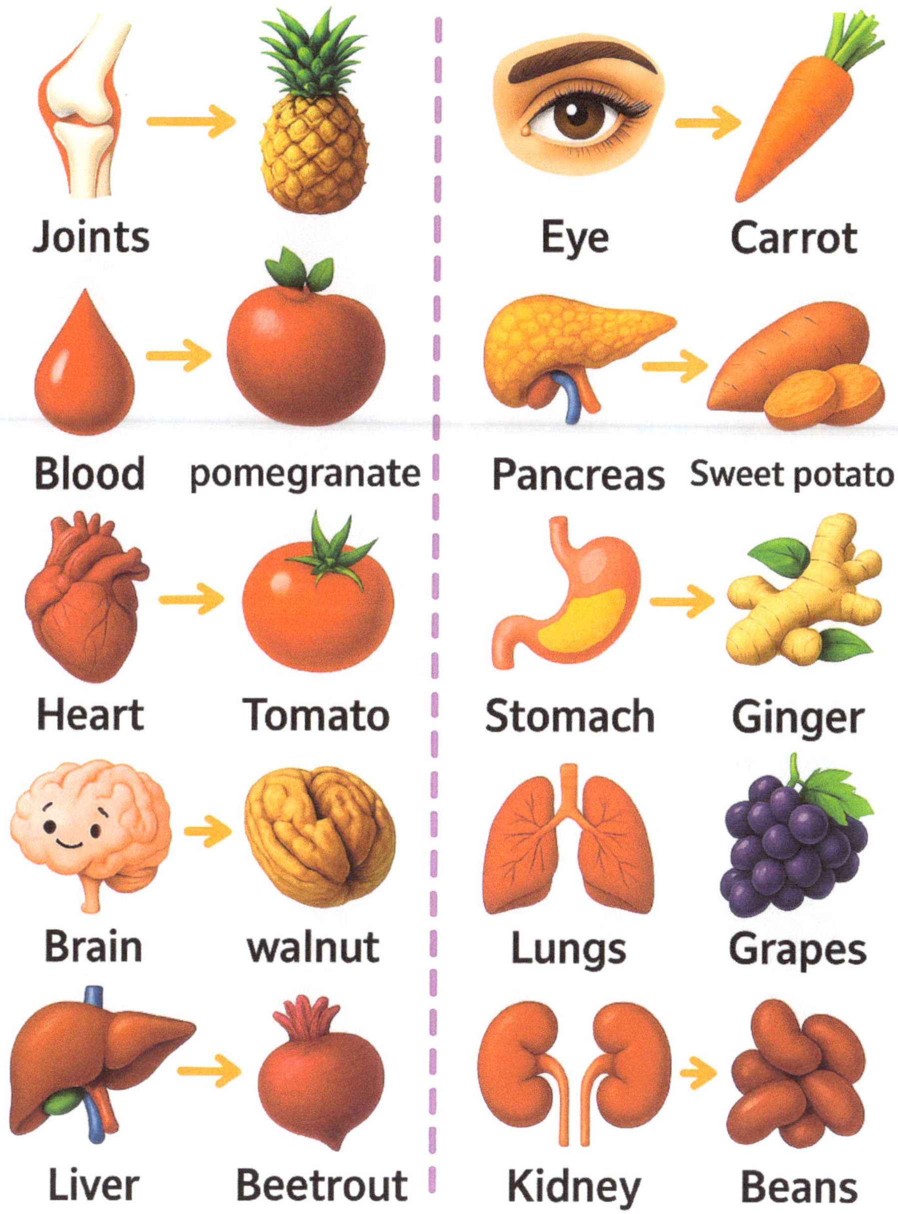

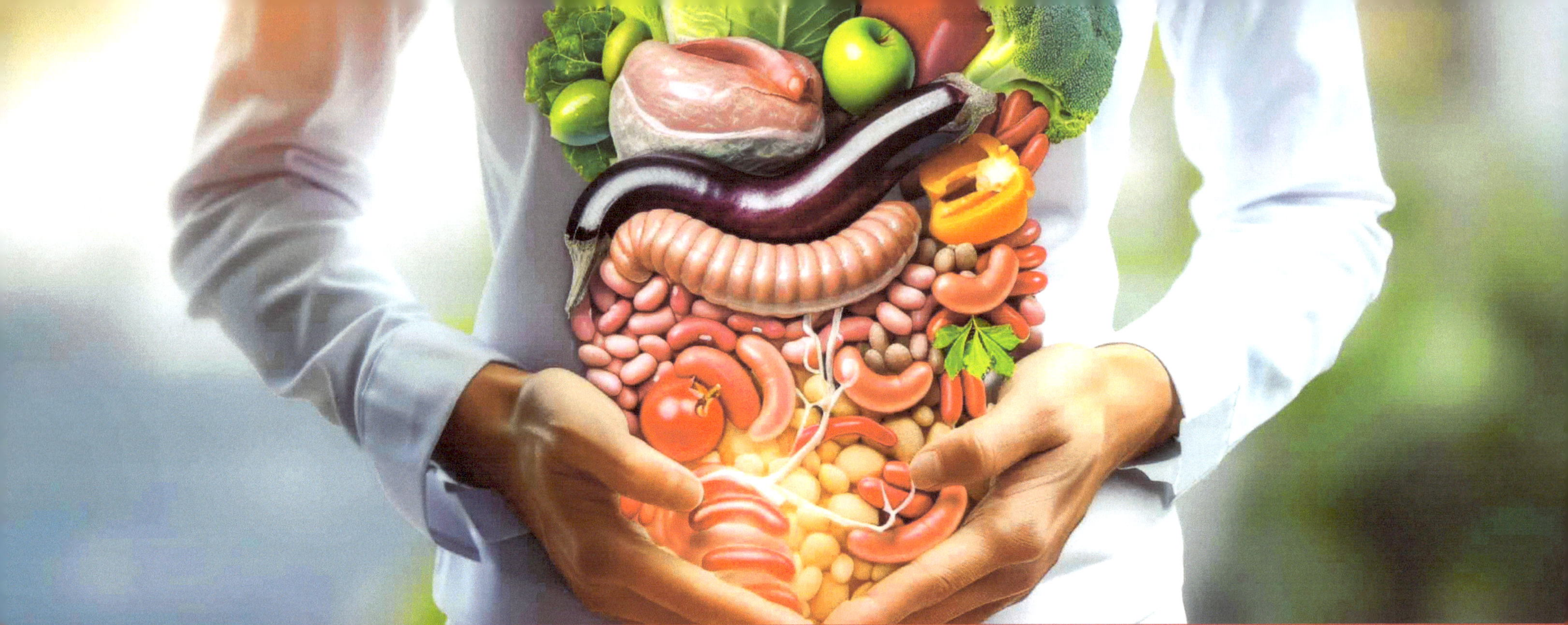

GUT (INTESTINAL) BIOME AND GUT HEALTH

An Important Life Factor

The human gut microbiome, consisting of trillions of bacteria, viruses, fungi, and other microorganisms residing in our digestive tract, has emerged as one of the most critical factors influencing overall health. This complex ecosystem, weighing approximately three pounds, contains more microbial cells than human cells in our body and plays fundamental roles far beyond digestion.

A healthy gut microbiome maintains delicate balance between beneficial and potentially harmful bacteria. Beneficial microbes like Lactobacillus and Bifidobacterium aid digestion, synthesize essential vitamins including B12 and K, and strengthen intestinal barrier function. They ferment fiber into short-chain fatty acids that nourish colon cells and reduce inflammation throughout the body.

The gut-brain axis reveals the microbiome's profound influence on mental health. Gut bacteria produce neurotransmitters like serotonin, with 90% of the body's serotonin manufactured in the intestines. This connection explains why gut health directly impacts mood, anxiety, and cognitive function, earning the gut the nickname "second brain."

Immune system function is intimately linked to gut health, as 70% of immune tissue resides in the digestive tract. A diverse microbiome trains immune cells to distinguish between harmful pathogens and beneficial organisms, preventing autoimmune responses while maintaining protection against infections.

Modern lifestyle factors threaten gut health. Processed foods, artificial sweeteners, excessive antibiotic use, chronic stress, and lack of sleep disrupt microbial balance, leading to dysbiosis—an imbalance that contributes to obesity, diabetes, inflammatory bowel disease, allergies, and mental health disorders.

Supporting gut health requires intentional dietary and lifestyle choices. Consuming diverse fiber-rich foods feeds beneficial bacteria, while fermented foods like yogurt, kefir, sauerkraut, and kimchi introduce helpful probiotics. Prebiotic foods such as garlic, onions, asparagus, and bananas nourish existing beneficial bacteria.

Limiting processed foods, managing stress through meditation or exercise, ensuring adequate sleep, and avoiding unnecessary antibiotics help maintain microbial diversity. Some individuals benefit from probiotic supplements, though whole food sources are generally preferable.

Understanding gut health as a cornerstone of wellness empowers individuals to make informed choices that support this vital ecosystem, ultimately enhancing physical health, mental well-being, and quality of life through the remarkable community of microorganisms within us.

GUT HEALTH FOODS

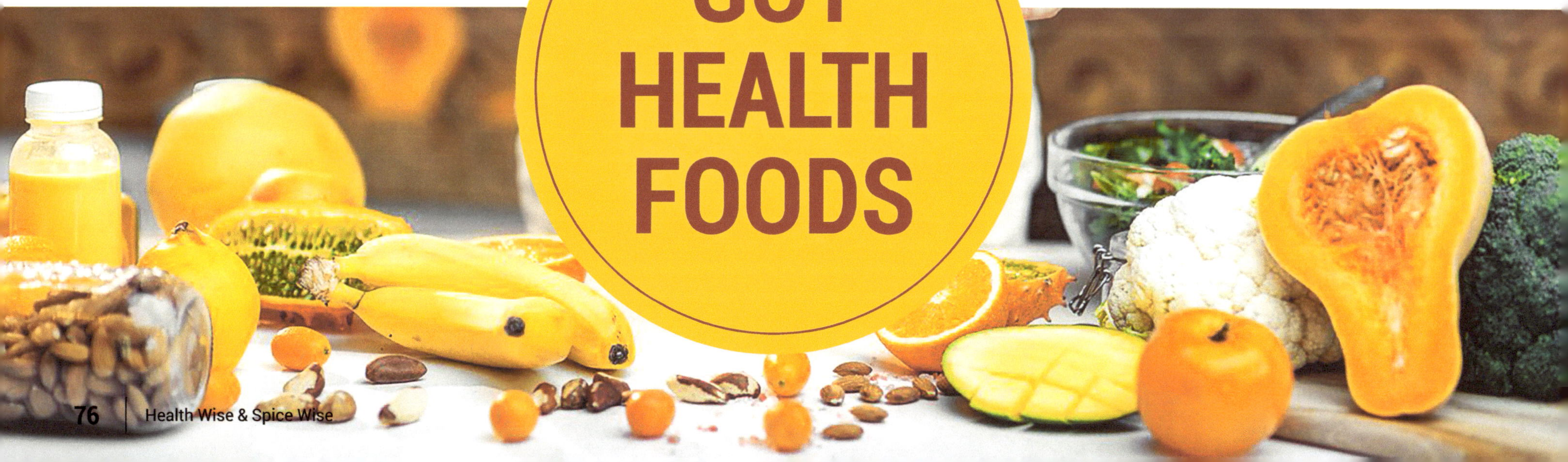

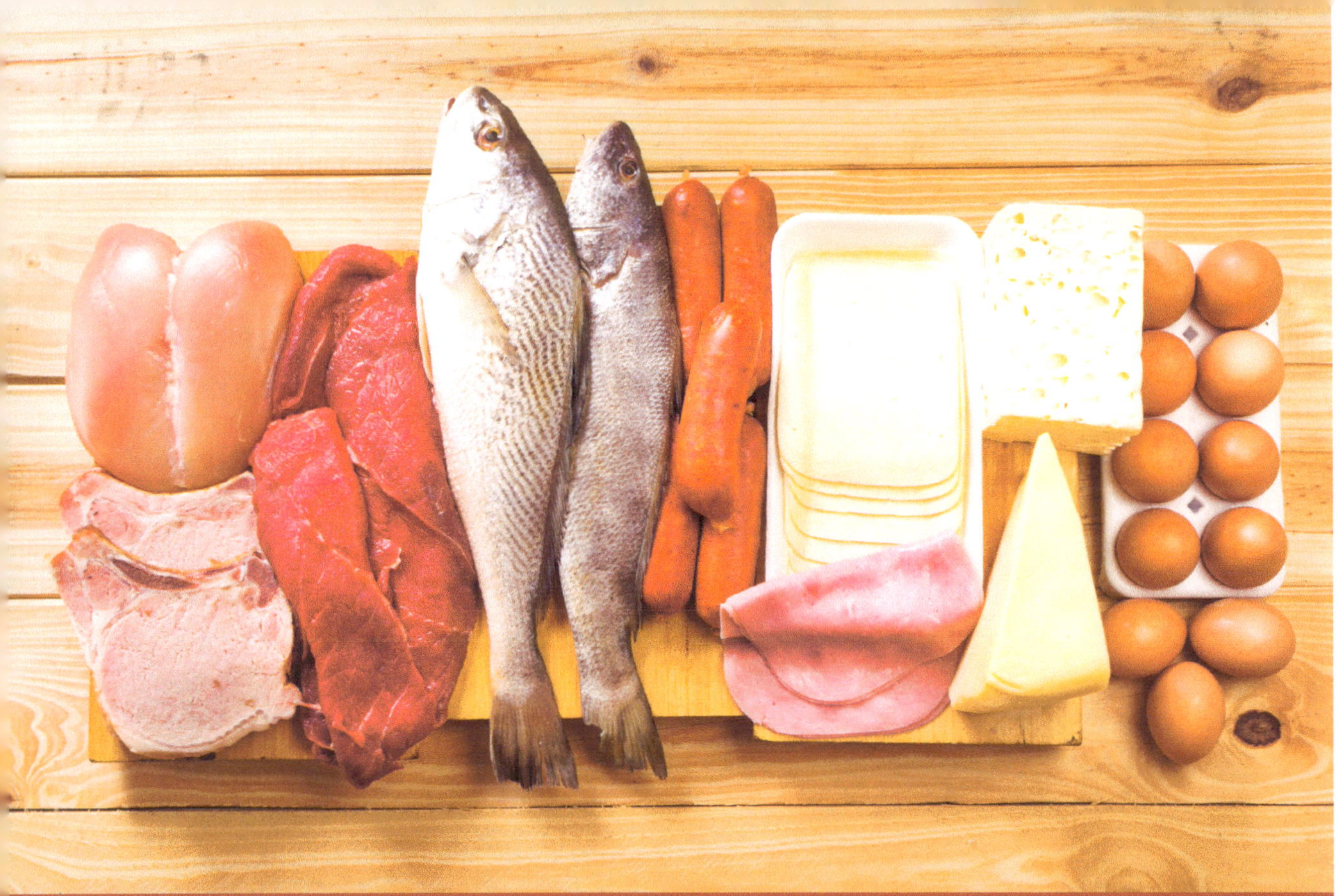

ACIDIC AND ALKALINE FOODS AND THE NEED TO BALANCE

The pH scale measures acidity and alkalinity from 0 to 14, with 7 being neutral. Foods below 7 are acidic, while those above are alkaline (basic). Understanding this balance is crucial for optimal health, as our bodies work tirelessly to maintain a slightly alkaline blood pH of 7.35-7.45 for proper cellular function.

Acidic foods include most proteins like meat, fish, eggs, and dairy products, along with grains, processed foods, sugar, coffee, and alcohol. These foods, while often nutritious, can create an acidic environment in the body when consumed excessively. Citrus fruits, though acidic in nature, actually have an alkalizing effect on the body once metabolized, demonstrating the difference between a food's initial pH and its effect on body chemistry.

Alkaline foods primarily consist of fresh vegetables, particularly leafy greens like spinach, kale, and broccoli, along with fruits such as avocados, melons, and bananas. Nuts like almonds, herbs, and certain seeds also promote alkalinity. These foods help neutralize acid buildup and support the body's natural pH balance.

When the diet becomes too acidic, the body must buffer this acidity by drawing alkaline minerals like calcium and magnesium from bones and tissues. This process can contribute to bone loss, muscle wasting, kidney stress, and chronic inflammation. An overly acidic environment may also impair immune function and cellular repair processes.

The ideal dietary approach follows the 80/20 rule: approximately 80% alkaline foods and 20% acidic foods. This doesn't mean eliminating acidic foods entirely, as many provide essential nutrients. Rather, it emphasizes increasing vegetable and fruit consumption while moderating processed foods, excessive animal proteins, and refined sugars.

Practical steps include starting meals with salads, incorporating green smoothies, choosing whole grains over refined ones, and drinking plenty of water with lemon. Adding alkaline foods like cucumber, celery, and leafy greens to daily meals helps counterbalance necessary acidic foods.

Maintaining this balance supports energy levels, immune function, bone health, and overall vitality, creating an internal environment where the body can thrive naturally.Balancing Acidic and Alkaline foods is crucial in diet control.

Common Acidic foods

(have a pH below 4.8) :

- Cheese and certain other dairy products
- Fish and other seafood
- Foods processed with high sodium
- Fresh meats and processed meats (fatty foods)
- Foods containing animal proteins
- Carbonated beverages such as soda
- Starchy foods such as all-purpose flour, brown rice, granola etc.
- Fried foods

Common Alkaline foods

(have a pH over 7.5) :

- Cucumbers
- Watermelon
- Avocado
- Various types of peppers
- Leafy vegetables, Celery, and root vegetables
- Bananas
- Almonds
- Sea Vegetables
- Citrus fruits, Pineapple, Ginger, Turmeric

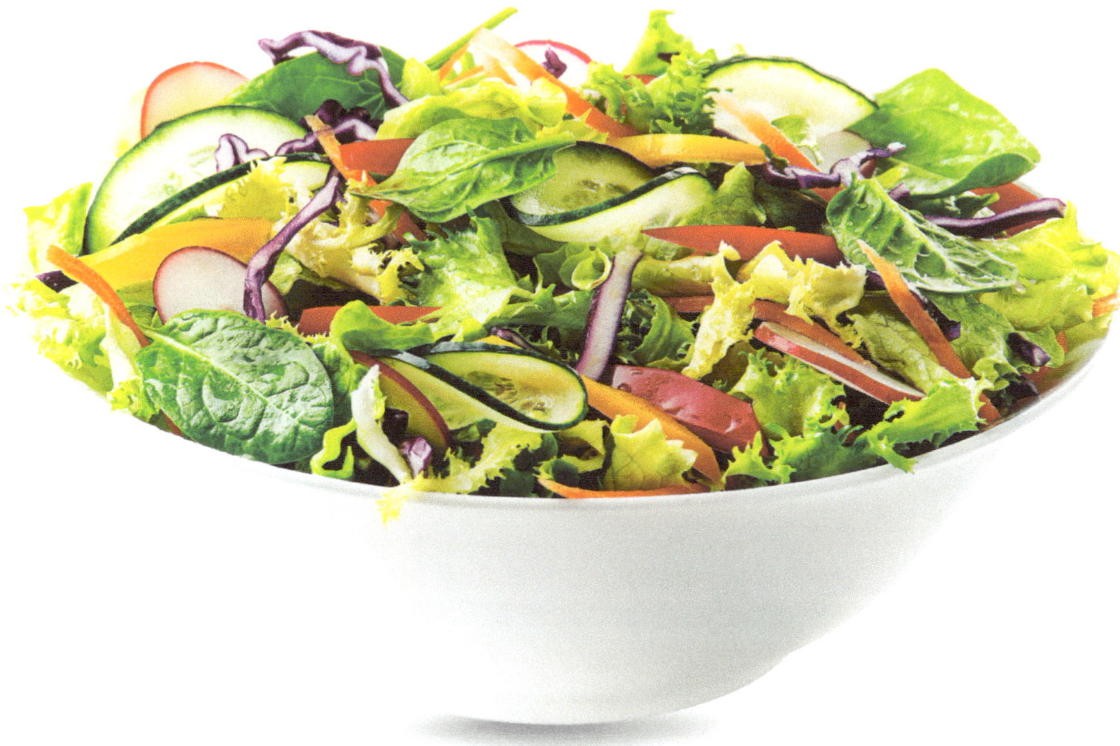

ORAL CARE

COMPREHENSIVE METHODS FOR CLEANING TEETH, GUMS, AND MOUTH

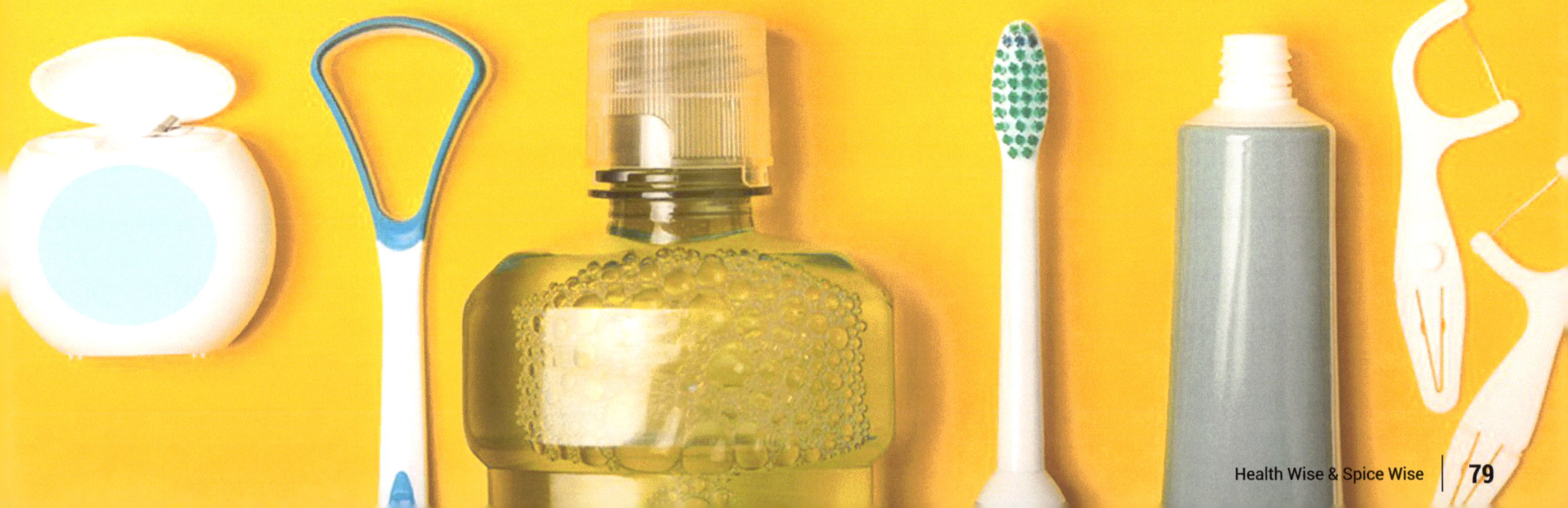

Oral health serves as a gateway to overall well-being, with poor dental hygiene linked to serious conditions, including heart disease, diabetes, and respiratory infections. The mouth harbors over 700 species of bacteria, making comprehensive oral care essential for preventing tooth decay, gum disease, and maintaining fresh breath. Understanding proper cleaning methods transforms daily hygiene routines into powerful preventive medicine.

Brushing Fundamentals

Effective toothbrushing requires proper technique, timing, and tools. Use a soft-bristled toothbrush sized appropriately for your mouth, replacing it every three to four months or after illness. Fluoride toothpaste strengthens enamel and fights cavity-causing bacteria. The American Dental Association recommends brushing twice daily for two minutes using gentle, circular motions rather than aggressive back-and-forth scrubbing that can damage enamel and irritate gums.

Hold the brush at a 45-degree angle to the gumline, allowing bristles to clean both teeth and gum pockets where bacteria accumulate. Clean all surfaces: outer, inner, and chewing surfaces of each tooth. Don't forget the tongue, which harbors bacteria contributing to bad breath and oral infections.

Flossing and Interdental Cleaning

Toothbrushes cannot reach the tight spaces between teeth where 40% of tooth surfaces reside. Daily flossing removes plaque and food particles from these areas, preventing gingivitis and cavities. Use 18 inches of floss, winding most around the middle fingers and leaving 1-2 inches for cleaning. Gently guide floss between teeth using a rubbing motion, avoiding snapping that can damage gums.

For those with difficulty using traditional floss, alternatives include floss picks, water flossers, and interdental brushes. Water flossers use pressurized water to remove debris and bacteria, particularly beneficial for people with braces, bridges, or implants.

Mouthwash and Rinses

Antimicrobial mouthwashes provide additional bacteria-fighting power and reach areas brushing and flossing might miss. Fluoride rinses offer extra cavity protection, while therapeutic mouthwashes target specific issues like gingivitis or dry mouth. However, mouthwash supplements don't replace brushing and flossing.

Oil pulling, an ancient Ayurvedic practice involving swishing coconut or sesame oil for 10-20 minutes, shows promise for reducing harmful bacteria and improving gum health, though more research is needed.

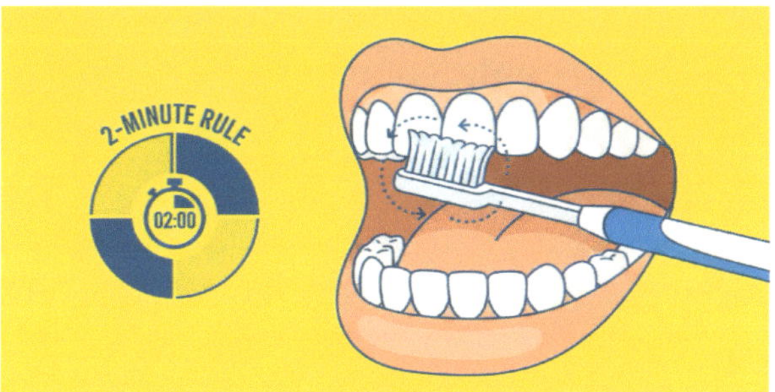

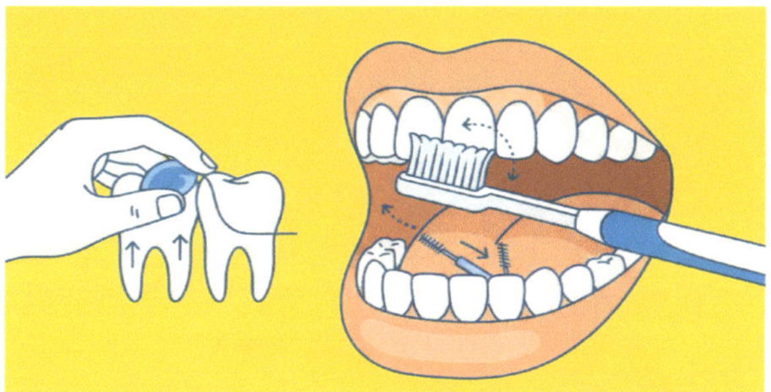

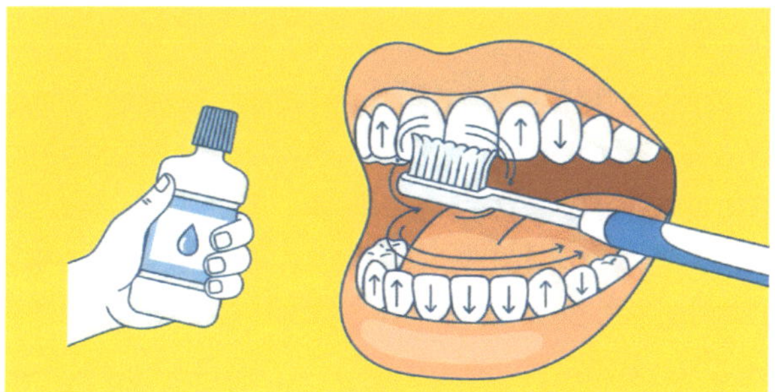

Gum Care Specifics

Healthy gums appear pink and firm, not red, swollen, or bleeding. Gentle gum massage during brushing stimulates circulation and strengthens gum tissue. For early gingivitis, focus on thorough plaque removal and consider antimicrobial rinses. Persistent bleeding, swelling, or recession requires professional evaluation.

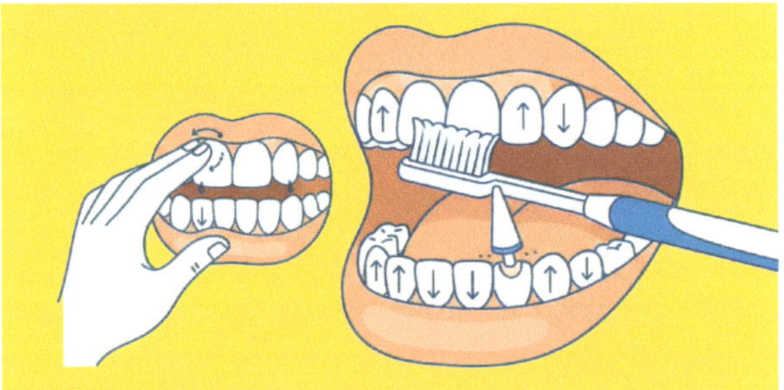

Advanced Techniques

Tongue cleaning using scrapers or toothbrush bristles removes bacteria and dead cells that cause halitosis. Clean from back to front with gentle pressure, rinsing the scraper between strokes.

Electric toothbrushes can be more effective than manual brushes, particularly for people with limited dexterity. Many feature timers and pressure sensors to optimize brushing techniques.

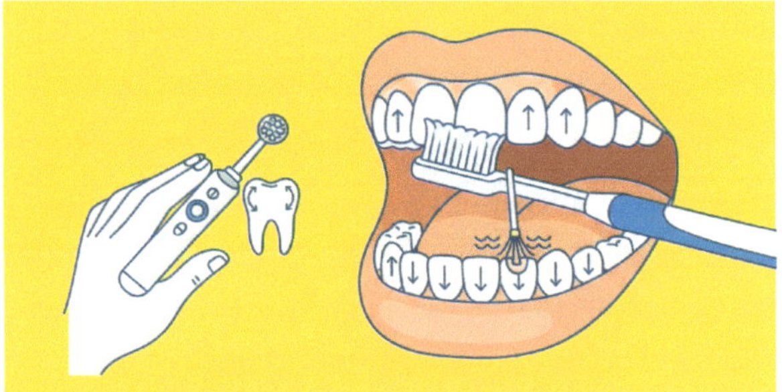

Professional Care Integration

Regular dental checkups and cleanings complement home care by removing tartar buildup that brushing cannot eliminate and detecting problems early. Most people benefit from biannual visits, though some may need more frequent cleaning.

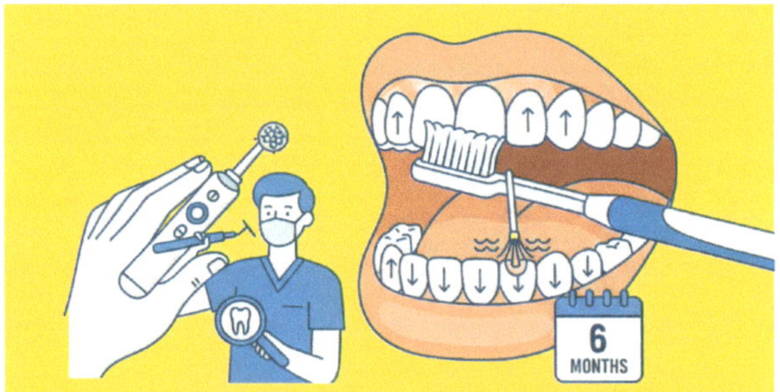

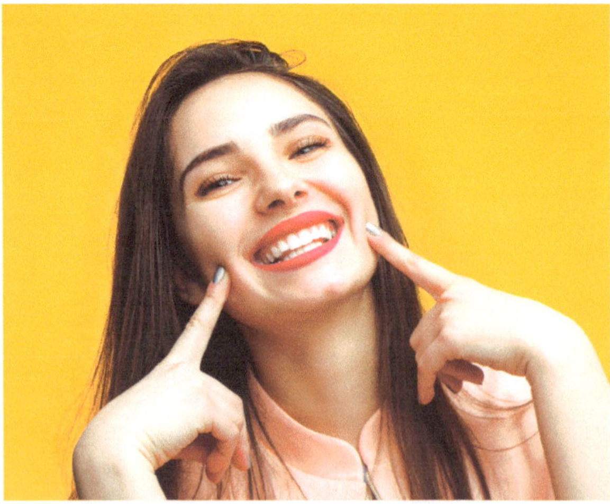

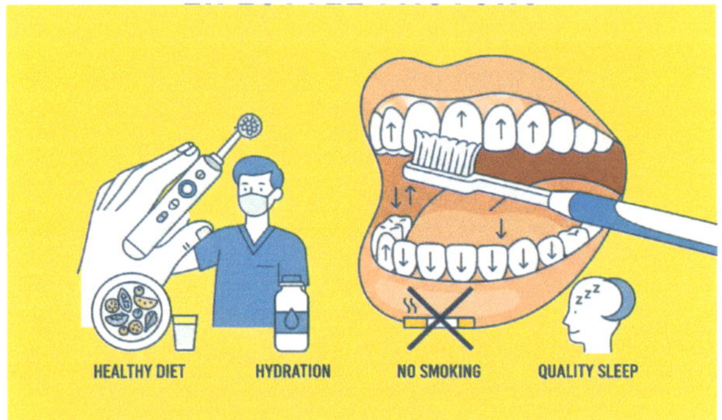

Lifestyle Factors

Diet significantly impacts oral health. Limit sugary and acidic foods that feed harmful bacteria and erode enamel. Stay hydrated to maintain saliva production, which naturally cleanses the mouth and neutralizes acids. Avoid tobacco products, which dramatically increasethe risks of gum disease and oral cancer.

Comprehensive oral care requires consistency and proper technique across multiple methods. This investment in daily hygiene pays dividends in preventing painful, expensive dental problems while supporting overall health and confidence through a healthy, attractive smile.

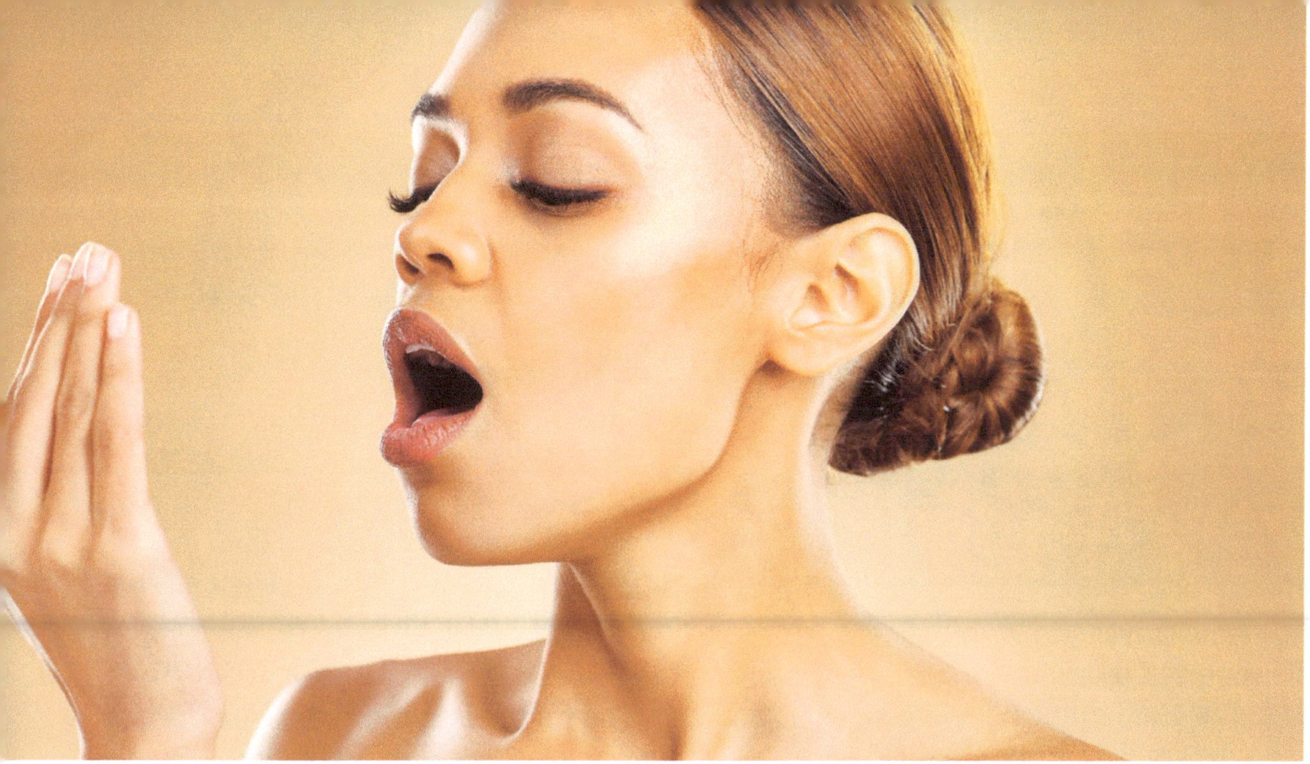

UNDERSTANDING BAD BREATH

COMMON CAUSES AND THROAT-RELATED ISSUES

Bad breath, or halitosis, affects millions and often stems from multiple sources. The most common culprit is poor oral hygiene, allowing bacteria to accumulate on teeth, gums, and tongue, producing foul-smelling compounds. Food particles trapped between teeth and certain foods like garlic and onions also contribute significantly.

Throat-related issues are major, often overlooked causes of bad breath. Tonsil stones, or tonsilloliths, form when debris calcifies in tonsil crevices, creating a persistent sulfur-like odor. Post-nasal drip from sinus infections or allergies allows mucus to accumulate in the throat, fostering bacterial growth and unpleasant smells. Chronic tonsillitis and pharyngitis create bacterial colonies that produce odor-causing compounds.

Dry mouth, whether from medications, mouth breathing, or dehydration, reduces saliva's natural cleansing action, allowing odor-causing bacteria to thrive. Respiratory infections like bronchitis and pneumonia can cause breath odor from infected lung tissue.

Systemic conditions also play roles: acid reflux brings stomach acids into the throat, creating sour breath, while diabetes, liver disease, and kidney problems can produce distinctive breath odors. Smoking and tobacco use damage oral tissues and dry the mouth, compounding the problem.

Addressing bad breath requires identifying the underlying cause, whether through improved oral hygiene, treating throat infections, or managing underlying health conditions.

HEALTH BENEFITS OF NASAL IRRIGATION

A Forgotten Home Remedy

Nasal irrigation, the practice of flushing nasal passages with saline solution, offers significant therapeutic benefits supported by clinical research. Studies demonstrate that patients with chronic sinus conditions experience symptom improvement of over 60% with daily nasal rinsing, making it as effective as many pharmaceutical treatments.

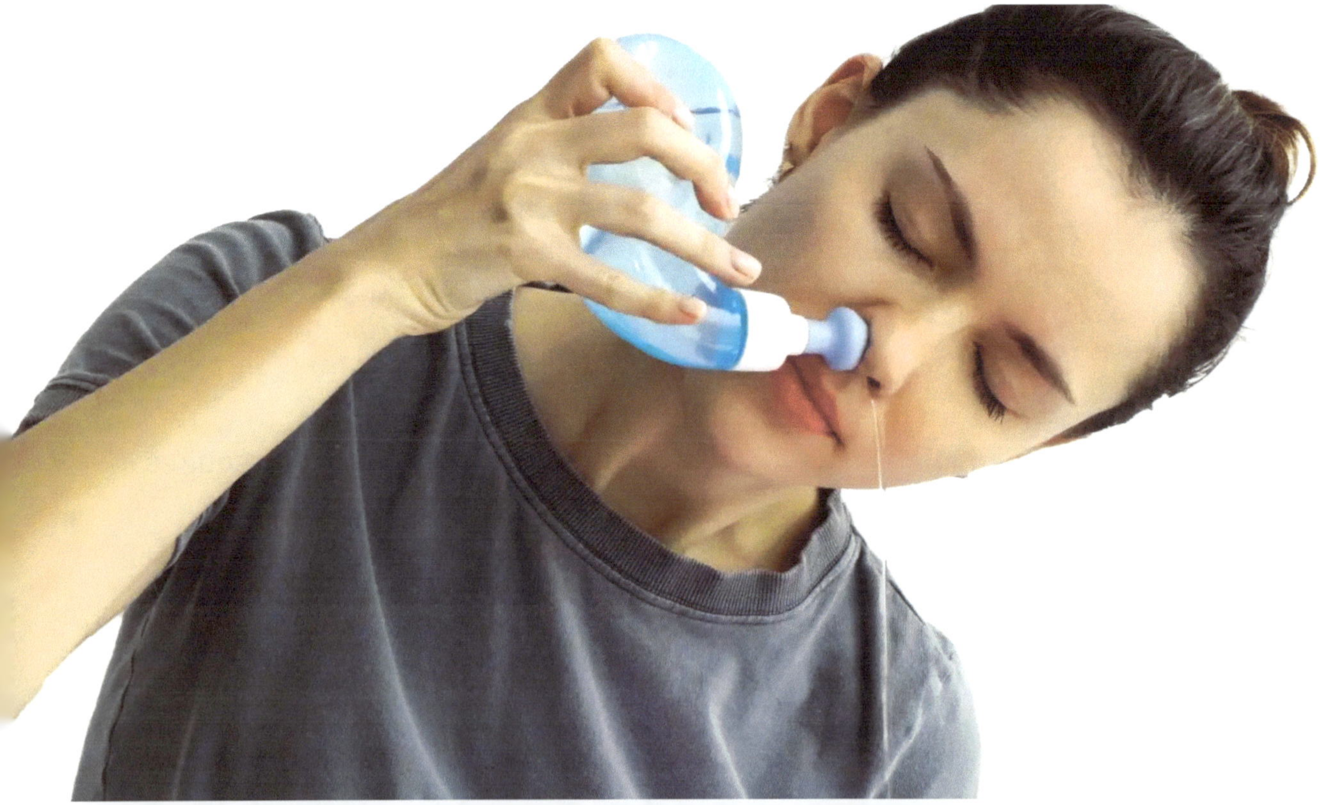

Primary Benefits

Infection Prevention and Treatment

Nasal irrigation removes bacteria, viruses, allergens, and debris from nasal passages, reducing infection risk. Recent research shows it can reduce SARS-CoV-2 viral loads and accelerate recovery from COVID-19 symptoms.

Enhanced Respiratory Function

The process promotes mucociliary clearance by moisturizing nasal cavities and removing encrusted material, improving the natural defense mechanisms of respiratory passages.

Allergy Relief

Regular irrigation flushes out allergens like pollen, dust, and pet dander, providing relief for allergic rhinitis sufferers without medication side effects.

Safety and Accessibility: Nasal irrigation has been used safely for adults and children with no documented serious adverse effects, making it suitable as a first-line treatment.

Common Methods of Nasal Irrigation

1. Neti Pot (Traditional Method)

The most widely recognized nasal irrigation device, the neti pot resembles a small teapot. Users fill it with saline solution, tilt their head over a sink, and pour the solution into one nostril, allowing it to flow through the nasal cavity and exit the other nostril. This gravity-fed method provides gentle, controlled irrigation.

2. Squeeze Bottles

Plastic squeeze bottles with specially designed tips allow users to control the pressure and flow rate of saline solutions. By gently squeezing the bottle, users can direct the irrigation stream into nasal passages. This method offers more pressure control than gravity-fed options.

3. Saline Nasal Sprays

Pre-made saline sprays provide convenient, portable nasal irrigation. Available over-the-counter, these sprays deliver measured amounts of sterile saline solution. While less thorough than other methods, they're ideal for travel and quick relief.

4. Electronic Irrigators

Battery-powered or electric devices provide pulsating saline irrigation with adjustable pressure settings. These units often include multiple tips for family use and offer consistent, controlled delivery of saline solution.

5. Bulb Syringes

Large rubber bulb syringes can be filled with saline and used to gently flush nasal passages. This method allows precise control over pressure and is often recommended for children under medical supervision.

6. Preparation Guidelines

All methods require proper saline solution preparation using distilled, sterile, or previously boiled water mixed with non-iodized salt in appropriate ratios (typically 1/4 teaspoon salt per cup of water). Other additives must be authorized and approved by your physician.

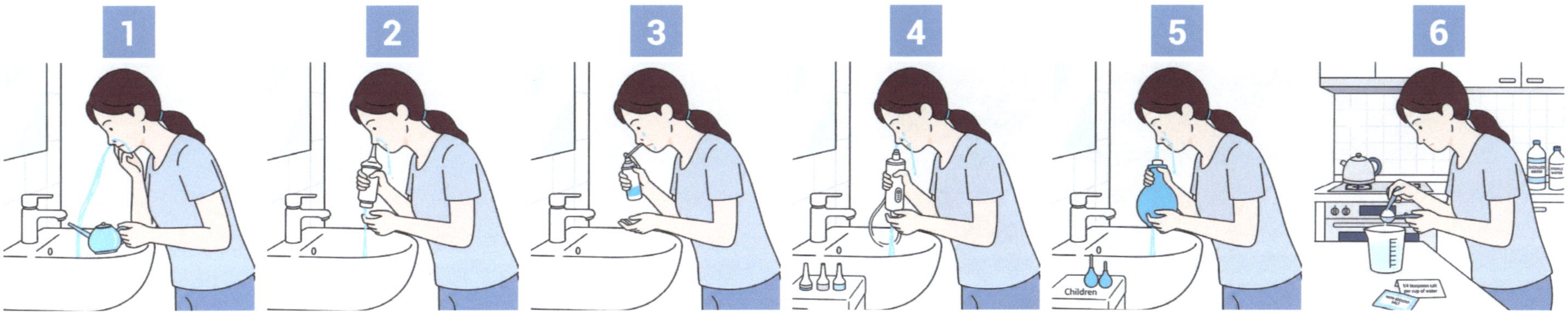

SLEEPING HABITS AND SLEEP SURFACES

THE FOUNDATION OF GENERAL HEALTH

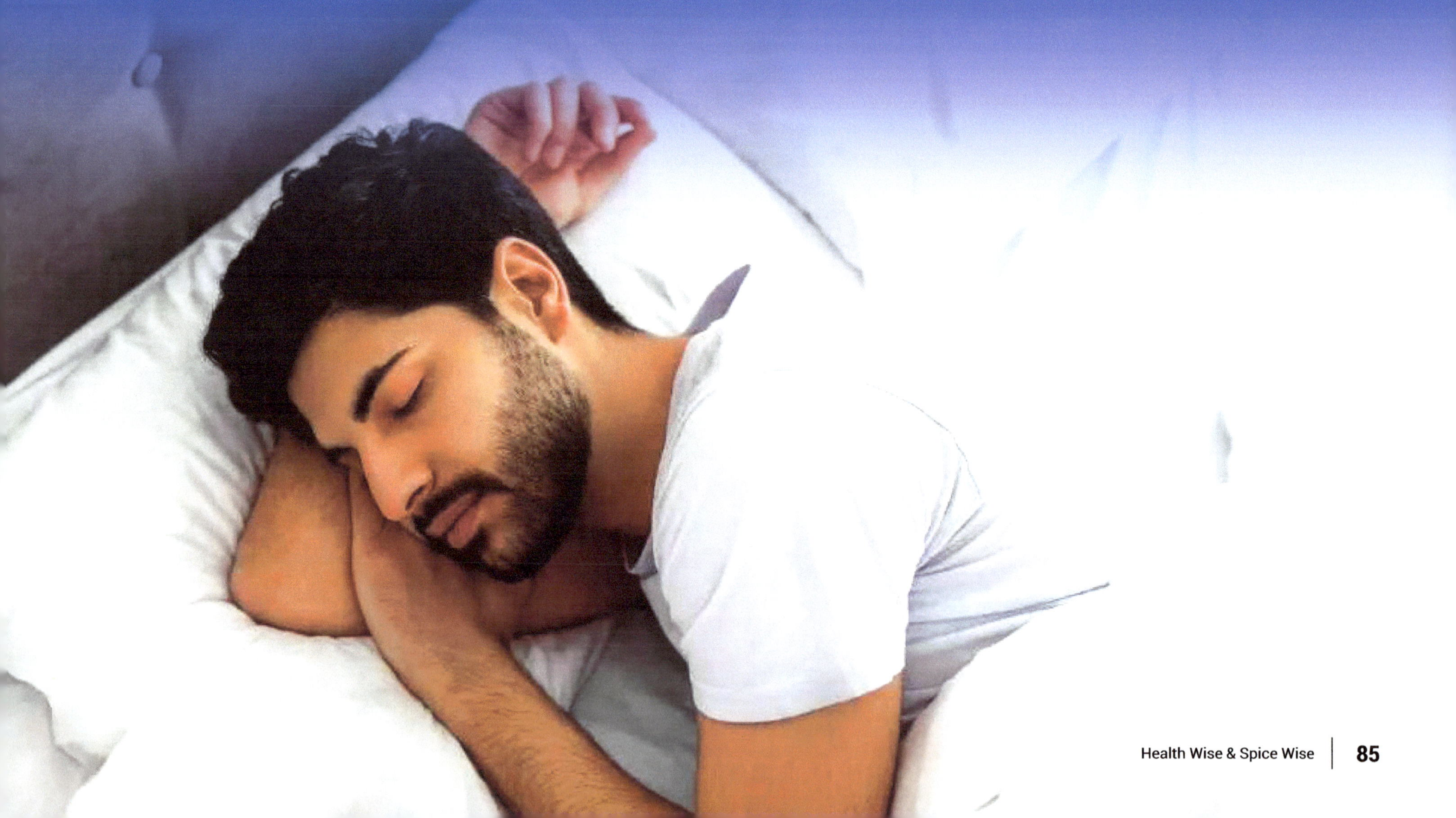

Sleep represents one of the most fundamental pillars of human health, yet it's often the first sacrifice made in our fast-paced society. Quality sleep directly impacts virtually every system in the body, from immune function and cognitive performance to cardiovascular health and emotional regulation. Understanding the intricate relationship between sleeping habits, sleep surfaces, and overall wellness reveals why prioritizing sleep quality is essential for optimal health.

The Science of Sleep's Health Impact

During sleep, the body undergoes critical restorative processes that cannot occur while awake. Growth hormone secretion peaks during deep sleep, facilitating tissue repair and muscle development. The glymphatic system, discovered relatively recently, flushes toxins from the brain during sleep, including amyloid plaques associated with Alzheimer's disease. Sleep deprivation disrupts these processes, contributing to accelerated aging, compromised immune function, and increased disease risk.

Chronic sleep insufficiency correlates with numerous health problems including obesity, diabetes, hypertension, and depression. Sleep-deprived individuals show impaired glucose metabolism, increased inflammation markers, and elevated cortisol levels. These physiological changes create a cascade of health consequences that extend far beyond daytime fatigue.

Optimal Sleep Habits for Health

Healthy sleep habits, collectively known as sleep hygiene, create conditions for restorative rest. Adults typically require 7-9 hours of sleep nightly, though individual needs vary. Consistency proves crucial—maintaining regular sleep and wake times, even on weekends, helps regulate the body's circadian rhythm.

The pre-sleep routine significantly impacts sleep quality. Creating a buffer zone between daily activities and bedtime allows the nervous system to transition from alertness to relaxation. Effective practices include dimming lights, avoiding screens for at least an hour before bed, engaging in calming activities like reading or gentle stretching, and maintaining cool bedroom temperatures between 60-67°F.

Dietary timing affects sleep quality. Heavy meals, caffeine, and alcohol within 3-4 hours of bedtime can disrupt sleep architecture. While alcohol may initially promote drowsiness, it fragments sleep later in the night, reducing restorative deep sleep and REM stages.

The Critical Role of Sleep Surfaces

Sleep surfaces dramatically influence sleep quality and physical health. The average person spends approximately one-third of their life in bed, making mattress selection a significant health investment. Proper spinal alignment during sleep prevents musculoskeletal pain and promotes healing.

Mattress firmness should accommodate individual body weight, sleep position, and comfort preferences while maintaining spinal neutrality. Side sleepers typically benefit from medium to medium-soft mattresses that contour to shoulder and hip curves. Back sleepers often prefer medium-firm support that maintains the spine's natural curvature. Stomach sleepers, though this position isn't ideal for spinal health, may need firmer surfaces to prevent excessive back arching.

Material composition affects sleep temperature regulation and allergen exposure. Memory foam provides excellent pressure relief but may retain heat. Latex offers responsiveness and natural cooling properties. Innerspring mattresses promote airflow but may not provide adequate pressure point relief. Hybrid designs combine multiple materials to address various sleep needs.

Pillows play an equally important role in spinal alignment and comfort. Proper pillow height maintains the neck's natural curve, preventing strain and tension headaches. Like mattresses, pillow selection should consider sleep position—side sleepers need higher loft to fill the space between shoulder and head, while stomach sleepers benefit from thin, soft pillows.

Environmental Factors and Sleep Surfaces

Beyond the mattress itself, the entire sleep environment influences rest quality. Bedding materials affect temperature regulation and comfort. Natural fibers like cotton, linen, and bamboo promote breathability, while synthetic materials may trap heat and moisture.

Regular mattress maintenance extends lifespan and maintains hygiene. Rotating mattresses every 3-6 months promotes even wear. Using mattress protectorsguards against allergens, dust mites, and moisture while preserving warranty coverage.

Investment in Long-term Health

Quality sleep surfaces represent an investment in long-term health rather than mere comfort purchases. Poor sleep quality costs individuals and society through increased healthcare utilization, reduced productivity, and accidents. Conversely, optimizing sleep habits and surfaces provides measurable returns through improved cognitive function, emotional stability, physical performance, and disease prevention.

Recognizing sleep as foundational to health—not a luxury—transforms our approach to rest and recovery, ultimately supporting vibrant, productive lives.

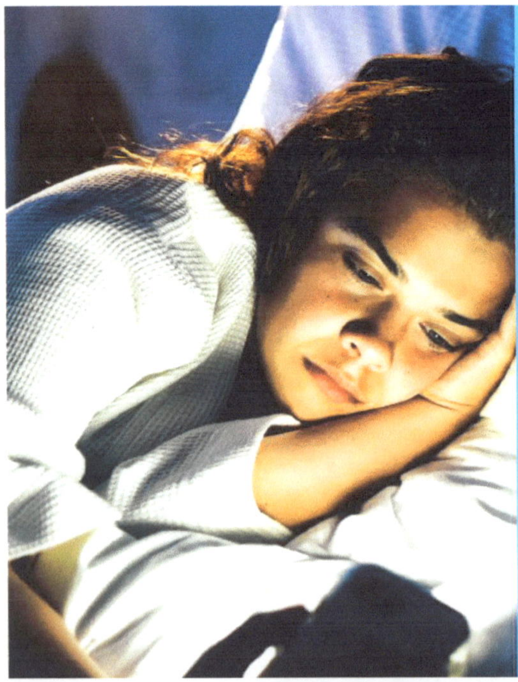

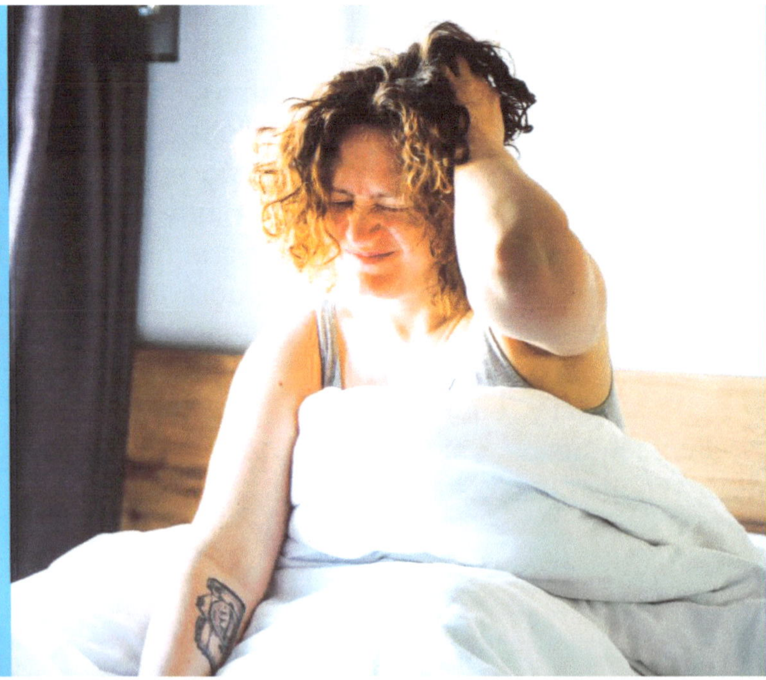

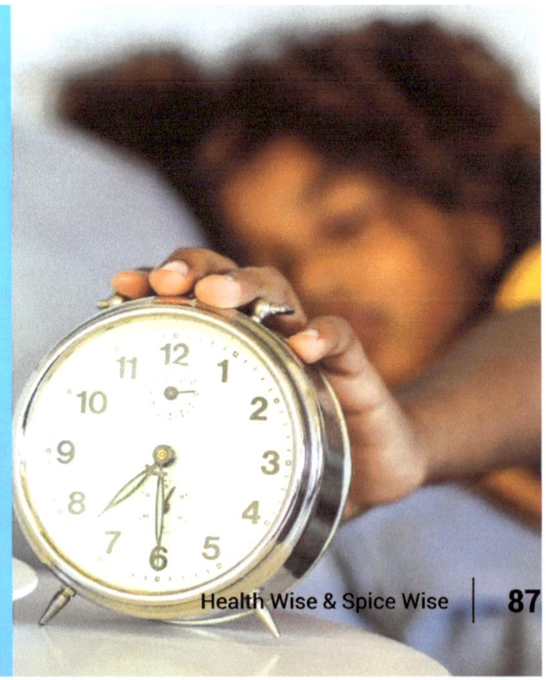

WALKING AND LIGHT EXERCISES

GREAT BOOSTERS OF GENERAL HEALTH

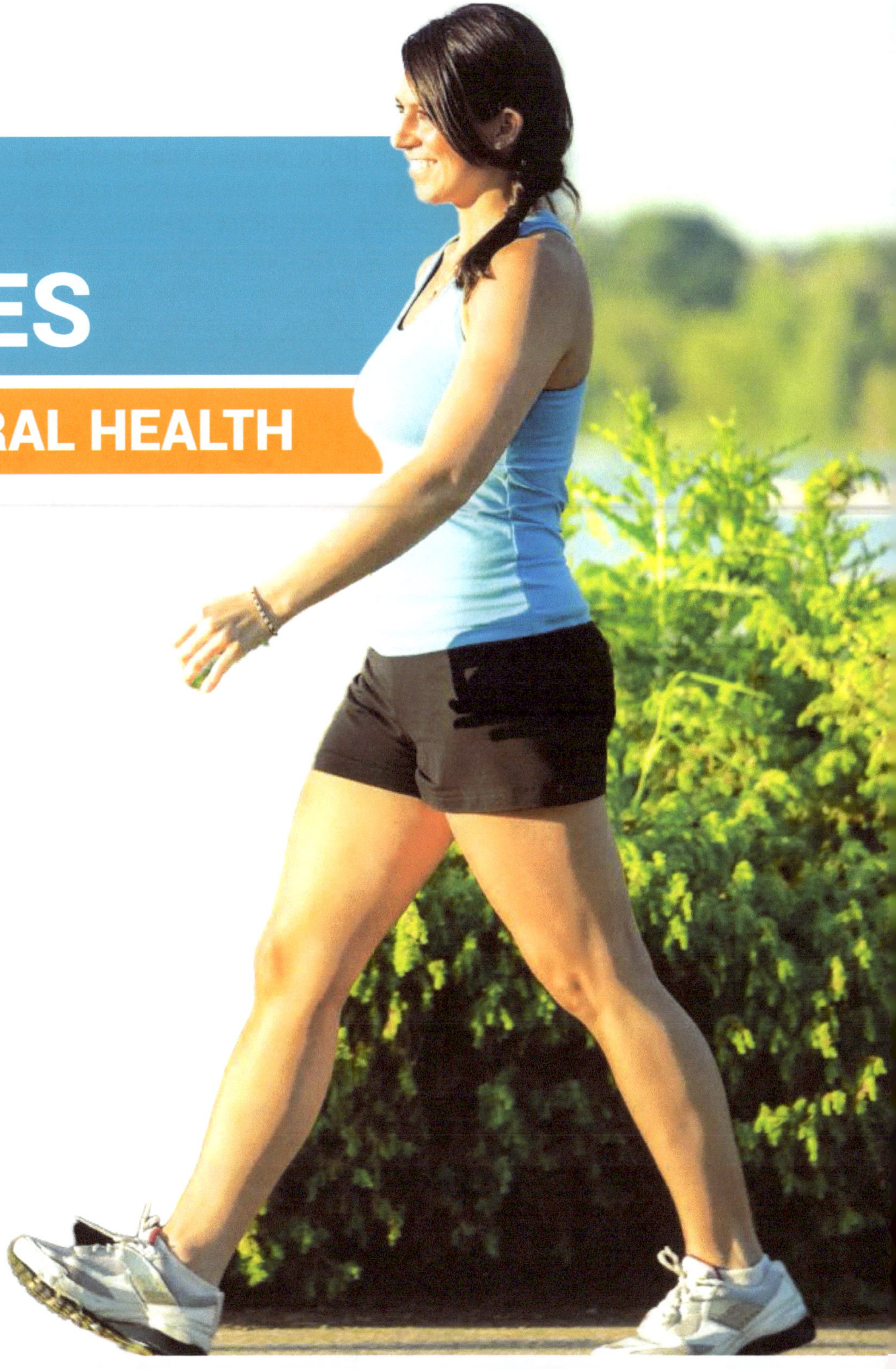

In a world obsessed with high-intensity workouts and extreme fitness regimens, the profound health benefits of simple walking and light exercise are often overlooked. Yet research consistently demonstrates that moderate, accessible forms of physical activity provide remarkable health improvements while being sustainable for people of all ages and fitness levels. Walking and light exercises represent the most democratic forms of health enhancement—requiring no expensive equipment, gym memberships, or specialized training.

The Science Behind Walking's Power

Walking activates nearly every system in the human body, triggering a cascade of beneficial physiological changes. Even a modest 30-minute daily walk stimulates cardiovascular improvements, including reduced blood pressure, improved circulation, and strengthened heart muscle. The rhythmic nature of walking promotes lymphatic drainage, supporting immune function and reducing inflammation throughout the body.

Neurologically, walking increases production of brain-derived neurotrophic factors (BDNF), a protein that supports neuron growth and connectivity. This explains why regular walkers show improved memory, enhanced creativity, and reduced risk of cognitive decline. The hippocampus, crucial for learning and memory, grows larger in people who walk regularly, providing protection against age-related mental decline.

Metabolic and Weight Management Benefits

Light exercises excel at promoting sustainable weight management through increased caloric expenditure and improved metabolic efficiency. Unlike intense workouts that can trigger excessive hunger responses, walking and gentle activities create manageable caloric deficits while preserving muscle mass. Regular walking improves insulin sensitivity, helping stabilize blood sugar levels and reducing diabetes risk. The "afterburn effect" from walking may be modest compared to high-intensity exercise, but its consistency and sustainability often yield superior long-term results. People who walk regularly tend to maintain their exercise habits for years, creating cumulative health benefits that surpass sporadic, intense workouts.

Mental Health and Stress Reduction

Walking serves as natural medicine for mental health conditions. The combination of rhythmic movement, fresh air, and often natural surroundings triggers endorphin release while reducing cortisol levels. Studies show that 30 minutes of daily walking can be as effective as antidepressant medications for mild to moderate depression.

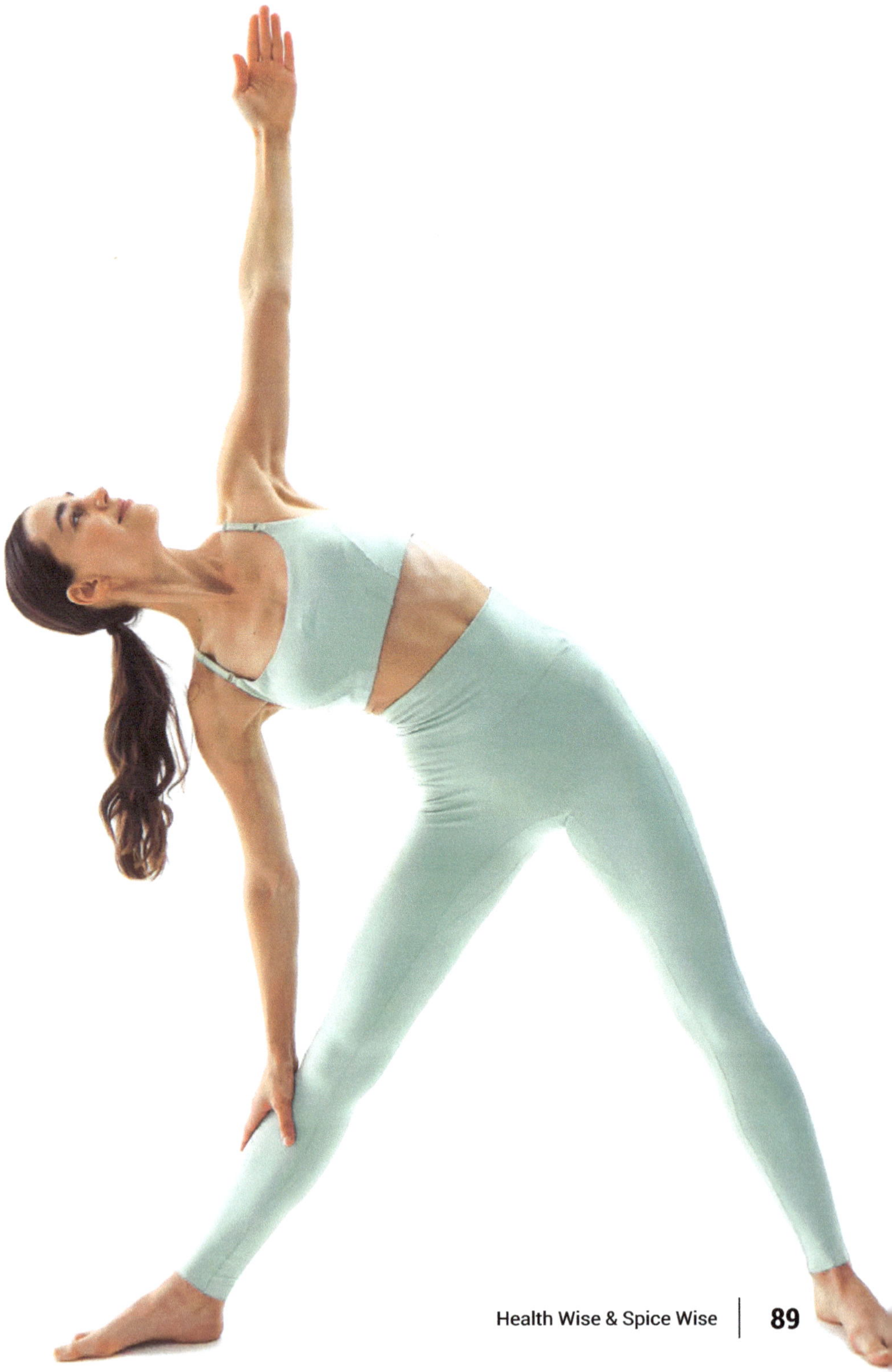

The meditative quality of walking promotes mindfulness and stress reduction. Walking outdoors particularly benefits mental health through exposure to natural light, which regulates circadian rhythms and supports mood stability. Even indoor walking provides mental health benefits through movement-induced neurochemical changes.

Bone Health and Musculoskeletal Benefits

Weight-bearing exercises like walking stimulate bone formation and density, crucial for preventing osteoporosis as we age. The gentle impact of walking strengthens bones without the joint stress associated with high-impact activities. Walking also improves balance and coordination, reducing fall risk in older adults.

Light resistance exercises complement walking by maintaining muscle mass and strength. Simple bodyweight movements, light weights, or resistance bands provide sufficient stimulus for muscle preservation without excessive fatigue or recovery demands.

Accessibility and Sustainability

The greatest advantage of walking and light exercises lies in their accessibility. These activities accommodate various physical limitations, fitness levels, and schedules. People with arthritis, heart conditions, or mobility issues can often participate when high-intensity exercises are contraindicated.

Walking requires minimal equipment, just comfortable shoes and weather-appropriate clothing. It can be performed anywhere: neighborhoods, parks, shopping malls, or even indoors. This flexibility eliminates common exercise barriers like gym intimidation, time constraints, or weather dependencies.

Practical Implementation Strategies

Starting a walking routine requires gradual progression and realistic goal-setting. Begin with 10–15-minute walks, gradually increasing duration and frequency. The "10,000 steps" guideline provides a useful target, though even 5,000-7,000 daily steps offer significant health benefits.

Incorporating walking into daily routines increases adherence. Park farther from destinations, take stairs instead of elevators, walk during phone calls, or establish walking meetings. Light exercises can be integrated throughout the day—wall push-ups during work breaks, gentle stretching while watching television, or bodyweight squats between household tasks.

Social and Community Benefits

Walking and light exercises often become social activities, enhancing relationships while improving health. Walking groups, family walks, or exercising with friends provide accountability and enjoyment. These social connections contribute to mental health benefits and exercise adherence.

The cumulative effect of consistent walking and light exercises creates profound health transformations. Rather than seeking dramatic fitness overhauls, embracing these gentle, sustainable practices provides lasting health improvements that enhance quality of life across all dimensions of wellness.

AVOIDING TENSION

STRATEGIES FOR A CALMER LIFE

Tension has become an epidemic in modern society, manifesting physically as muscle tightness, headaches, and fatigue, while emotionally presenting as anxiety, irritability, and overwhelm. Understanding tension's sources and implementing effective prevention strategies can dramatically improve both physical comfort and mental well-being.

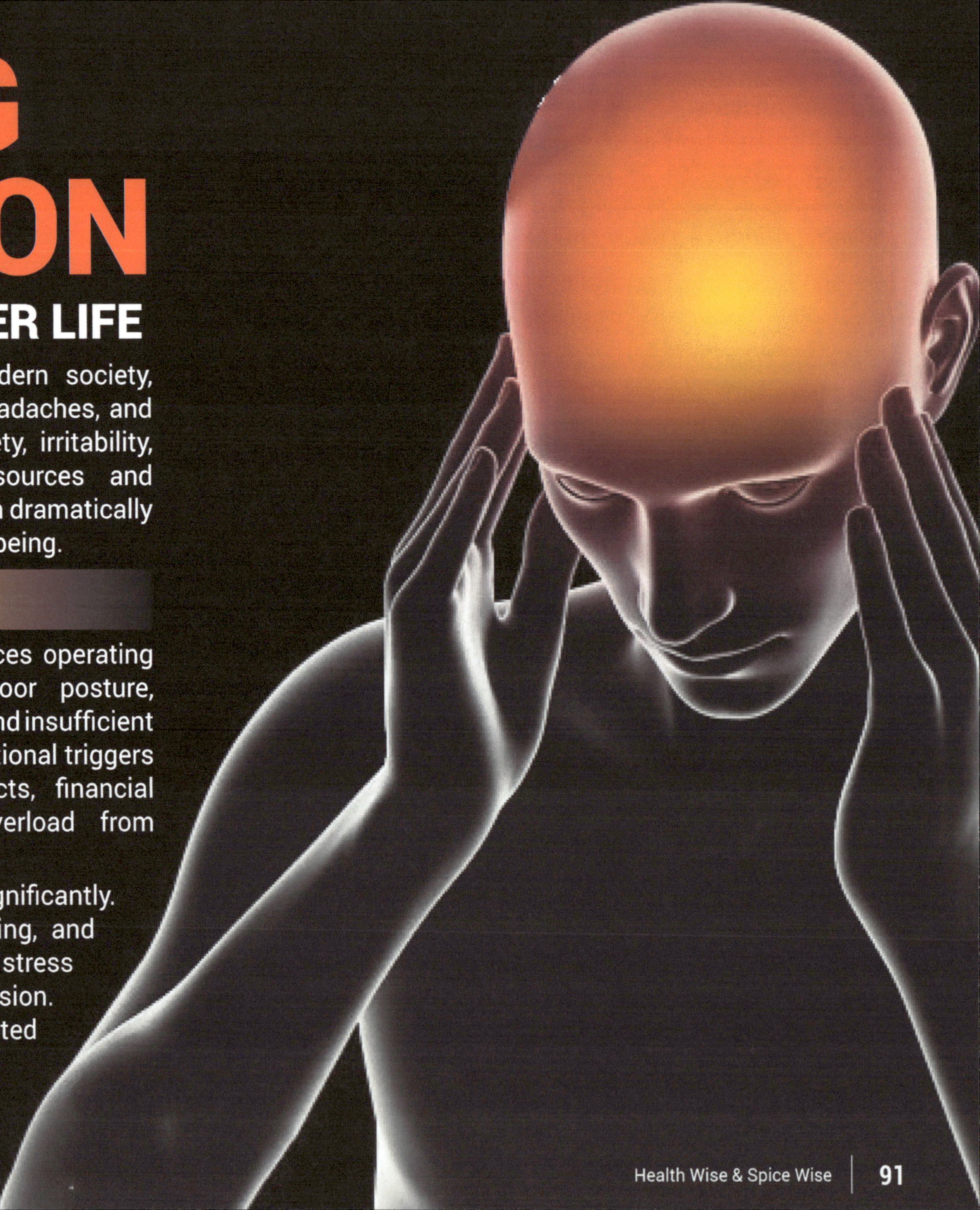

Identifying Tension Sources

Tension typically stems from multiple sources operating simultaneously. Physical causes include poor posture, repetitive movements, inadequate ergonomics, and insufficient movement throughout the day. Mental and emotional triggers encompass work stress, relationship conflicts, financial worries, perfectionism, and information overload from constant connectivity.

Environmental factors also contribute significantly. Noise pollution, cluttered spaces, harsh lighting, and time pressures create subtle but persistent stress that accumulates physical and mental tension. Recognizing these varied sources enables targeted intervention strategies.

Physical Prevention Techniques

Regular movement prevents tension buildup by promoting circulation and muscle flexibility. Simple desk stretches, shoulder rolls, and neck rotations performed throughout the day interrupt tension patterns before they become problematic. Progressive muscle relaxation, systematically tensing and releasing muscle groups, helps identify and release unconscious tension.

Proper ergonomics significantly reduces physical stress. Adjusting computer screens to eye level, using supportive seating, and maintaining neutral wrist positions prevent repetitive strain. Taking breaks, every 30-60 minutes, allows muscles to reset and prevents cumulative stress.

Breathing techniques provide immediate tension relief. Deep diaphragmatic breathing activates the parasympathetic nervous system, naturally counteracting stress responses. The 4-7-8 technique—inhaling for 4 counts, holding for 7, exhaling for 8—quickly reduces both physical and mental tension.

Mental and Emotional Strategies

Time management reduces the pressure that creates tension. Prioritizing tasks, setting realistic expectations, and building buffer time into schedules prevent the rush that generates stress. Learning to say "no" to non-essential commitments protects time and energy resources.

Mindfulness practices help identify tension early, enabling intervention before escalation. Brief meditation sessions, mindful walking, or simply pausing to notice physical sensations create awareness that facilitates release.

Lifestyle Modifications

Sleep quality directly impacts tension levels. Maintaining consistent sleep schedules, creating restful environments, and addressing sleep disorders prevents the accumulated stress that poor rest creates.

Regular exercise serves as both prevention and treatment for tension. Physical activity releases endorphins, improves circulation, and provides healthy outlets for stress energy. Even light activities like walking or gentle yoga provide significant benefits.

Nutrition affects tension levels through blood sugar stability and inflammation. Limiting caffeine, staying hydrated, and maintaining steady energy through balanced meals prevents physiological stress that manifests as tension.

Creating boundaries around technology use reduces information overload and mental stimulation that contributes to tension. Designated phone-free times and spaces allow the nervous system to truly rest and recover.

Avoiding tension requires proactive, consistent attention to both physical and mental well-being through simple, sustainable daily practices.

ISOLATION VS ENGAGING *with Others*

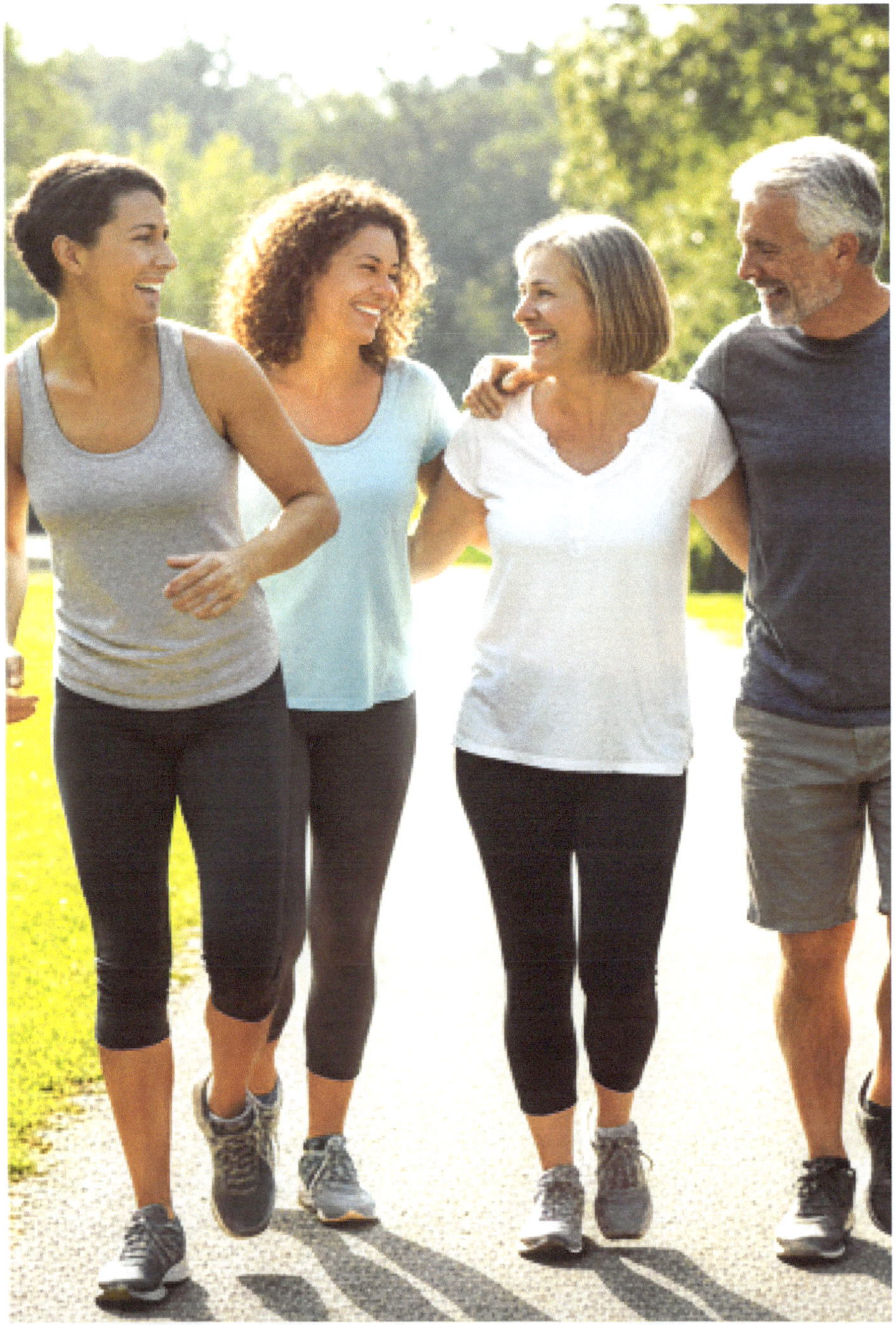

The Health Benefits of Social Connection

Human beings are fundamentally social creatures, evolved to thrive within communities and relationships. The choice between isolation and social engagement profoundly impacts both physical and mental health, with mounting scientific evidence revealing that meaningful social connections are as vital to well-being as proper nutrition, exercise, and adequate sleep.

The Hidden Dangers of Isolation

Social isolation has emerged as a significant public health crisis, with effects comparable to smoking 15 cigarettes daily or consuming excessive alcohol. Chronic loneliness triggers inflammatory responses in the body, elevating cortisol levels and weakening immune function. Isolated individuals face increased risks of cardiovascular disease, stroke, dementia, and premature death.

The psychological toll of isolation is equally devastating. Without regular social interaction, cognitive function declines more rapidly, depression and anxiety symptoms intensify, and self-esteem deteriorates. The absence of external perspectives can lead to rumination, distorted thinking patterns, and loss of motivation for self-care activities.

Isolation also disrupts sleep patterns and appetite regulation. The stress of loneliness affects neurotransmitter balance, particularly serotonin and dopamine, which govern mood, motivation, and overall life satisfaction. These changes create a downward spiral where isolation breeds more isolation.

The Healing Power of Social Engagement

Conversely, meaningful social connections provide profound health benefits across multiple dimensions. Regular social interaction stimulates the release of oxytocin, often called the "bonding hormone," which reduces stress, lowers blood pressure, and promotes healing. Social engagement also triggers endorphin release, creating natural mood elevation and pain relief.

Strong social networks provide crucial support during challenging times, offering practical assistance, emotional comfort, and different perspectives on problems. This support buffer helps individuals navigate stress more effectively, reducing its harmful health impact. People with robust social connections recover faster from illnesses, cope better with chronic conditions, and maintain independence longer as they age.

Social engagement promotes cognitive health by providing mental stimulation through conversation, shared activities, and exposure to new ideas. Regular interaction exercises memory, language skills, and problem-solving abilities, helping maintain cognitive sharpness throughout life.

Quality Over Quantity

The health benefits of social connection depend more on relationship quality than quantity. A few deep, meaningful relationships provide greater health benefits than numerous superficial acquaintances. Authentic connections characterized by trust, mutual support, and genuine care create the strongest protective effects against illness and mental health challenges.

Toxic relationships, however, can be more harmful than beneficial isolation. Relationships marked by criticism, manipulation, or chronic conflict generate stress that undermines health. Learning to cultivate healthy relationships while setting boundaries with harmful ones is crucial for maximizing social connection benefits.

Practical Strategies for Healthy Engagement

Building and maintaining social connections requires intentional effort, especially in our digital world. Joining clubs, volunteering, attending community events, or pursuing shared interests creates opportunities for meaningful interaction. Regular communication with family and friends, whether through calls, visits, or shared activities, maintains important bonds.

Even small social interactions provide benefits. Greeting neighbors, chatting with cashiers, or participating in group fitness classes creates micro-connections that contribute to overall social well-being. For those struggling with social anxiety, starting with low-pressure situations and gradually building confidence helps develop social skills.

Finding Balance

While social connection is vital, some solitude is also necessary for reflection, creativity, and personal growth. The key lies in choosing solitude rather than experiencing forced isolation and ensuring that alone time enhances rather than replaces social connections.

The evidence is clear: investing in relationships and social engagement represents one of the most powerful strategies for maintaining health, happiness, and longevity throughout life.

HOW YOUR HOME SETTINGS IMPACT YOUR MOODS AND GENERAL HEALTH

Your home environment serves as more than shelter; it's a powerful determinant of physical health, mental well-being, and emotional stability. The spaces where we spend most of our time profoundly influence our stress levels, sleep quality, productivity, and overall life satisfaction. Understanding these connections empowers us to create healing, supportive environments that promote wellness.

Light and Its Psychological Impact

Natural light exposure regulates circadian rhythms, influencing sleep patterns, hormone production, and mood regulation. Homes with ample natural light reduce symptoms of Seasonal Affective Disorder and depression while boosting vitamin D synthesis. Dark, poorly lit spaces can trigger feelings of lethargy, sadness, and disconnection.

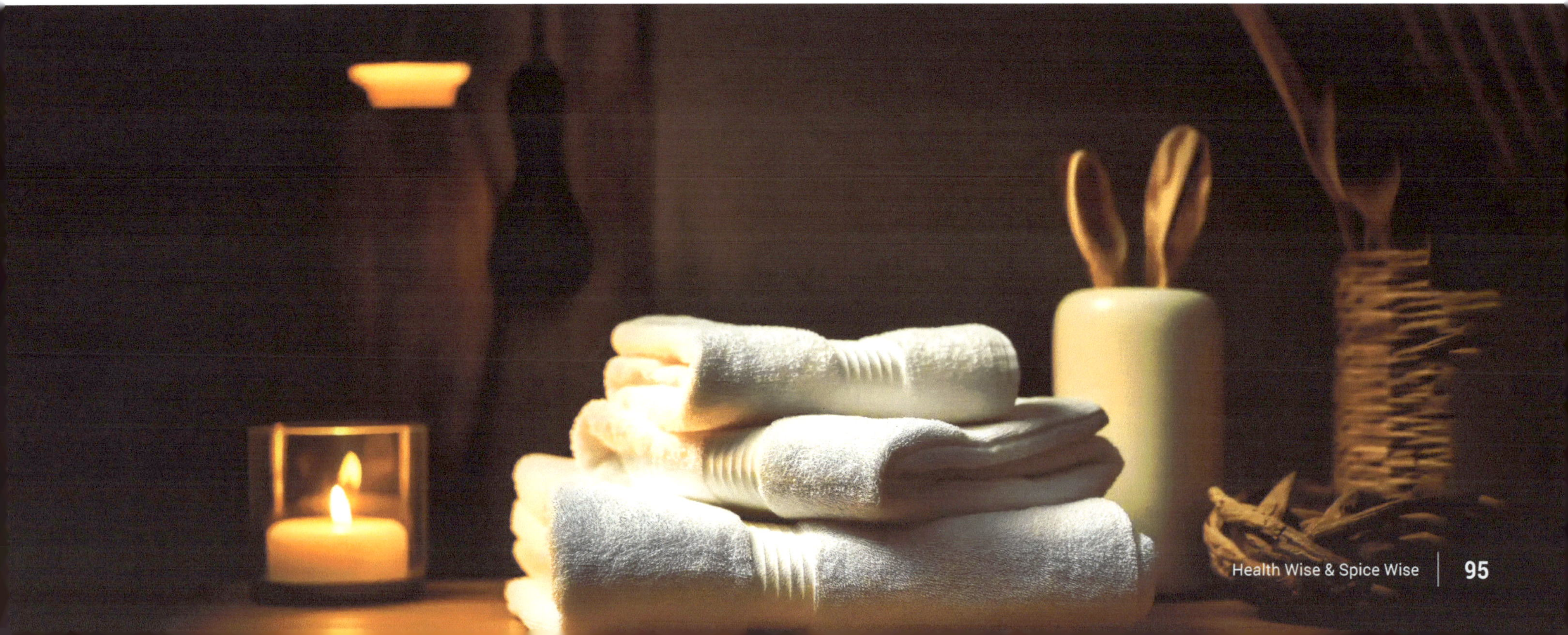

Artificial lighting quality matters equally. Harsh fluorescent lights can cause eye strain and headaches, while warm, soft lighting promotes relaxation. Blue light from electronic devices disrupts sleep when used in bedrooms, making lighting choices crucial for different rooms' functions.

Color Psychology and Emotional Responses

Colors dramatically affect mood and behavior through psychological and physiological mechanisms. Blue tones promote calmness and reduce blood pressure, making them ideal for bedrooms and relaxation areas. Green, associated with nature, reduces eye strain and promotes healing. Warm colors like yellow and orange can boost energy and creativity, but may become overwhelming in large quantities.

Red stimulates appetite and conversation, suitable for dining areas but potentially problematic in bedrooms where it might increase agitation. Neutral colors provide versatility and create peaceful, timeless environments that don't overwhelm the senses.

Clutter and Mental Health

Cluttered environments create visual chaos that translates to mental stress. Studies show that people living in disorganized homes have elevated cortisol levels throughout the day. Clutter competes for attention, making it difficult to focus and relax. The constant visual reminders of unfinished tasks create a psychological burden even during rest periods.

Conversely, organized, minimalist spaces promote mental clarity and emotional calm. The process of decluttering itself provides therapeutic benefits, creating a sense of control and accomplishment while reducing decision fatigue from managing excess possessions.

Air Quality and Physical Health

Indoor air quality significantly impacts respiratory health, cognitive function, and overall well-being. Poor ventilation, chemical pollutants from cleaning products, and allergens like dust mites can trigger asthma, allergies, and headaches. Plants improve air quality by filtering toxins and adding oxygen, while also providing psychological benefits through connection with nature.

Temperature and humidity levels affect comfort, sleep quality, and immune function. Overly dry air irritates respiratory systems, while excessive humidity promotes mold growth. Maintaining 30-50% humidity and comfortable temperatures supports optimal health.

Noise and Stress Levels

Chronic noise exposure elevates stress hormones, disrupts sleep, and impairs concentration. Traffic, loud neighbors, or mechanical sounds create persistent low-level stress that accumulates over time. Sound-absorbing materials, white noise machines, or strategic furniture placement can mitigate unwanted sounds.

Creating Healing Spaces

Intentional home design considers how each space affects occupants' well-being. Bedrooms optimized for sleep feature blackout curtains, comfortable temperatures, and minimal electronics. Living areas that promote relaxation include comfortable seating, soft lighting, and personal touches that create an emotional connection.

Your home environment either supports or undermines your health goals. By thoughtfully addressing lighting, color, organization, air quality, and noise, you create spaces that nurture rather than stress your mind and body.

THE IMPACT OF RELIGION AND FAITH PRACTICES ON OVERALL LIFE SATISFACTION

Religion and faith practices have been integral to human civilization for millennia, offering frameworks for meaning, community, and personal growth. Extensive research across diverse cultures and belief systems consistently demonstrates that religious and spiritual engagement correlates with higher levels of life satisfaction, psychological well-being, and overall happiness. Understanding these connections reveals how faith practices contribute to human flourishing beyond their theological significance.

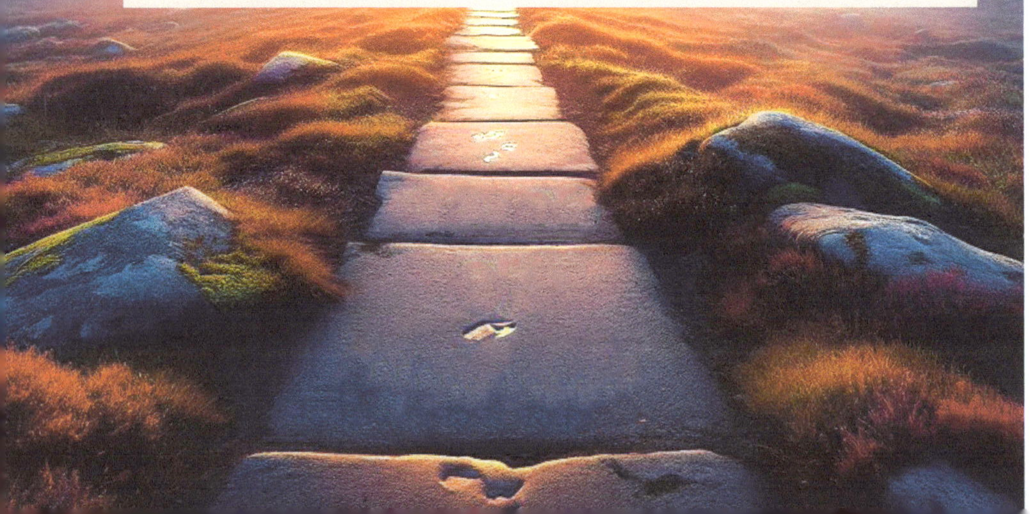

Psychological Benefits of Faith

Religious and spiritual practices provide powerful psychological anchors that enhance emotional resilience and life satisfaction. Faith traditions typically offer comprehensive worldviews that help individuals find meaning and purpose, particularly during challenging circumstances. This sense of meaning acts as a protective factor against depression, anxiety, and existential despair.

Prayer, meditation, and other contemplative practices common across religions promote stress reduction and emotional regulation. These activities activate the parasympathetic nervous system, reducing cortisol levels and promoting feelings of peace and well-being. Regular spiritual practices also enhance self-reflection and personal growth, contributing to greater self-awareness and emotional maturity.

Faith provides hope and optimism through beliefs in divine providence, the afterlife, or universal justice. This hope sustains individuals through difficulties and contributes to greater life satisfaction. Religious frameworks often emphasize gratitude, forgiveness, and compassion,which research strongly links to increased happiness and psychological well-being.

Community and Social Connection

Perhaps the most significant benefit of religious participation lies in the social connections it fosters. Faith communities provide built-in support networks that offer practical assistance, emotional comfort, and shared experiences. These relationships often transcend superficial interactions, creating deep bonds based on shared values and mutual care.

Regular religious gatherings combat loneliness and isolation, which are significant risk factors for depression and poor health. Faith communities typically provide structured opportunities for service and giving, activities that boost happiness through helping others. The intergenerational nature of many religious communities also provides wisdom exchange and mentorship opportunities that enrich participants' lives.

Religious social networks often demonstrate remarkable resilience during crises, mobilizing quickly to provide support during illness, loss, or other difficulties. This reliable social safety net contributes significantly to overall life satisfaction and security.

Behavioral and Lifestyle Benefits

Many religious traditions promote lifestyle choices that directly contribute to happiness and well-being. Dietary guidelines, substance restrictions, and emphasis on self-discipline often result in better physical health outcomes. Regular worship schedules create structure and rhythm that many find comforting and organizing.

Religious teachings typically emphasize virtues like kindness, honesty, and patience—character traits that improve relationships and social interactions. The practice of tithing or charitable giving, common across faiths, has been shown to increase personal happiness through the joy of generosity.

Coping Mechanisms and Resilience

Faith provides robust coping mechanisms for life's inevitable challenges. Religious frameworks help individuals process suffering, loss, and disappointment within broader contexts of meaning. Prayers, ritual, and community support offer multiple avenues for processing grief and trauma.

The emphasis on surrender, acceptance, or divine will found in many traditions can reduce anxiety about controlling outcomes, leading to greater peace of mind. Faith practices often encourage long-term perspectives that help individuals weather temporary difficulties with greater equanimity.

Individual Variations and Authenticity

The happiness benefits of religion and faith practices are most pronounced when engagement is authentic and personally meaningful rather than merely social or obligatory. Individuals who genuinely embrace their faith traditions typically experience greater benefits than those who participate superficially.

Different personality types may find happiness through various aspects of religious practices, through contemplative practices, others through community service, and still others through intellectual study of sacred texts.

Research consistently demonstrates that genuine religious and spiritual engagement contributes significantly to life happiness through meaning-making, community connection, beneficial lifestyle practices, and resilient coping mechanisms that enhance overall well-being across life's seasons.

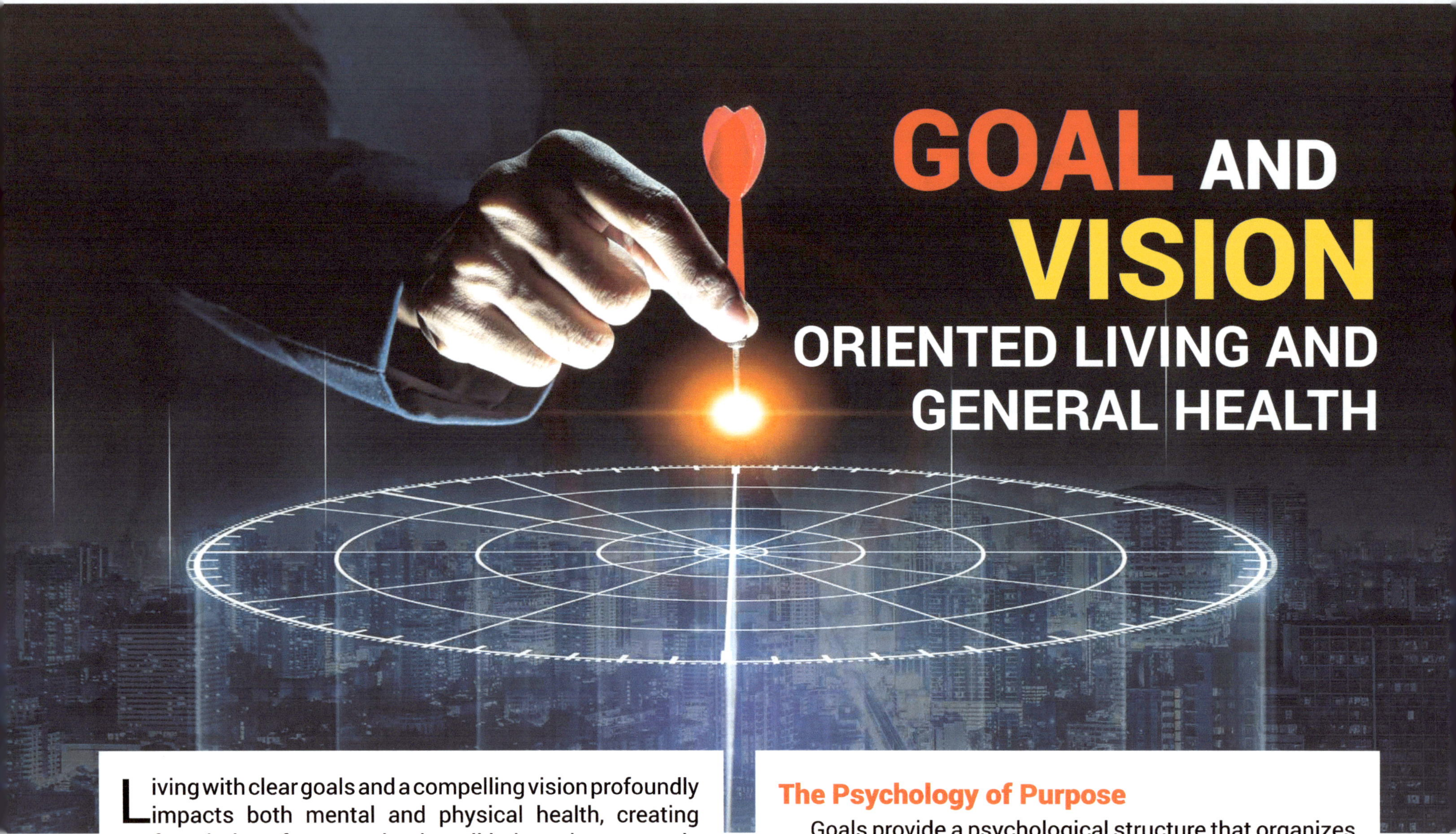

GOAL AND VISION ORIENTED LIVING AND GENERAL HEALTH

Living with clear goals and a compelling vision profoundly impacts both mental and physical health, creating a foundation for sustained well-being that extends far beyond mere achievement. Research consistently demonstrates that individuals with defined purposes and directional clarity experience lower rates of depression, enhanced immune function, and increased longevity compared to those drifting without clear objectives.

The Psychology of Purpose

Goals provide a psychological structure that organizes thoughts, emotions, and behaviors toward meaningful outcomes. This sense of direction reduces anxiety and decision fatigue by creating clear priorities and frameworks for daily choices. When aligned with personal values, goals generate intrinsic motivation that sustains energy and enthusiasm even during challenging periods.

Vision-oriented living activates the brain's reward systems through anticipation and progress recognition. Each step toward meaningful goals triggers dopamine release, creating natural mood elevation and motivation reinforcement. This neurochemical process counters depression and builds resilience against life's inevitable setbacks.

Physical Health Benefits

Purposeful living directly impacts physical health through multiple pathways. Goal-oriented individuals typically maintain better self-care practices, viewing healthy habits as investments in their ability to achieve desired outcomes. Regular exercise, nutritious eating, and adequate sleep become means to ends rather than burdensome obligations.

Research shows that people with strong life purposes have lower inflammation markers, reduced cortisol levels, and stronger cardiovascular health. The stress-buffering effects of meaningful goals help regulate blood pressure and improve immune function. Studies of older adults reveal that those with clear purposes live longer and maintain cognitive function better than their aimless counterparts.

Behavioral Organization and Habits

Clear goals create a natural behavioral organization that supports health-promoting routines. When daily activities align with larger purposes, time management improves, and energy is directed efficiently toward priorities. This reduces the scattered living that often leads to poor health choices and chronic stress.

Vision-oriented individuals typically develop better coping strategies and problem-solving skills, viewing obstacles as challenges to overcome rather than insurmountable barriers. This mindset promotes adaptive responses to stress that protect both mental and physical health.

Implementation Strategies

Effective goal-setting balances ambition with realism, creating steppingstones toward larger visions. SMART goals (Specific, Measurable, Achievable, Relevant, Time-bound) provide frameworks that generate progress and maintain motivation. Regular review and adjustment ensure goals remain aligned with evolving values and circumstances.

Connecting daily actions to larger purposes transforms routine activities into meaningful contributions toward desired futures. This connection infuses ordinary moments with significance, enhancing overall life satisfaction and health-supporting behaviors.

Goal and vision-oriented living creates upward spirals where purpose drives healthy choices, which in turn provide the energy and capacity to pursue meaningful objectives, establishing sustainable patterns of well-being and fulfillment.

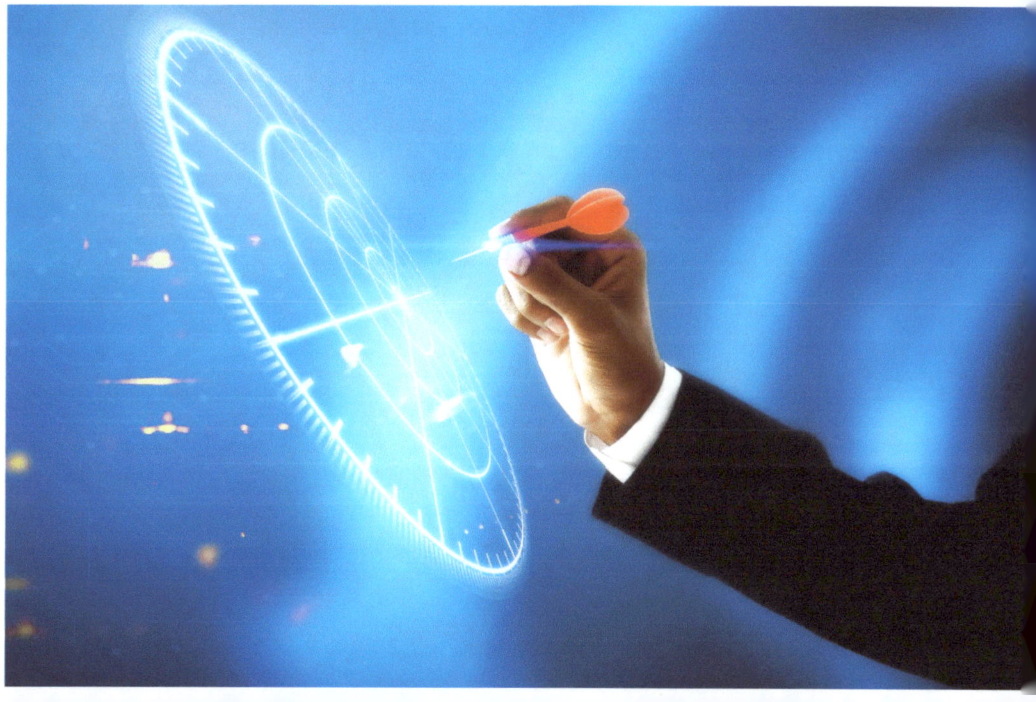

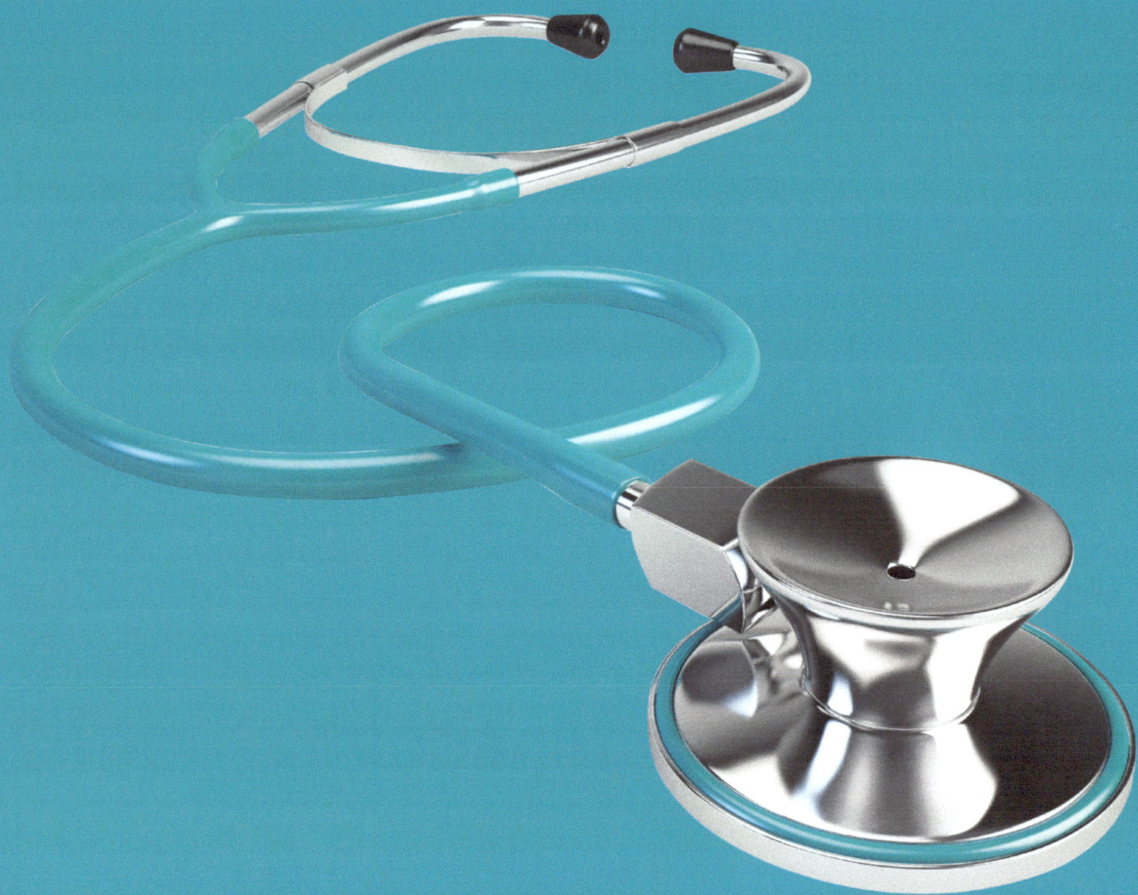

THE IMPORTANCE OF REGULAR HEALTH CHECKS

Regular health checks represent one of the most powerful tools in preventive medicine, yet they're often overlooked until problems arise. These routine examinations serve as early warning systems, detecting potential health issues before they develop into serious, costly, or life-threatening conditions. The well-known phrase "prevention is better than cure" finds its most practical application in consistent health monitoring.

Early Detection Saves Lives

Many serious diseases, including heart disease, diabetes, cancer, and hypertension, develop silently without obvious symptoms in their early stages. Regular screenings can identify these conditions when they're most treatable. For example, mammograms detect breast cancer years before lumps become palpable, while colonoscopies can identify and remove precancerous polyps before they become malignant. Blood pressure checks catch hypertension before it damages organs, and cholesterol screenings reveal cardiovascular risks long before heart attacks occur.

Early intervention dramatically improves treatment outcomes and survival rates. Catching diabetes in its pre-diabetic stage allows for lifestyle modifications that can prevent or delay full disease development. Similarly, identifying heart disease risk factors enables interventions that can prevent heart attacks and strokes.

Cost-Effectiveness and Quality of Life

Preventive care through regular check-ups proves far more cost-effective than emergency treatments. Treating early-stage cancer costs significantly less than advanced-stage interventions, while managing controlled hypertension prevents expensive complications like kidney failure or stroke rehabilitation.

Beyond financial considerations, early detection preserves quality of life. Conditions managed from their onset typically require less invasive treatments and cause fewer long-term complications. Patients maintain independence, mobility, and normal activities longer when health issues are caught and addressed early.

Establishing Health Baselines

Regular check-ups establish personal health baselines that help detect subtle changes over time. What's normal for one individual may be concerning for another. Tracking trends in blood pressure, cholesterol, weight, and other markers provides valuable insights that single measurements cannot offer.

Age-Appropriate Screening Guidelines

Different life stages require specific screening focuses. Young adults need baseline measurements and lifestyle counseling, middle-aged individuals require increased cancer screenings, while older adults need comprehensive assessments for multiple chronic conditions.

Building Healthcare Partnerships

Regular visits foster relationships with healthcare providers who understand individual health histories, family backgrounds, and personal risk factors. This continuity enables more personalized care and better communication about health concerns.

Regular health checks transform healthcare from reactive crisis management to proactive wellness maintenance, ultimately supporting longer, healthier, more fulfilling lives through informed prevention and early intervention strategies.

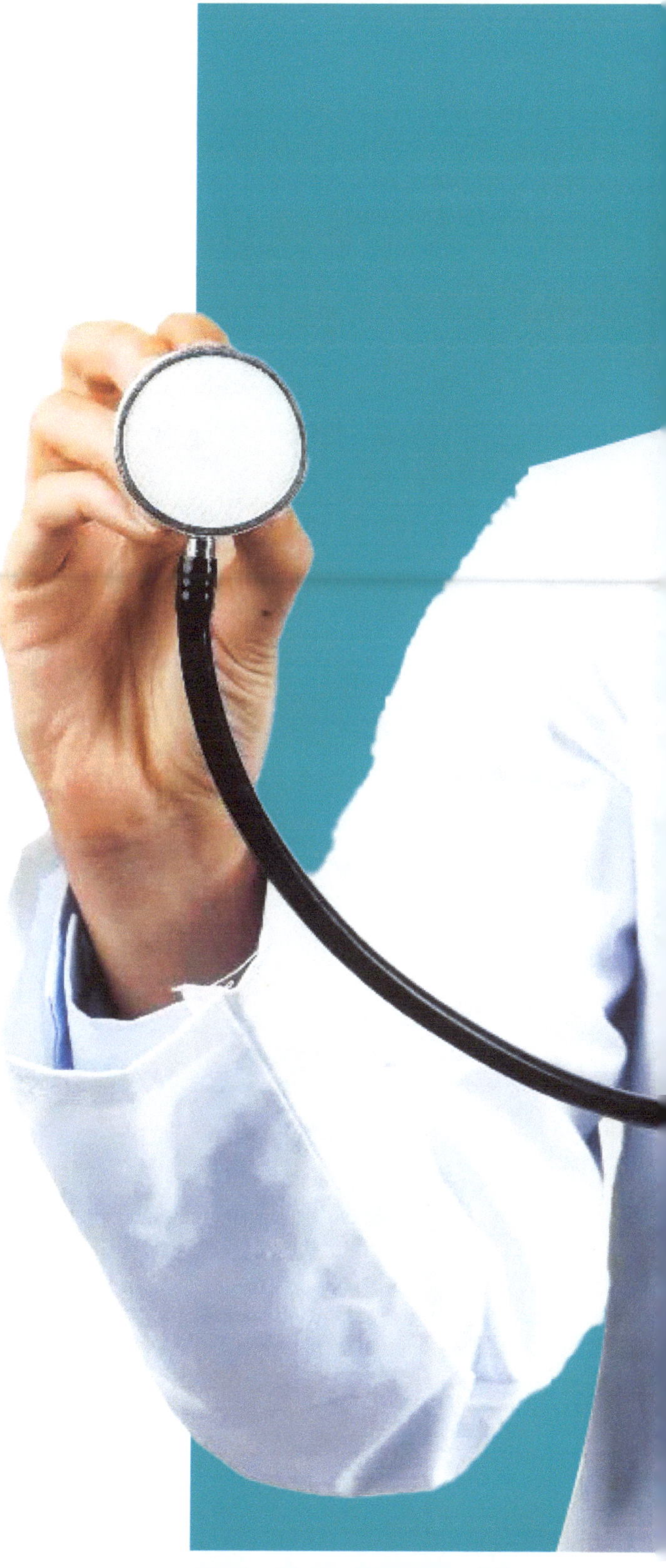

IMPORTANCE OF KEEPING A DAILY ROUTINE AND PLANNING

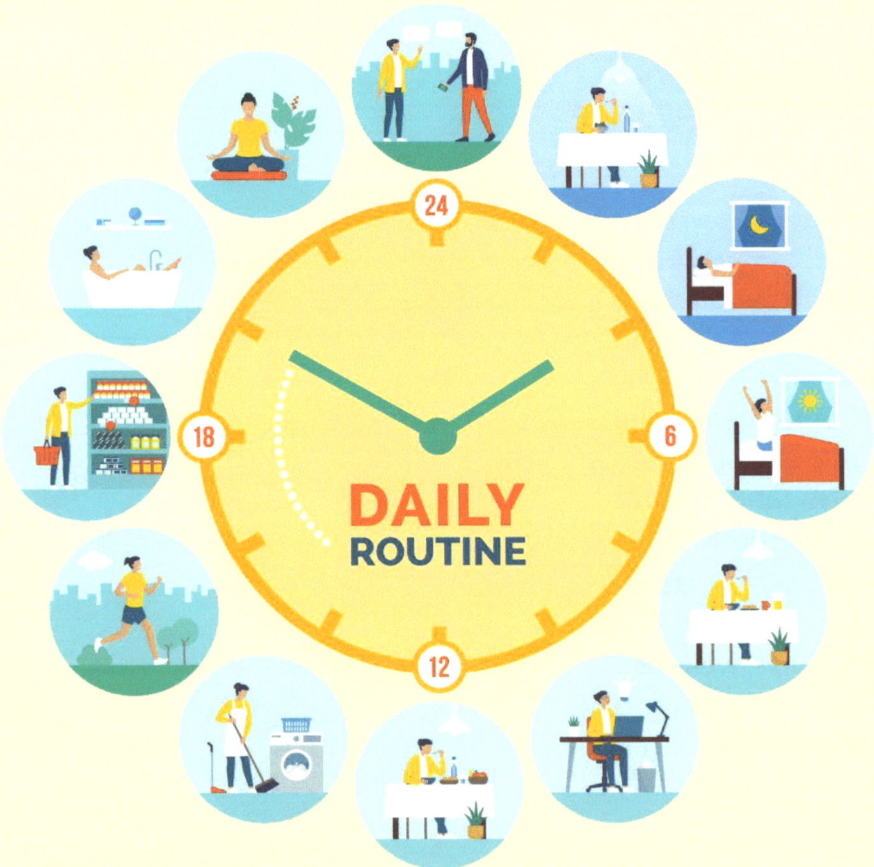

Daily routines and systematic planning form the invisible architecture of successful, healthy, and fulfilling lives. Far from restricting freedom, well-structured routines create the foundation that actually enables greater spontaneity, productivity, and peace of mind. Understanding the profound impact of organized living reveals why the most successful individuals across all fields consistently emphasize the power of intentional daily habits and forward-thinking planning.

Neurological Benefits of Routine

The human brain thrives on predictable patterns that reduce cognitive load and decision fatigue. When daily activities become automatic through routine, the brain conserves mental energy for more important decisions and creative tasks. This neurological efficiency explains why successful entrepreneurs often wear similar clothing daily or eat identical breakfasts—eliminating trivial decisions, which preserves mental resources for significant choices.

Routines activate the brain's reward systems through completion of familiar patterns, creating small doses of satisfaction throughout the day. This steady stream of micro-achievements builds confidence and momentum that carries into larger goals and challenges.

Stress Reduction and Mental Health

Structured routines provide psychological anchors that reduce anxiety and uncertainty. Knowing what comes next eliminates the stress of constant decision-making while creating a sense of control over daily life. This predictability becomes especially valuable during challenging periods when external circumstances feel chaotic or overwhelming.

Consistent sleep, meals, and exercise routines regulate circadian rhythms and hormone production, directly impacting mood stability and mental health. People with regular schedules typically experience better sleep quality, more stable energy levels, and reduced symptoms of anxiety and depression.

Physical Health Optimization

Daily routines naturally incorporate health-promoting behaviors into consistent patterns. Regular mealtimes support healthy digestion and metabolism, while scheduled exercise becomes a non-negotiable habit rather than an optional activity dependent on motivation. Consistent sleep schedules improve recovery, immune function, and cognitive performance.

Routine medical care, including medication timing, preventive appointments, and self-monitoring activities, becomes seamlessly integrated into daily patterns rather than requiring constant reminders or motivation.

Productivity and Goal Achievement

Planning transforms abstract aspirations into concrete, actionable steps. Daily, weekly, and monthly planning sessions create roadmaps that connect daily activities to larger objectives. This alignment ensures that time and energy investment move individuals consistently toward their goals rather than allowing days to pass without meaningful progress.

Routines eliminate the friction that prevents action. When behaviors become habitual, they require less willpower and motivation to maintain. This automation of positive behaviors creates compound effects where small daily actions accumulate into significant long-term achievements.

Time Management and Efficiency

Structured planning reveals time allocation patterns and identifies inefficiencies. Many people underestimate how much time routine activities require or overestimate available discretionary time. Realistic planning based on actual time requirements enables more accurate scheduling and reduces the stress of running behind schedule.

Batch processing similar activities within routines increases efficiency. Responding to emails during designated times, meal preparation sessions, or scheduled communication blocks reduce task-switching overhead and improve focus quality.

Flexibility Within Structure

Effective routines provide structure while maintaining flexibility for unexpected opportunities or changing circumstances. The key lies in distinguishing between non-negotiable core activities that support health and goals versus adaptable elements that can shift based on circumstances.

Well-designed routines include buffer time for unexpected events and regular review periods to assess and adjust patterns based on changing needs or priorities.

Implementation Strategies

Successful routine development starts small with one or two keystone habits that naturally support other positive behaviors. Morning routines often serve as daily foundation-setters that influence energy and focus throughout the remaining hours.

Regular planning sessions—weekly reviews and daily prioritization—maintain alignment between daily actions and longer-term objectives while allowing for course corrections and adaptations.

The discipline of routine and planning ultimately creates the freedom to pursue meaningful goals with confidence, energy, and sustained progress toward fulfilling lives.

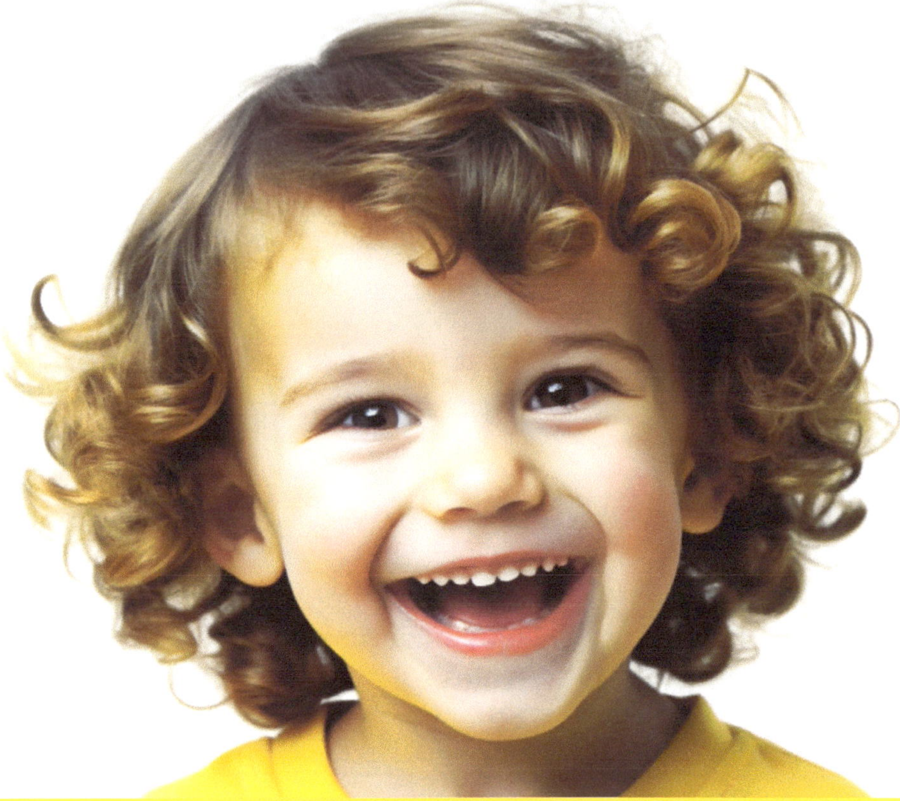

LAUGHTER IS THE BEST MEDICINE

The age-old adage "laughter is the best medicine" has proven to be more than just a cheerful saying – it's a scientifically-backed truth that reveals the profound healing power of humor. When we laugh, our bodies undergo remarkable physiological changes that promote both physical and mental well-being.

Laughter triggers the release of endorphins, our body's natural feel-good chemicals, which act as powerful mood elevators and natural painkillers. These neurochemicals help reduce stress hormones like cortisol and adrenaline, creating an immediate sense of relaxation and joy. The physical act of laughing also provides a mini workout for our cardiovascular system, improving blood circulation and temporarily boosting heart rate in a healthy way.

Beyond the immediate effects, regular laughter strengthens the immune system by increasing the production of antibodies and activating protective cells like T-cells and natural killer cells. This enhanced immune response helps the body better fight off infections and diseases. Laughter also serves as a natural stress reliever, helping people cope with difficult situations and maintain perspective during challenging times.

The social benefits of laughter are equally important. Shared humor creates bonds between people, reduces social anxiety, and fosters a sense of community and belonging. In healthcare settings, laughter therapy has shown promising results in improving patient outcomes, reducing recovery times, and enhancing overall quality of life.

Whether through comedy shows, time with friends, or simply finding humor in everyday situations, incorporating more laughter into our daily lives is a simple yet powerful prescription for better health and happiness.

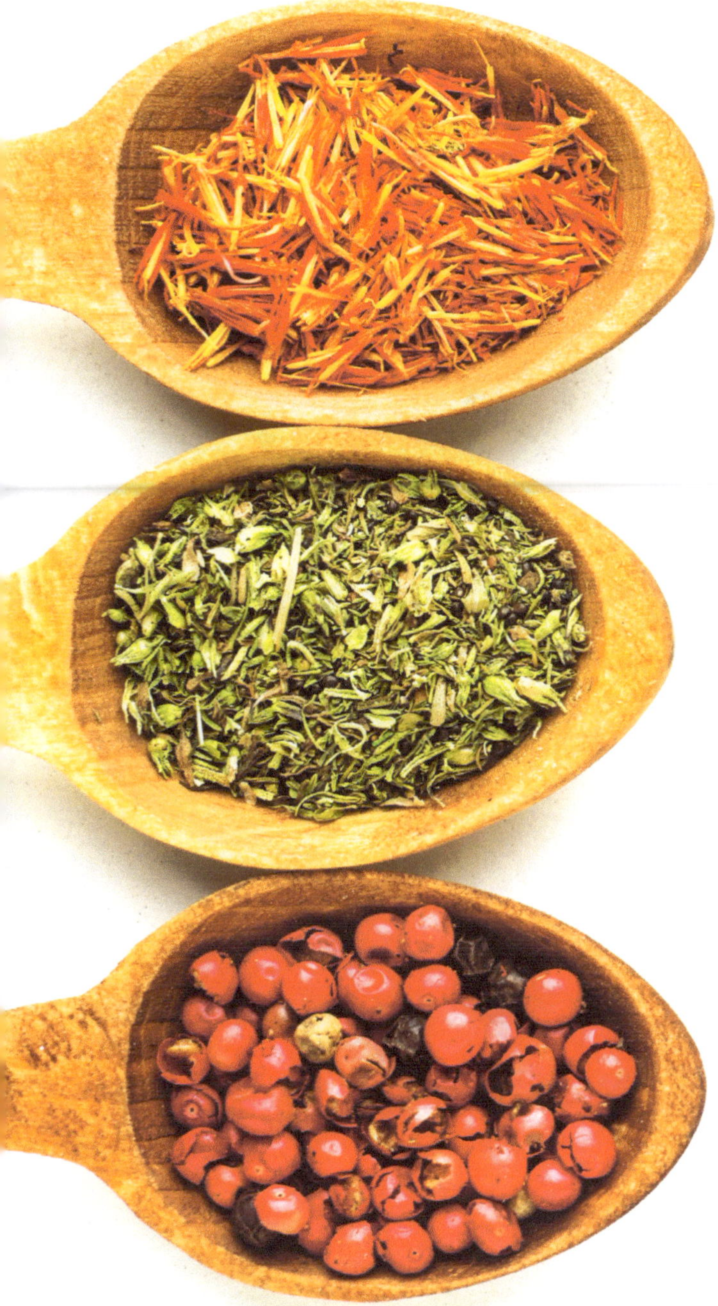

SPICE WISE

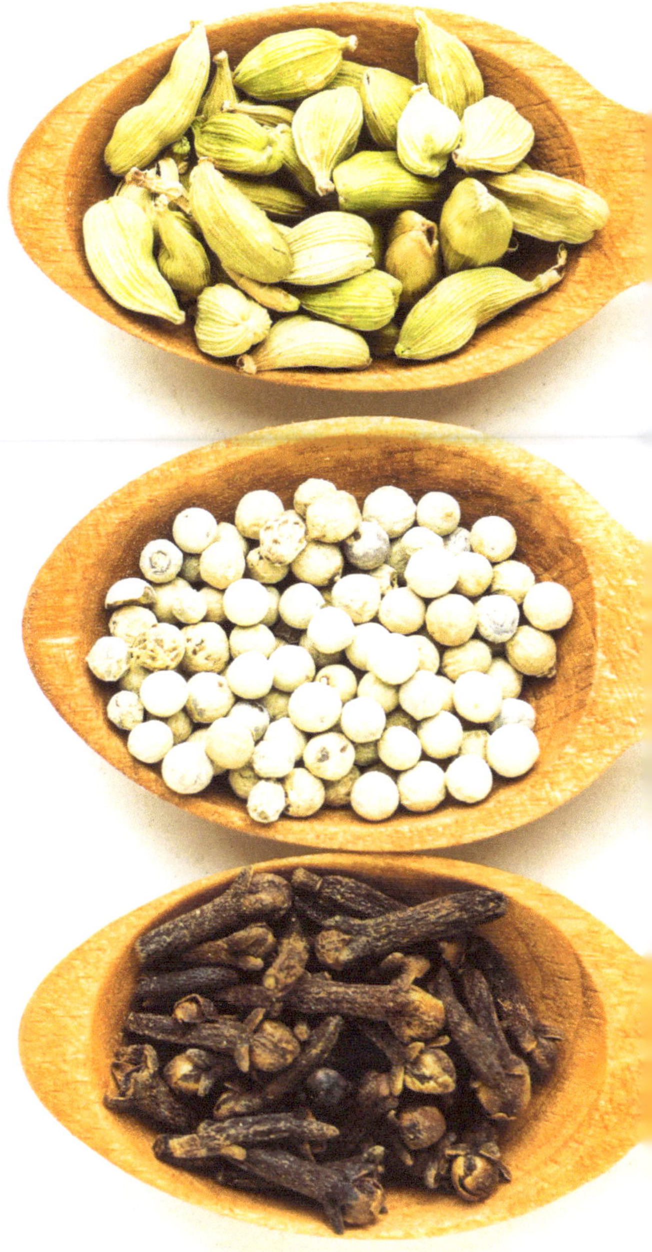

Around 6 million years ago, early humans co-evolved with flowering plants. They discovered that wrapping meat in leaves of bushes enhanced its taste. Certain nuts, seeds, berries, and bark also contributed to flavor. Spices and herbs were initially used to mask unpleasant tastes and odors of food and later to keep food fresh. Ancient civilizations didn't differentiate between spices for flavoring and those for medicinal purposes.

Biblical Times

Spices held great importance in biblical times (around 17th century BC). The Song of Solomon mentions culinary spices like cinnamon and saffron. Queen Sheba gifted King Solomon gold and spices. The New Testament refers to tithing of spices like mint, dill, and cumin.

Spices we use today have a rich and fascinating history spanning thousands of years and multiple continents. Here's a brief overview:

Ancient Egypt

The Ebers Papyrus (1500 BC) lists medicinal treatments using spices like caraway, coriander, fennel, garlic, mint, and onion. Onion and garlic were particularly important for health and stamina. Egyptians sourced flavor-enhancing spices like cardamom and cinnamon from Ethiopia.

Early Chinese Influence

Shen Nung, an ancient Chinese figure, compiled the Pen Ts'ao Ching (The Classic Herbal) around 2700 BC. It mentioned over a hundred medicinal plants, including spice cassia (similar to cinnamon).

Early History

- **Ancient Civilizations:** Spices date to ancient civilizations such as Egypt, China, and South Asia. Spices like cinnamon, black pepper, and ginger were used for culinary, medicinal, and even embalming purposes.

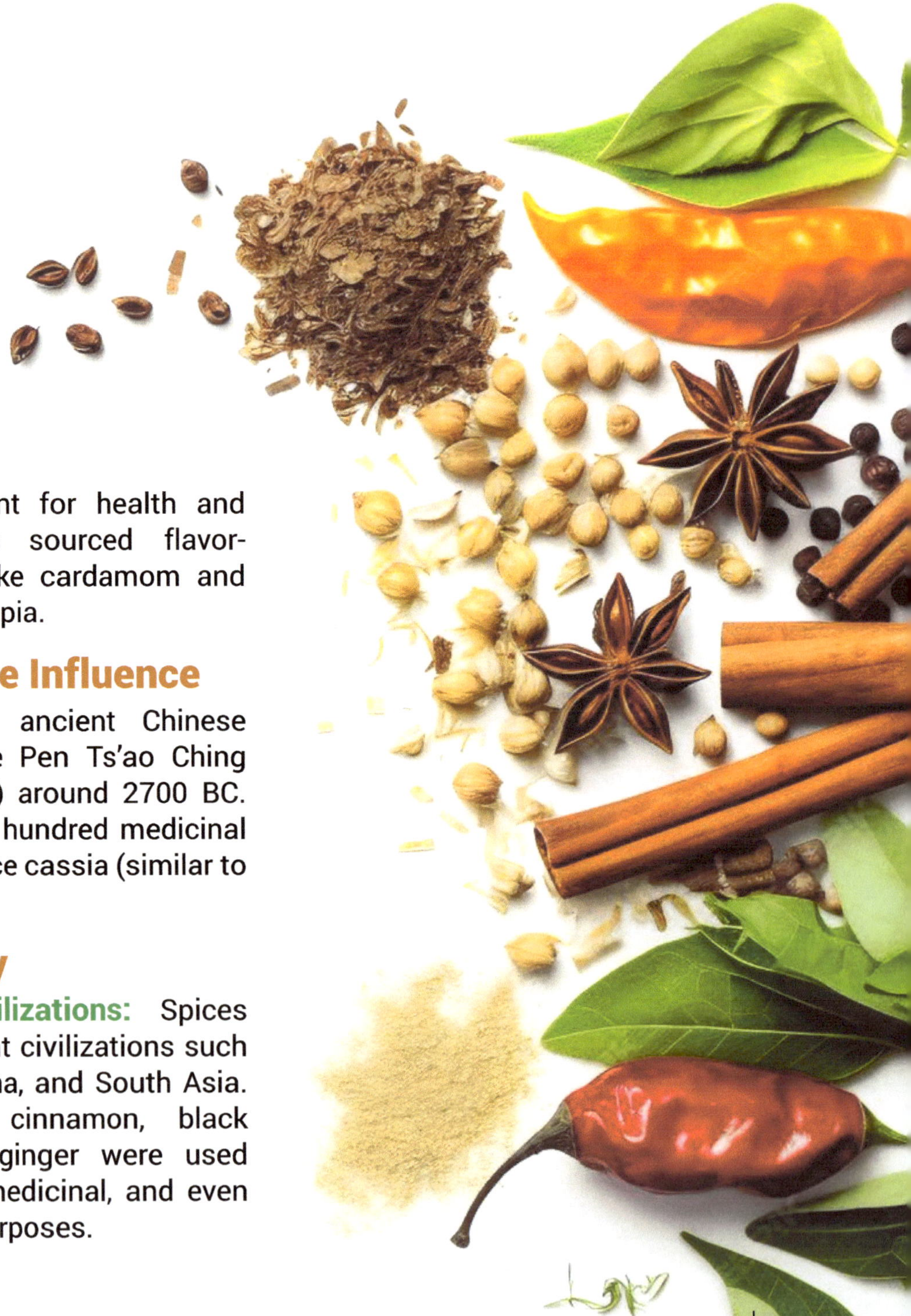

- **Trade Routes:** Strategic location on ancient trade routes, including the Silk Road, facilitated the exchange of spices with other civilizations. Spices like black pepper, cardamom, and cinnamon were highly sought after.

Medieval Period

- **Arab and Persian Influence:** During the medieval period, Arab and Persian traders played a crucial role in disseminating Asian spices to the West. Spices became luxury commodities in Europe.
- **European Exploration:** In the 15th century, European powers, particularly the Portuguese, Dutch, and later the British, sought direct access to many spice-producing regions. This led to the exploration and establishment of maritime trade routes.

Colonial Era

- **British East India Company:** The British East India Company played a significant role in monopolizing the spice trade during the colonial period. They controlled spice production, distribution, and trade routes, impacting the livelihoods of local spice farmers.
- **Spice Plantations:** The British introduced large-scale spice plantations in South Asia, particularly in regions like Kerala and Karnataka, in India.

Modern Era

- **Post-Independence Revival:** India became a major player in the global spice market. Government policies supported spice cultivation, and India remained a significant exporter of various spices.
- **Diverse Spice Production:** Today, many countries produce and process many spices that have become part of many favorite dishes we enjoy. Spices have added flavor to our food and played a significant role in cultural exchange, economic prosperity, and even exploration.

Spices are mainly natural plant products, deriving from seeds, roots, fruits, flowers, leaves, and barks. Many have medicinal values and cosmetic uses, rather than just flavoring ingredients.

As stated earlier, most spices originate in Eastern countries and have been used for thousands of years, as some are mentioned in the Vedas and other religious books, including the Bible. They do have a tropical background in many aspects. Initially, most spices were added to mask any unpleasant smell or taste of certain food items. Later, it was discovered (probably from trial and error of thousands of years) that many spices add to a healthy, longer life, due to their antioxidant and other favorable qualities. Ancient Egyptian historical records from 1500 BC have recorded the medicinal use of caraway, coriander, fennel, garlic, mint, and onion. Onion and Garlic were given special importance in stamina and vitality. From the early historic era, Cinnamon and Cardamom were traded between eastern and western nations. Some of the oldest Chinese historical records also mention the importance of many species used in their daily lives.

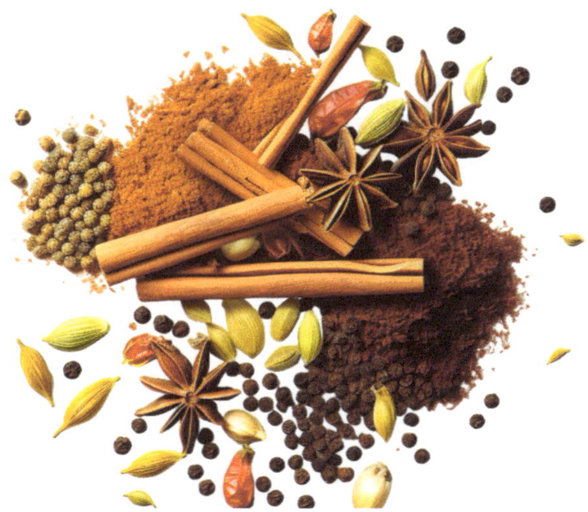

BRIEF HISTORY

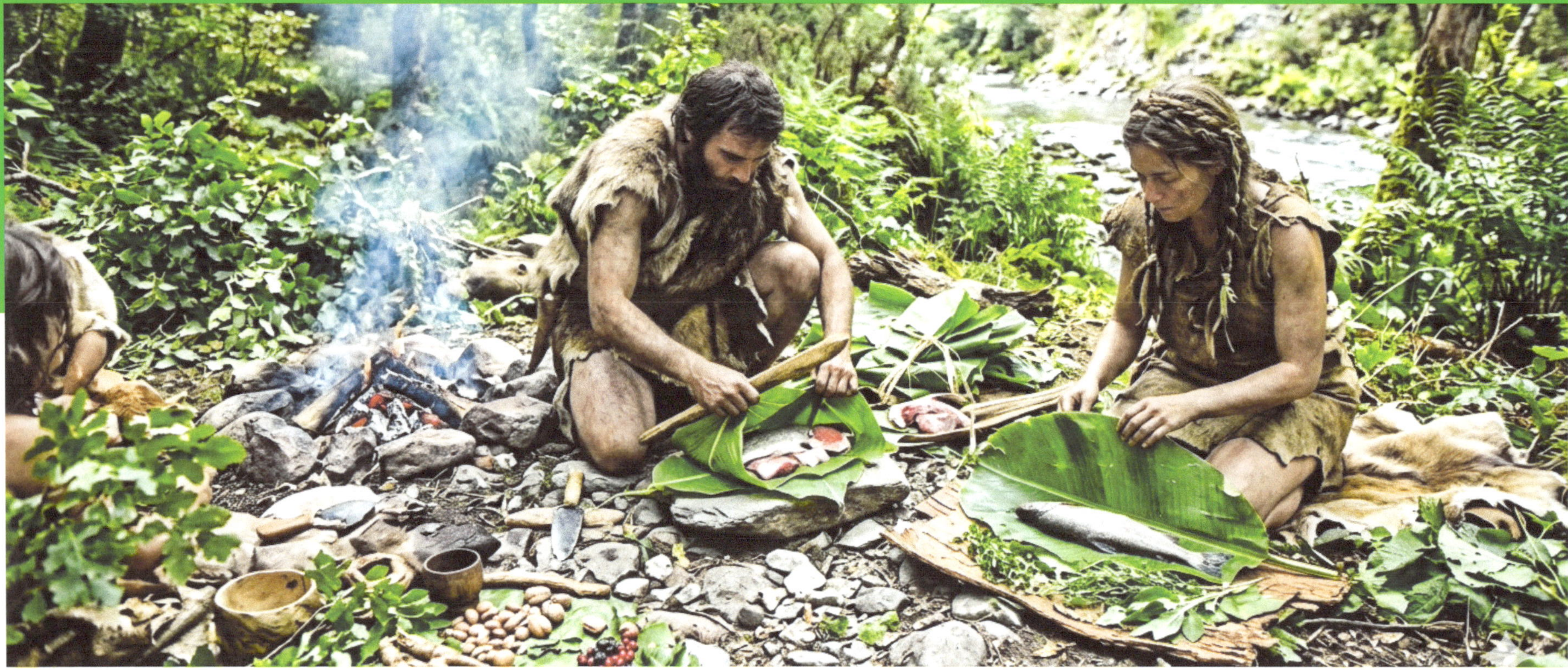

Early Humans' lives revolved around nature, plants, and animals. They depended on nature for all their daily needs, including health aspects. They discovered from trials that wrapping food, including fish and meat, in fresh leaves of bushes around added flavor and taste to the food.

Some spices were used to mask the unpleasant taste or odor of the food item.

Ancient Hindu Vedas, such as Rigveda and Atharvaveda, refer to many plants and plant products, which were the basis of Ayurvedic medicines. Since there are too many numbers, I will avoid listing them here.

Hippocrates, the father of medicine, has documented the healing properties of different spices and herbal products, emphasizing careful preparation.

Historically, Greek medical practitioners used a lot of herbs and spices found in the countryside to treat many ailments. Some wore herbs such as marjoram and parsley as head crowns to avoid drunkenness.

MOST COMMON SPICES AND

- Allspice (Pimenta dioica)
- Annatto seeds (Bixa orellana)
- Asafetida (Ferula assa-foetida)
- Anise (Pimpinella anisum)
- Basil (Ocimum basilicum)
- Bay leaf (Laurus nobilis)
- Black cardamom (Amomum subulatum)
- Black cumin (Bunium persicum)
- Black mustard seed (Brassica nigra)
- Black pepper (Piper nigrum)
- Boldo leaves (Peumus boldo)
- Cardamom (Elettaria cardamomum)
- Chameleon plant (Houttuynia cordata)
- Cinnamon (Cinnamomum zeylanicum)
- Cloves (Syzygium aromaticum)
- Coconut (Cocos nucifera)
- Coriander (Coriandrum sativum)
- Cubeb pepper (Piper cubeba)
- Cumin (Cuminum cyminum)
- Curry leaf (Murraya koenigii)
- Dill seed (Anethum graveolens)
- Epazote (Chenopodium ambrosioides)
- Fennel (Foeniculum vulgare)
- Fenugreek (Trigonella foenum-graecum)
- Filè (sassafras) (Sassafras albidum)
- Fingerroot (Boesenbergia pandurata)
- Garden cress (Lepidium sativum)
- Garlic (Allium sativum)
- Ginger (Zingiger officinale)
- Grains of Paradise (Melegueta Pepper) (Aframomum melegueta)
- Greater galanga (Alpinia galanga)
- Hyssop (Hyssopus officinalis)
- Indian bay leaf (Cinnamomum tamala)
- Kaffir lime (Citrus hystrix)
- Lavender (Lavandula angustifolia)
- Lemon grass (Cymbopogon citratus)
- Lemon verbena (Lippia citriodora)
- Lemon (Citrus limon)
- Lesser galanga (Kaempferia galanga)
- Lime (Citrus aurantifolia)
- Nutmeg and Mace (Myristica fragrans)
- Long pepper (Piper longum)
- Mahaleb cherry (Prunus mahaleb)

THEIR BOTANICAL NAMES

- Mango (Mangifera indica)
- Mexican tarragon (Tagetes lucida)
- Marjoram (Majorana hortensis)
- Myrtle (Myrtus communis)
- Nasturtium (Tropaeolum majus)
- Nigella (Nigella sativa)
- Olive (Olea europaea)
- Olive Oil
- Onion (Allium cepa)
- Oregano (Origanum vulgare)
- Paracress (Spilanthes acmella)
- Perilla (Perilla frutescens)
- Pink pepper (Schinus terebinthifolius)
- Poppy (Papaver somniferum)
- Rocket (Eruca sativa)
- Rose (Rosa damascena)
- Rosemary (Rosmarinus officinalis)
- Rue (Ruta graveolens)
- Saffron (Crocus sativus)
- Sage (Salvia officinalis)
- Savory (Satureja hortensis)
- Screw pine (pandanus) flower (Pandanus odoratissimus)
- Sesame (Sesamum indicum)
- Sichuan pepper (Zanthoxylum piperitum)
- Silphion (Silphium)
- Star anise (Illicium verum)
- Sumac (Rhus coriaria)
- Tamarind (Tamarindus indica)
- Tarragon (Artemisia daracunculus)
- Thyme (Thyumus vulgaris)
- Tonka beans (Dipteryx odorata)
- Turmeric (Curcuma longa)
- Vanilla (Vanilla planifolia)
- Wasabi (Wasabia japonica)
- Most common Peppers used in Cooking
- Wines
- Citrus Juice and Rind
- Vinegars
- Soy Sauce
- Honey
- Maple Syrup
- Worcestershire sauce
- Miso Paste
- Common Nuts Used in Cooking

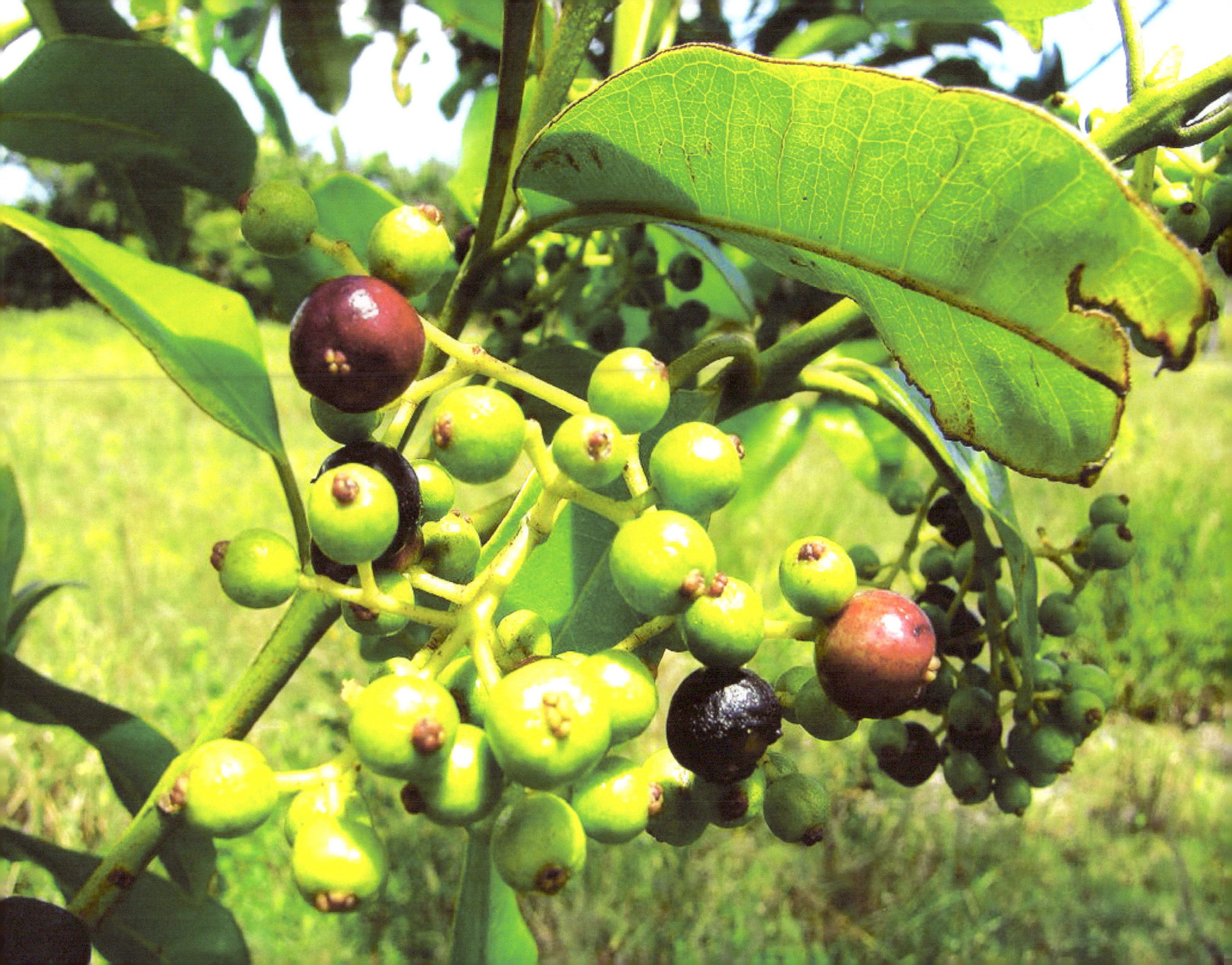

ALLSPICE (PIMENTA DIOICA)

Allspice (Pimenta dioica), also known as Jamaica pepper, is a versatile spice that combines the flavors of cinnamon, nutmeg, and cloves. It's known as a versatile spice that adds depth and complexity to your dishes while offering numerous health benefits.

Here are some key properties and health benefits of allspice

NUTRITIONAL CONTENT

- **Essential Oils :** It contains essential oils such as eugenol, which gives it its characteristic aroma and flavor.
- **Vitamins and Minerals :** Rich in vitamins A, C, and B-complex vitamins, as well as minerals like calcium, iron, magnesium, and manganese.
- **Antioxidants :** High in antioxidants that help protect cells from oxidative stress and damage.
- **Fiber :** Contains dietary fiber, which aids in digestion and promotes gut health.

HEALTH BENEFITS

- **Digestive Health :** Aids in digestion, relieves gas and bloating, and can help alleviate indigestion.
- **Anti-inflammatory :** Reduces inflammation and can help alleviate conditions like arthritis and muscle pain.
- **Pain Relief :** Known for its analgesic properties, providing relief from headaches and joint pain.
- **Antimicrobial Properties :** Has antibacterial and antifungal properties that help fight infections.
- **Immune System Support :** High vitamin C content helps boost the immune system and protect against infections.
- **Respiratory Health :** Used to treat respiratory conditions like colds, coughs, and bronchitis due to its expectorant properties.
- **Antioxidant Properties :** Contains compounds that help neutralize free radicals, promoting overall health and reducing the risk of chronic diseases.

USAGE

- **Culinary Uses :** Allspice is used to flavor a wide variety of dishes, including meats, stews, soups, sauces, and baked goods. It's a key ingredient in Jamaican jerk seasoning and Middle Eastern cuisine.
- **Medicinal Uses :** Can be consumed as tea, a supplement, or essential oil for its health benefits.
- **Aromatherapy :** Allspice essential oil is used in aromatherapy for its warming and invigorating effects.

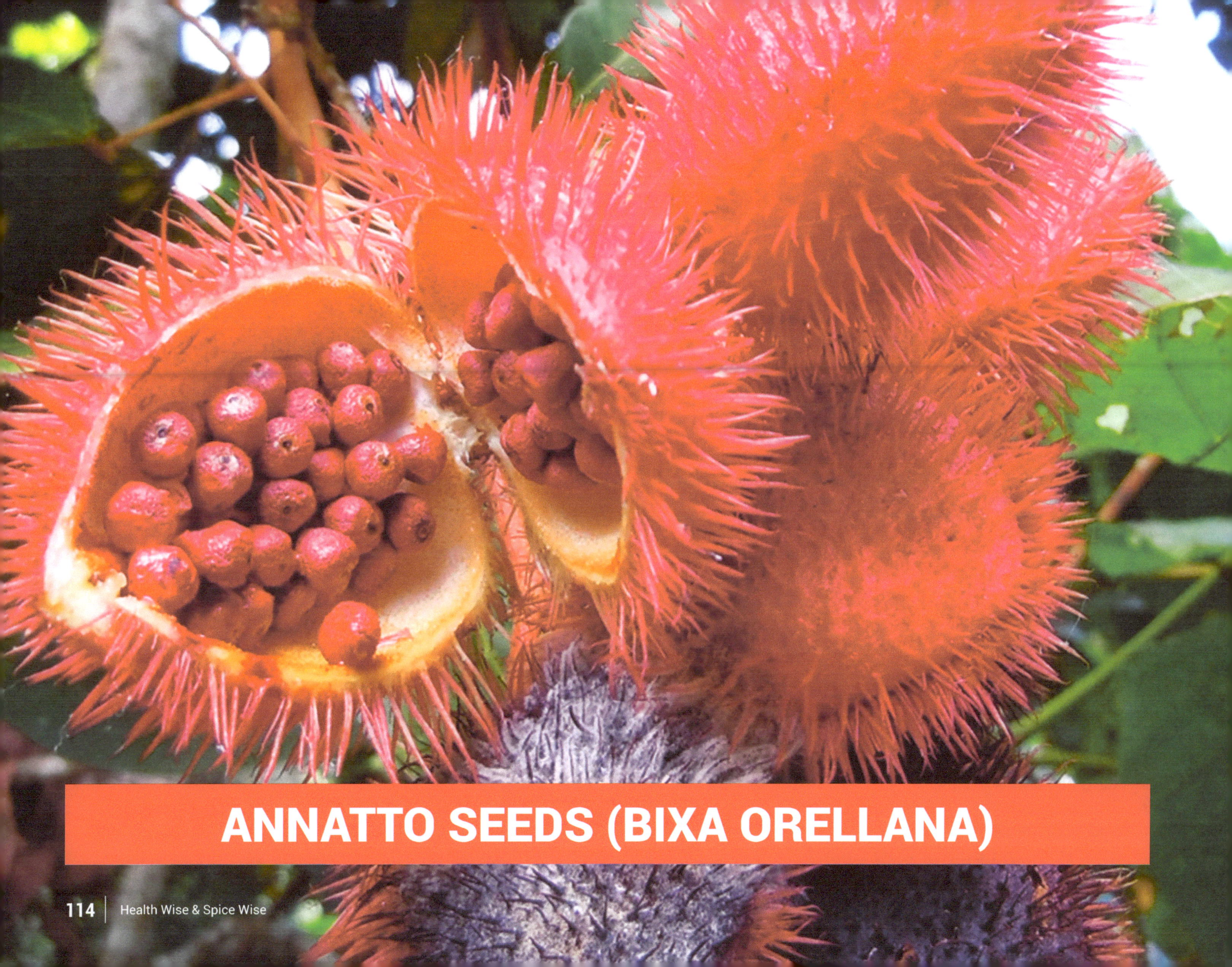

ANNATTO SEEDS (BIXA ORELLANA)

BOTANICAL INFORMATION

Scientific Name: Bixa orellana Family: Bixaceae Common Names: Achiote, Roucou, Lipstick tree, Achiotillo, Urucum Plant Type: Tropical and subtropical perennial shrub or small tree Description: Taprooted, perennial, evergreen or deciduous shrub that reaches up to 3 m in height with distinctive large pink flowers and round crown

COUNTRY OF ORIGIN

Primary Origin : Native to Mexico, Central America, South America, and the Caribbean, particularly tropical Central and Amazonian South America Current Cultivation: Grown in tropical countries such as Peru, Mexico, Ecuador, Indonesia, India, Kenya, and East Africa Global Distribution: Now grown throughout the world in suitable tropical climates Historical Note: Principally distributed through intentional introduction for use as a source of annatto dye

PART USED

Primary : Seeds - produce one of the dyes most frequently used worldwide Secondary: Leaves (used to make medicine) Seed Characteristics: Furry, heart-shaped seeds Active Compounds: Carotenoid pigments (bixin and norbixin), tocotrienols Processing: Seeds processed into powder, paste, oil, or extract

CULINARY USES

Flavor Profile: "Slightly peppery with a hint of nutmeg" scent and "slightly nutty, sweet, and peppery" flavor Primary Applications:

- Traditional dishes in Central and South America, Mexico, and the Caribbean, such as cochinita pibil, chicken in achiote, caldo de olla, and nacatamal
- Natural food coloring agent
- Impart yellow to red-orange color to foods
- Spice and seasoning paste
- Rice and meat dishes
- Latin American and Caribbean cuisine

HEALTH BENEFITS

Traditional Uses : Diabetes, diarrhea, fevers, fluid retention, heartburn, malaria, and hepatitis Modern Research-Backed Benefits:

- Reduced inflammation, improved eye and heart health, antioxidant, antimicrobial, and anticancer properties
- Rich in anti-inflammatories and antioxidants like carotenoids and tocotrienols, which prevent cellular damage and maintain good brain health
- Liver detoxification and protection from oxidative damage
- Anti-inflammatory properties for skin health and hydrating properties
- Used as antioxidant and bowel cleanser Topical Applications: Applied directly to treat burns

COMMERCIAL APPLICATIONS

Food Industry : Industrial food coloring to add yellow or orange color to butter, cheese, margarine, ice creams, meats, and condiments Textile Industry: Natural dye for textiles and fabric coloring Cosmetics Industry: Natural coloring and ingredients in cosmetic products Paint Industry: Natural pigment for paint production Pharmaceutical: Used in drugs and as natural coloring agent Livestock Feed: Spent seeds after pigment extraction used for livestock feeding as protein and energy source.

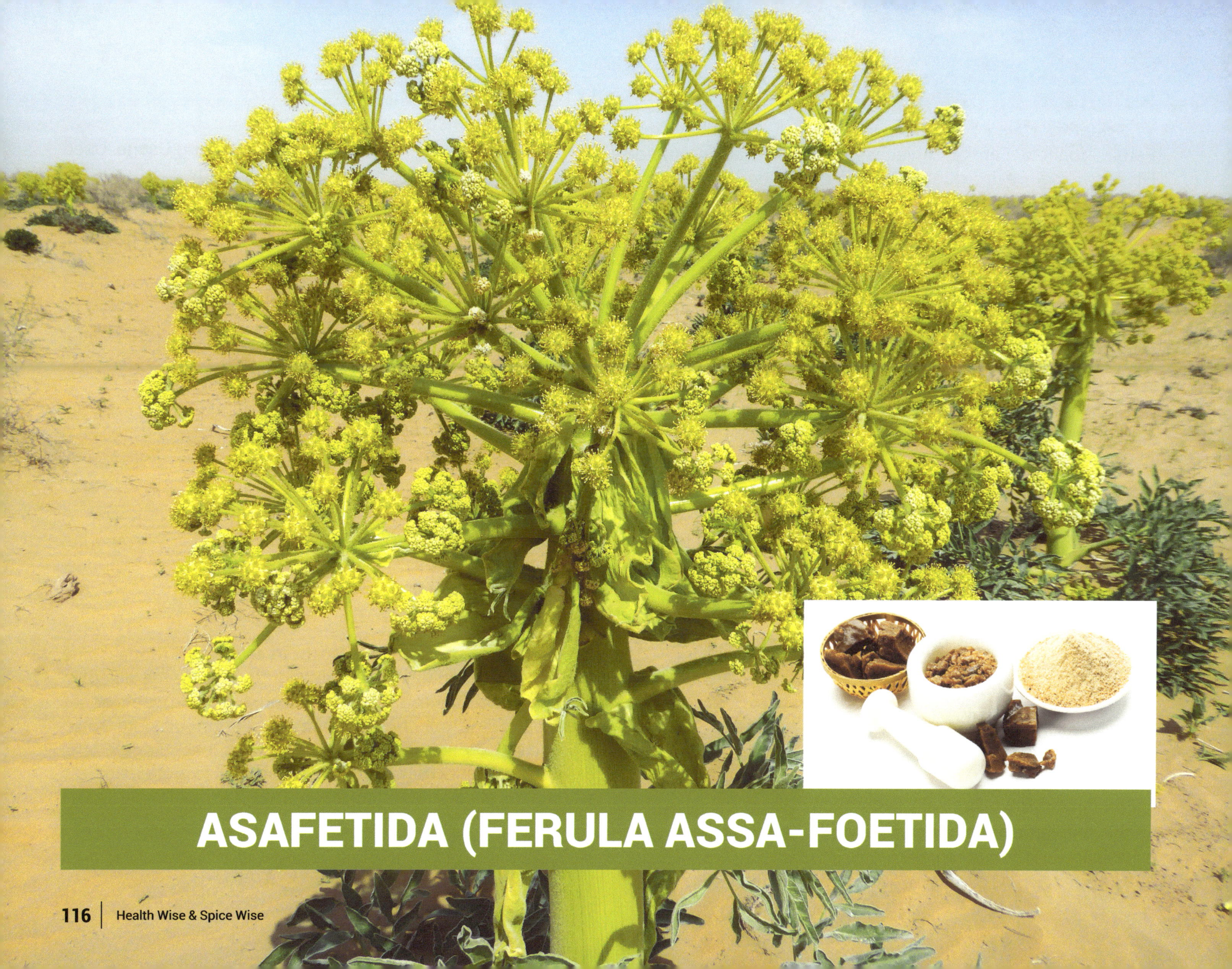

ASAFETIDA (FERULA ASSA-FOETIDA)

BOTANICAL INFORMATION

Scientific Name : Ferula assa-foetida L. (main species), Ferula foetida Family: Apiaceae (Umbelliferae) Common Names: Hing, Devil's dung, Stinking gum, Food of the gods Plant Type: Herbaceous perennial plant Description: Large perennial herb that can grow up to 2 meters tall with thick taproot and compound umbellate flowers

COUNTRY OF ORIGIN

Primary Origin : Native to Iran, Afghanistan, and Central Asia Main Production Regions: Southern Iran (especially near Lar), Eastern Iran, western Afghanistan, western Pakistan, Central Asia (Karakum Desert, Kyzylkum Desert) Current Cultivation: Mainly wild-harvested rather than cultivated Historical Note: Brought to Europe by Alexander the Great's expedition, familiar in early Mediterranean through land trade across Iran

PART USED

Primary : Oleo-gum-resin extracted from taproots and rhizomes Extraction Method: Resin produced by solidifying juice from cuts made in living roots Processing: Available as crude resin, compounded (mixed with starch/gum), or powdered form Active Compounds: Sulfur-containing compounds, essential oils, ferulic acid esters Appearance: Brownish or yellowish resin with strong sulfurous odor

CULINARY USES

Flavor Profile : Acrid taste with strong onion-like odor due to organic sulfur compounds, mellows when cooked Primary Applications:

- Indian cuisine (especially vegetarian dishes)
- Flavoring agent in curries, dal, and meatballs
- Pickles and condiments
- Spice mixtures and masalas
- Enhances umami flavors in dishes
- Traditional Persian and Central Asian cooking Usage: Used in very small quantities due to potent aroma and flavor

HEALTH BENEFITS

Traditional Uses : Digestive aid, flatulence, bloating, indigestion, asthma, whooping cough, bronchitis, epilepsy, stomachache, intestinal parasites Modern Research-Backed Benefits:

- Antioxidant properties that protect cells from free radical damage
- Anti-inflammatory and antimicrobial effects
- Digestive support and relief from bloating and gas
- Antispasmodic properties for muscle relaxation
- Expectorant for respiratory conditions
- Natural laxative effects
- Sedative properties for nervous system
- Potential antiviral and antibacterial activities Therapeutic Properties: Spasmolytic, anti-coagulant, vermifuge, stimulant, emmenagogue

COMMERCIAL APPLICATIONS

Food Industry : Flavoring agent in processed foods, spice blends, and condiments Pharmaceutical Industry: Used in traditional medicine preparations and as therapeutic agent Essential Oil Production: Steam distillation of gum resin produces essential oil for flavoring International Spice Trade: Exported primarily from Iran and Afghanistan to global markets Traditional Medicine: Incorporated into Ayurvedic and Unani medicine systems Culinary Export: Major ingredient in Indian spice exports worldwide

ANISE (PIMPINELLA ANISUM)

BOTANICAL BACKGROUND

- Anise is a tender annual herb from the Apiaceae family, native to the eastern Mediterranean and Southwest Asia.
- The plant grows about 1 meter tall, with finely divided feathery leaves and umbels of small white flowers.
- Its seeds are small, oval, grayish-brown, and possess a sweet licorice aroma.

COMMON CULINARY APPLICATIONS

- Anise seeds are sweet and aromatic, with a flavor profile similar to fennel and star anise but lighter.
- Used extensively in Mediterranean, Middle Eastern, and European baking (like biscotti, breads).
- Essential in flavoring liquors such as ouzo, absinthe, and anisette.

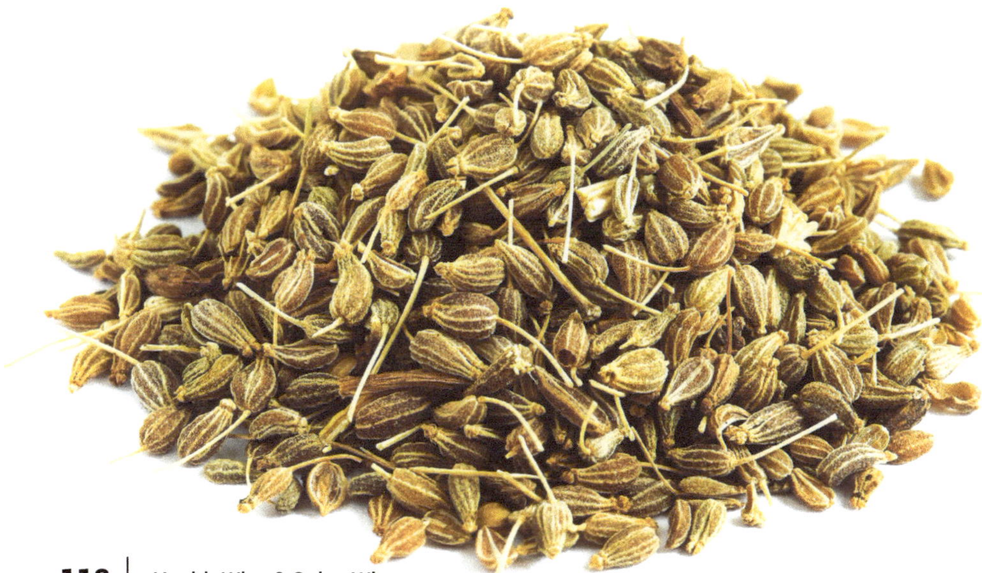

TYPES / VARIETIES

- Typically, only one species widely cultivated, but seed quality varies by region, affecting oil content and sweetness.

CULINARY USES

- Used whole or ground in baked goods, herbal teas, and spice blends.
- Adds complexity to sausages, stews, and sauces.
- Anise oil is extracted for flavoring sweets and beverages.

HEALTH BENEFITS

- Known for carminative and digestive benefits, reducing bloating and gas.
- Antispasmodic effects help soothe gastrointestinal cramps.
- Traditionally used to increase breast milk production and ease coughs.

"Anise soothes the stomach and lifts the spirit with its sweet, calming embrace." — **Dr. Lina Hassan**

BASIL (OCIMUM BASILICUM)

BOTANICAL BACKGROUND

- Annual/short-lived perennial herb, family Lamiaceae.
- Native to tropical Asia & Africa; widely cultivated.
- Aromatic, glossy green leaves; square stems; small white/ purple flowers.
- Grows 30–60 cm; prefers warm, sunny, well-drained soil.
- Historically used in culinary, medicinal, ceremonial contexts.

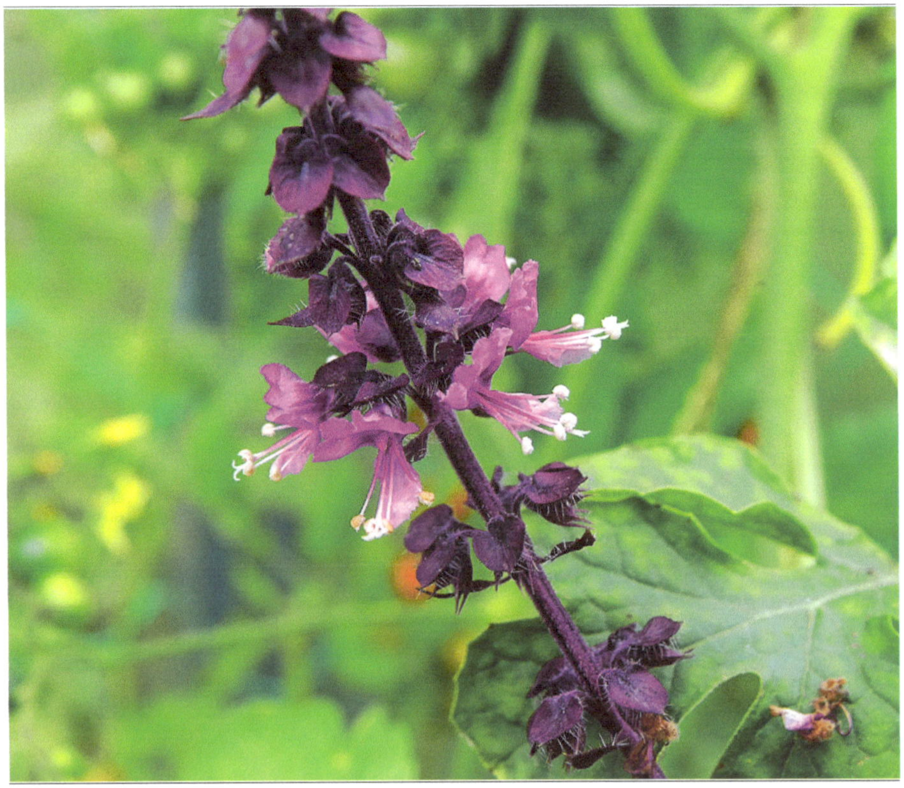

COMMON CULINARY APPLICATIONS

- Fresh in salads, sandwiches, caprese dishes.
- Key in pesto, sauces, tomato-based dishes.
- Flavoring for soups, stews, pizzas, pasta.
- Infused in oils, vinegars, beverages.
- Sweet, aromatic, slightly peppery or anise-like flavor.

TYPES / VARIETIES

- Sweet Basil (O. basilicum var. basilicum) – common culinary basil.
- Thai Basil (O. basilicum var. thyrsiflora) – anise/licorice flavor.
- Lemon Basil (O. basilicum citriodorum) – citrusy aroma.
- Purple Basil (O. basilicum 'Purpurascens') – mild clove flavor, ornamental.
- Holy Basil (O. tenuiflorum/Tulsi) – medicinal and ceremonial use.

CULINARY:

- Fresh/dried in salads, sauces, pesto, soups; infused in oils or beverages; garnish for meats, seafood, vegetables.

HEALTH BENEFITS

- Rich in antioxidants, vitamins A, K, C, minerals; aids digestion, reduces inflammation; supports immunity; antibacterial, stress-relieving; supports cardiovascular health and blood sugar regulation; historically used for respiratory and skin support.

BAY LEAF (LAURUS NOBILIS)

- Common Name and Botanical Name Indian bay leaf - Cinnamomum tamala
- Part of the Plant Used Leaf
- Country or Region of Origin South Asia

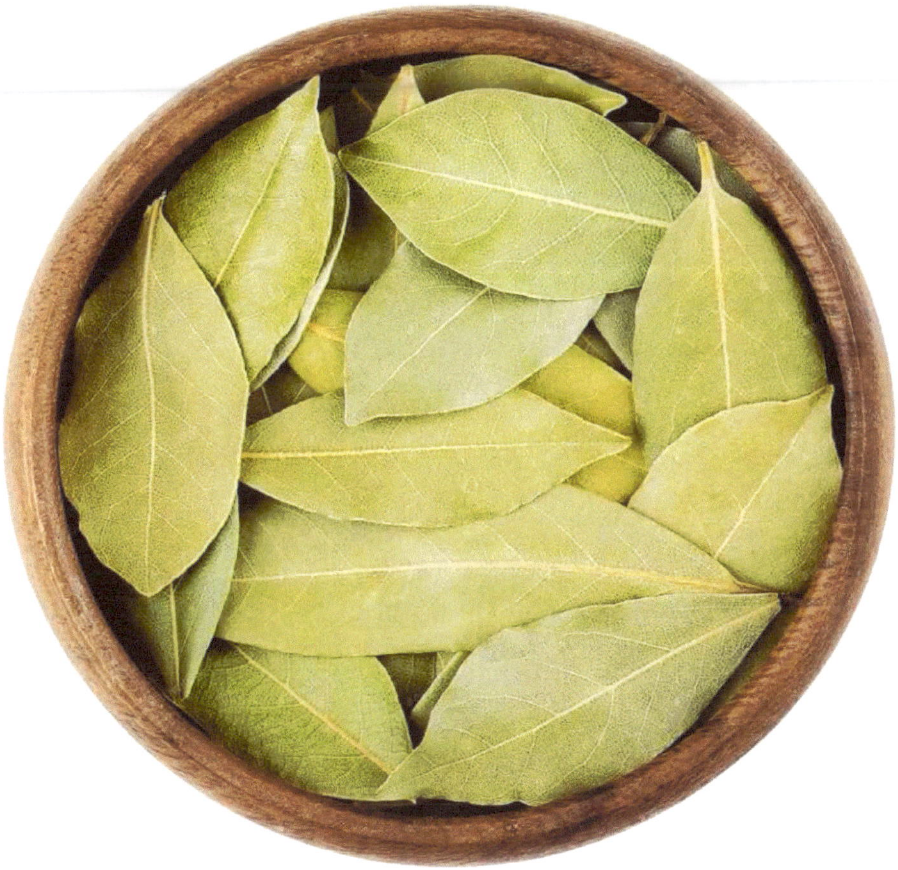

Bay leaves are commonly used in cooking, especially in garam masala and biryani. They are also used in pickling, soups, stews, rice dishes, brines for meat, and seafood

Indian bay leaves, also known as cassia leaves, have many properties, including:

- **Antimicrobial :** Bay leaves contain eugenol, which inhibits the growth of bacteria and fungi.
- **Anti-inflammatory :** Bay leaves contain compounds like linalool, eugenol, and myrcene, which can reduce inflammation and pain.
- **Antioxidant :** Bay leaves are packed with antioxidants, which can help protect cells from oxidative stress.
- **Wound healing :** Bay leaves can accelerate wound healing and alleviate pain and irritation.
- **Stress and anxiety reduction :** When burned, bay leaves release a calming aroma that can relax the nerves and reduce tension.
- **Immune system support :** Bay leaves may support the immune system.
- **Chemical protection :** Bay leaves may protect against chemicals that can cause genetic mutations.
- **Insecticidal :** Bay leaves may help repel insects.

BLACK CARDAMOM (AMOMUM SUBULATUM)

BOTANICAL BACKGROUND

- Perennial herb, family Zingiberaceae.
- Native to Himalayas (India, Nepal, Bhutan).
- Large brown pods (2–5 cm) with aromatic seeds.
- Grows in shady, humid, high-altitude areas (800–2,000 m).
- Pods dried over open flames smoky aroma.

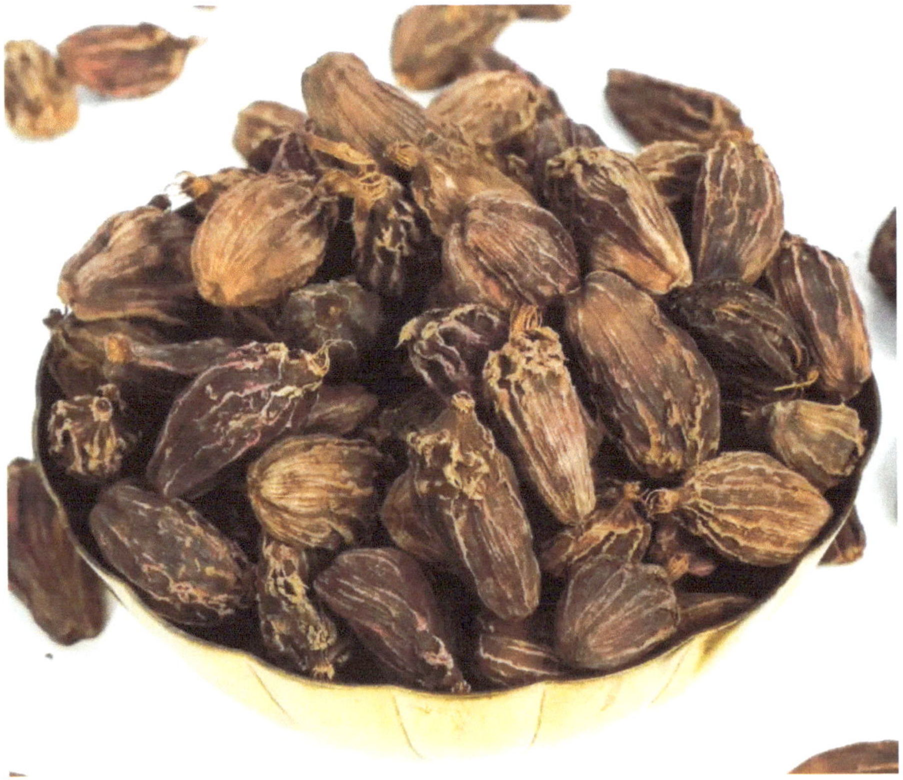

COMMON CULINARY APPLICATIONS

- Whole pods in curries, stews, biryanis.
- Key in garam masala, Nepali spice mixes.
- Infused in dals, soups, rice dishes.
- Added to marinades, slow-cooked meats.
- Smoky, earthy, resinous, menthol flavor.

TYPES / VARIETIES

- A. subulatum – Nepali cardamom, main type.
- A. tsao-ko – Chinese black cardamom, larger, camphor flavor.
- A. costatum – regional, limited use.
- Flavor intensity varies with altitude/climate.

CULINARY

- adds depth to curries, rice, meats; used in blends; infused in teas/liqueurs.

HEALTH

- aids digestion, relieves bloating; supports respiratory health; antimicrobial, antioxidant; mild diuretic; traditional oral health use.

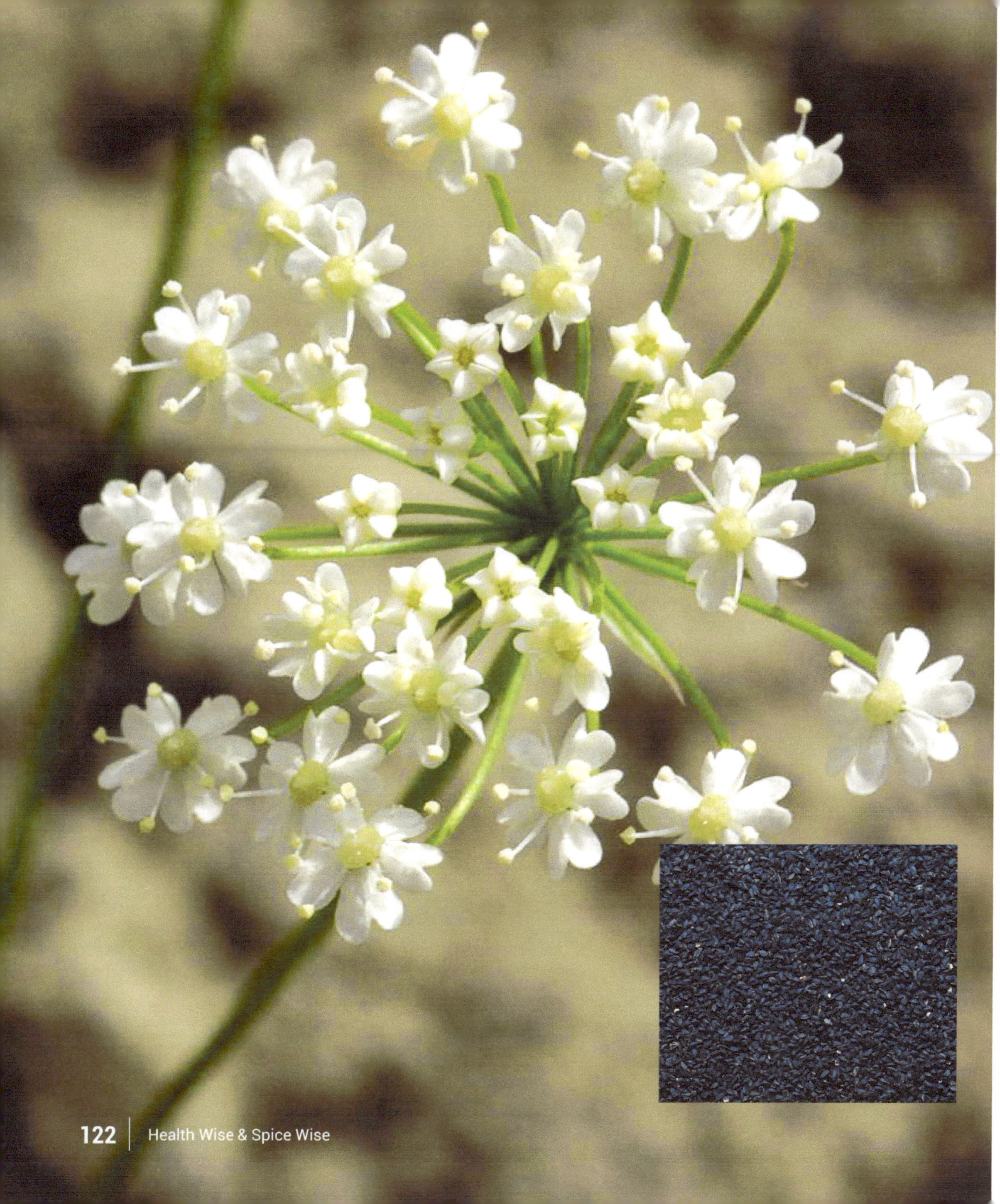

BOTANICAL BACKGROUND

- Biennial/perennial, family Apiaceae.
- Native to Iran, Afghanistan, Central & South Asia.
- Slender stems, feathery leaves, small white umbels.
- Tiny crescent-shaped black seeds, aromatic.
- Distinct from Nigella sativa ("black seed").

COMMON CULINARY APPLICATIONS

- Whole/ground seeds in spice blends.
- Key in Persian, Afghan, North Indian cuisine.
- Seasoning for breads, rice, curries, pickles.
- Added to soups, stews, vegetables.
- Warm, earthy, nutty, slightly bitter flavor.

TYPES / VARIETIES

- B. persicum – true black cumin, prized in Persian/Afghan cooking.
- B. cylindricum – smaller seeds, less common.
- Local landraces vary in aroma, oil content.
- Often confused with Nigella sativa and caraway.

BLACK CUMIN (BUNIUM PERSICUM)

CULINARY

- used in pilafs, breads, curries, pickles, spice mixes.

HEALTH

- rich in oils, antioxidants, minerals; aids digestion; relieves bloating; supports respiratory health; antimicrobial; traditional tonic & appetite stimulant.
- Boldo leaves (Peumus boldus) are an aromatic herb native to Chile that's used as a culinary spice throughout South America. Here's comprehensive information about boldo as a cooking ingredient:

CULINARY APPLICATIONS

- Boldo leaves are versatile in savory cooking applications. They're commonly used to season fish, mushrooms, vegetables, and meat dishes. The leaves work particularly well as a component in sauces and marinades. In Brazilian and other South American cuisines, cooks often wrap fish or meat in boldo leaves before frying, which imparts flavor while protecting the protein during cooking.
- The dried fruits of the boldo plant can be processed into spicy condiments, adding another dimension to the plant's culinary uses.

FLAVOR PROFILE

- Boldo leaves have a distinctive taste that becomes more palatable after drying and cooking. The flavor profile includes notes of camphor, pepper, and mint. Fresh boldo can have a somewhat strong, medicinal quality, but proper preparation mellows these characteristics into a more appealing aromatic profile.

COOKING METHODS AND SUBSTITUTIONS

- Boldo leaves function similarly to bay leaves in cooking applications. They can be used as a wrap for slow-roasting meats like lamb, or incorporated into accompanying sauces. The leaves work well as a substitute for Indian bay leaves in dishes like Northern Indian kormas and can be included in spice blends similar to garam masala.
- Boldo is sometimes mixed with yerba mate to modify that herb's strong flavor, showing its ability to complement and balance other ingredients.

PREPARATION AND USAGE

- Like bay leaves, boldo leaves are typically removed from dishes before serving, as they can be tough and unpleasant to eat whole. They're best used whole during cooking to infuse flavor, then discarded. The leaves can be used fresh but are more commonly used dried, which concentrates their flavor and makes them easier to store and handle.

ORIGIN AND AVAILABILITY

- Native to Chile's coastal regions, boldo has become popular throughout Latin America and is increasingly available in specialty spice shops and online retailers catering to South American cuisine.

BLACK MUSTARD SEED (BRASSICA NIGRA)

Grown commercially in India, Pakistan, Canada, and parts of Europe.

CULINARY USES

- The seeds are the primary source of pungent, sharp-flavored mustard used in cooking and condiments.
- Widely used in Indian cuisine — seeds are tempered in hot oil to release a nutty, spicy flavor in curries, dals, pickles, and chutneys.
- Used to make Dijon mustard and other whole-grain mustard preparations.
- Young leaves and shoots are edible and used as greens in salads or cooked dishes.
- Mustard oil, extracted from the seeds, is a staple cooking oil in South Asian and Eastern European cuisines.

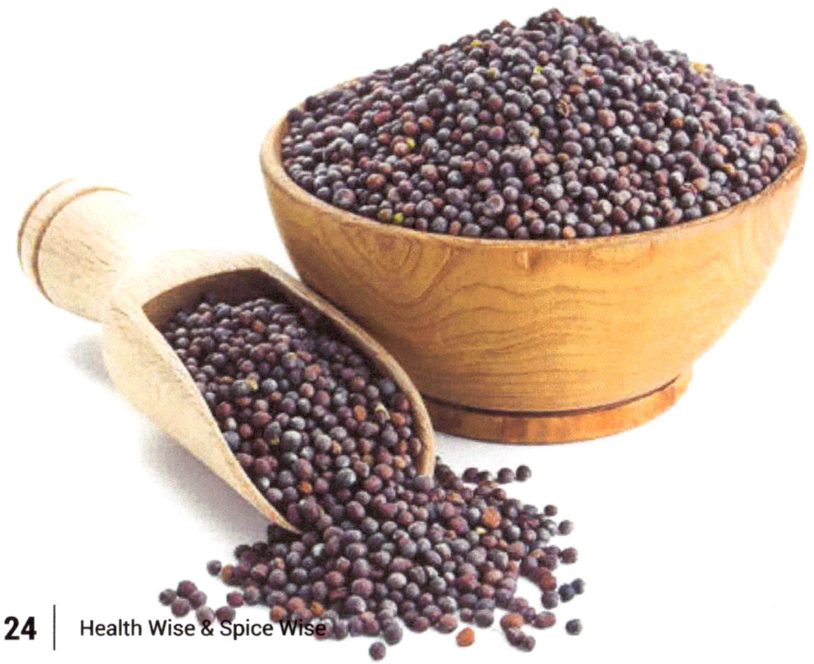

MEDICINAL & TRADITIONAL USES:

- It has a long history in Ayurvedic and traditional medicine.
- Seeds contain glucosinolates, which break down into allyl isothiocyanate — the compound responsible for its heat and medicinal properties.
- Traditionally used as a rubefacient (applied to skin to increase blood flow) in mustard plasters for muscle pain, arthritis, and respiratory congestion.
- May have antimicrobial and anti-inflammatory properties.
- Used historically to stimulate digestion and appetite.

NUTRITIONAL PROFILE (SEEDS)

- Black mustard seeds are rich in:
  - Fatty acids (erucic acid, oleic acid)
  - Glucosinolates (sinigrin)
  - Selenium, magnesium, and phosphorus
  - Omega-3 fatty acids
  - Vitamin E and antioxidants

CULTURAL & HISTORICAL SIGNIFICANCE

- Referenced in the Bible — the Parable of the Mustard Seed (Matthew 13:31–32) is widely believed to refer to Brassica nigra, which was common in the Holy Land.
- Used in ancient Greek and Roman medicine — Hippocrates and Pliny the Elder both documented its therapeutic uses.
- One of the oldest cultivated spice plants, with records going back over 5,000 years

BLACK PEPPER (PIPER NIGRUM)

BOTANICAL BACKGROUND

- Perennial climbing vine, family Piperaceae.
- Native to South India; now grown in tropics.
- Produces green berries (peppercorns) dried to black pepper.
- Green, white, and red forms from same plant.
- "King of Spices," traded since antiquity.

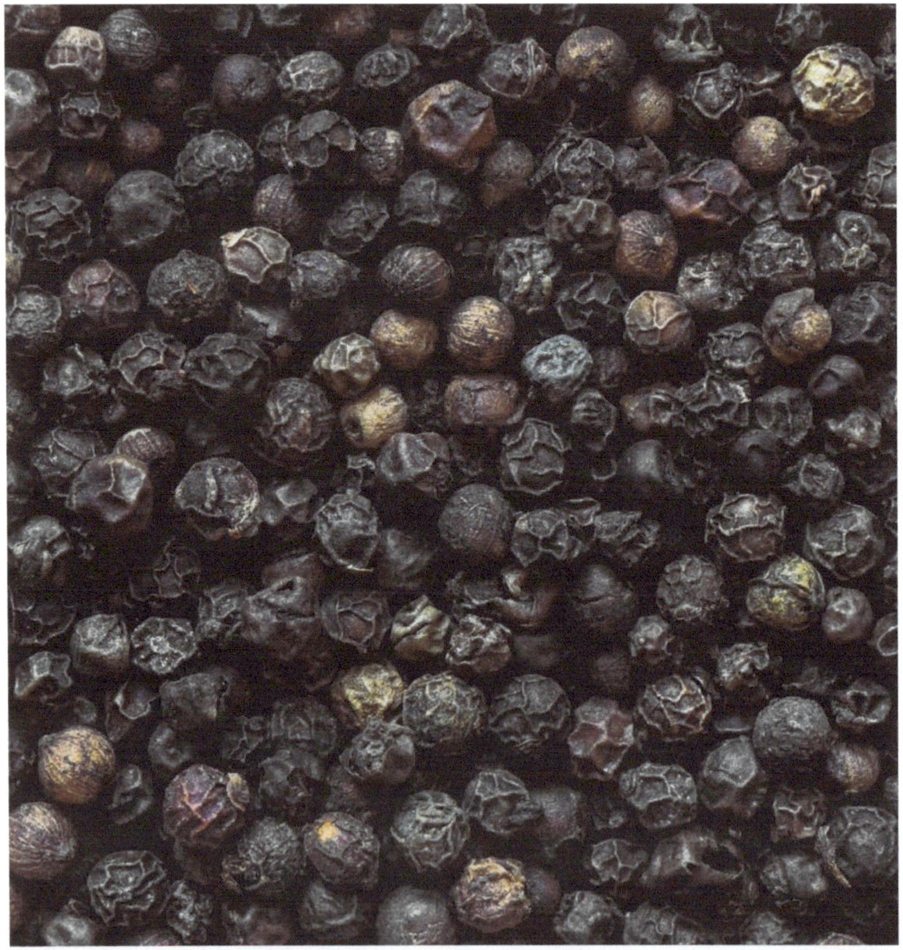

COMMON CULINARY APPLICATIONS

- Ground/cracked as universal seasoning.
- Key in spice blends (garam masala, curry, steak rubs).
- Adds flavor to soups, sauces, meats, vegetables.
- Used in pickling, sausages, cheeses.
- Pungent, sharp, mildly spicy, aromatic.

TYPES / VARIETIES

- Malabar – mild, aromatic.
- Tellicherry – large, bold, prized.
- Lampong (Indonesia) – sharp, smoky.
- Sarawak (Malaysia) – mild, fruity.
- Vietnamese – widely produced, balanced.

CULINARY

- seasoning worldwide; spice rubs, sauces, soups, marinades, pickles.

HEALTH

- piperine enhances nutrient absorption; aids digestion; antioxidants reduce inflammation; supports respiratory health; may boost metabolism.

BOLDO LEAVES (PEUMUS BOLDO)

a fascinating herbal plant long prized for its digestive, liver-protective, and detoxifying properties.

BOTANICAL OVERVIEW

- Common Name: Boldo
- Scientific Name:Peumus boldus
- Family: Monimiaceae
- Plant Type: Evergreen shrub or small tree
- Native to: Central Chile (South America)

OTHER NAMES:

- Spanish: Boldo del Chile
- Portuguese: Boldo-do-Chile, Boldo verdadeiro
- French: Boldo du Chili
- Hindi (sometimes marketed as): Chilean Boldo

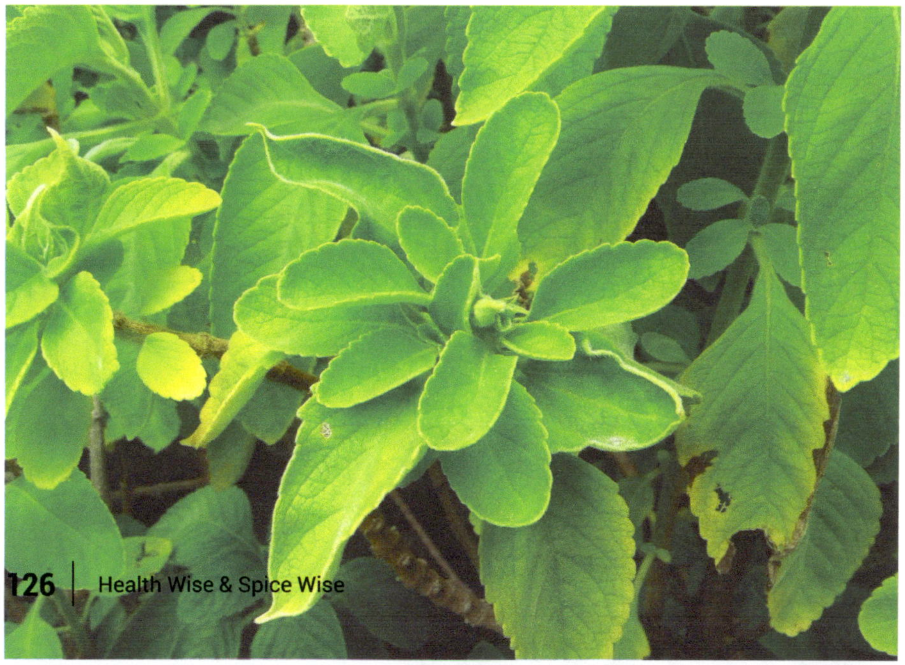

TRADITIONAL AND CULINARY USES

CULINARY USES:

- Herbal tea (Boldo tea): The most common form; used after meals to aid digestion.
- Occasionally used as a seasoning herb in South American dishes, though sparingly because of its strong flavor.

FLAVOR PROFILE:

- • Bitter, herbal, slightly minty and camphorous.
- • Blends well with mint, lemongrass, or anise in herbal infusions.

MEDICINAL AND THERAPEUTIC BENEFITS

Boldo is one of the most respected traditional herbs in South American and European herbal medicine, especially for the liver, gallbladder, and digestive system.

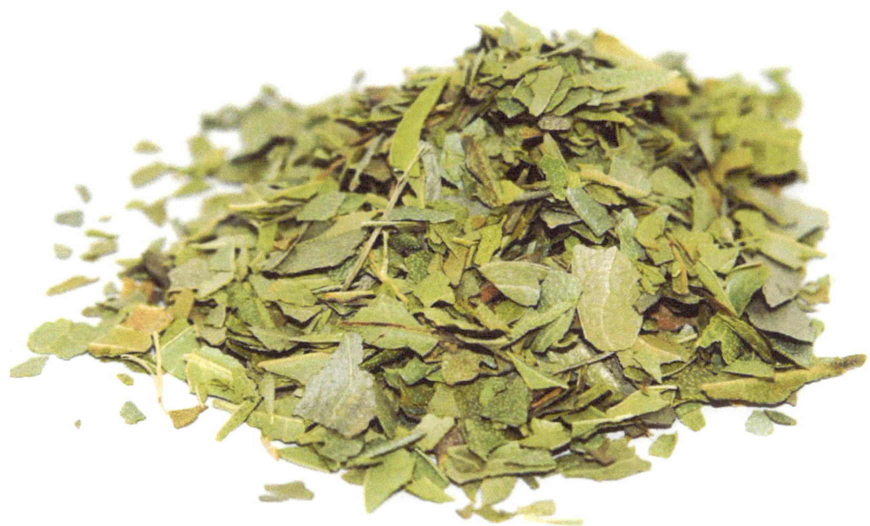

CARDAMOM (ELETTARIA CARDAMOMUM)

BOTANICAL BACKGROUND

- Perennial herb, family Zingiberaceae.
- Native to South India & Sri Lanka; grown in Guatemala/ tropics.
- Tall plant (2–4 m), rhizomes, small green pods (1–2 cm) with seeds.
- "Queen of Spices," valued since ancient trade.

COMMON CULINARY APPLICATIONS

- Sweet & savory dishes worldwide.
- Flavoring for curries, rice, stews, spice blends.
- Key in Indian/Middle Eastern sweets, chai, desserts.
- Infused in coffee, teas, liqueurs.
- Warm, sweet, floral, citrusy flavor.

TYPES / VARIETIES

- Green Cardamom – common, aromatic, sweet.
- Malabar – smaller, subtle flavor.
- Mysore – larger, strong aroma, high oil.
- Guatemalan – major export, robust flavor.

CULINARY

- pods, seeds, or ground in curries, biryanis, teas, coffees, desserts, spice blends.

HEALTH

aids digestion, relieves bloating; freshens breath, oral health; antioxidants reduce inflammation; supports respiratory health; may help regulate blood sugar & heart health.

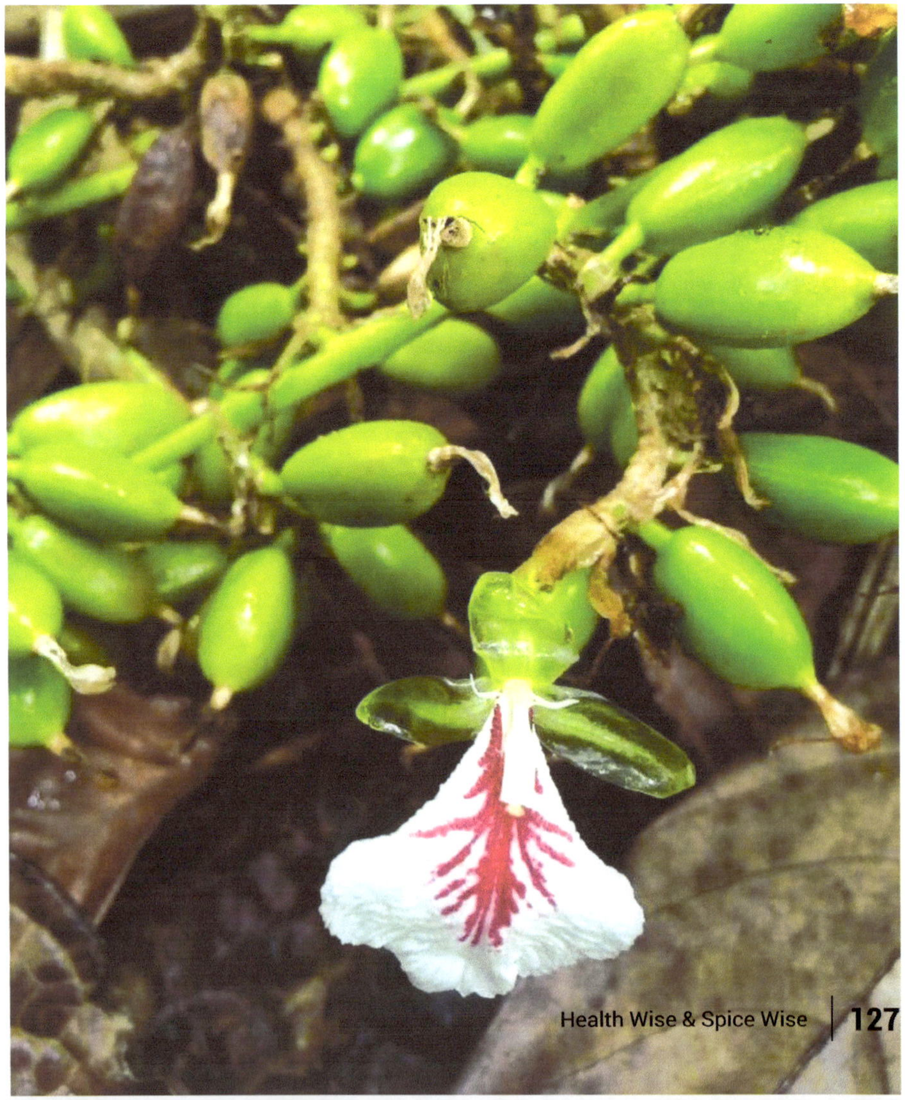

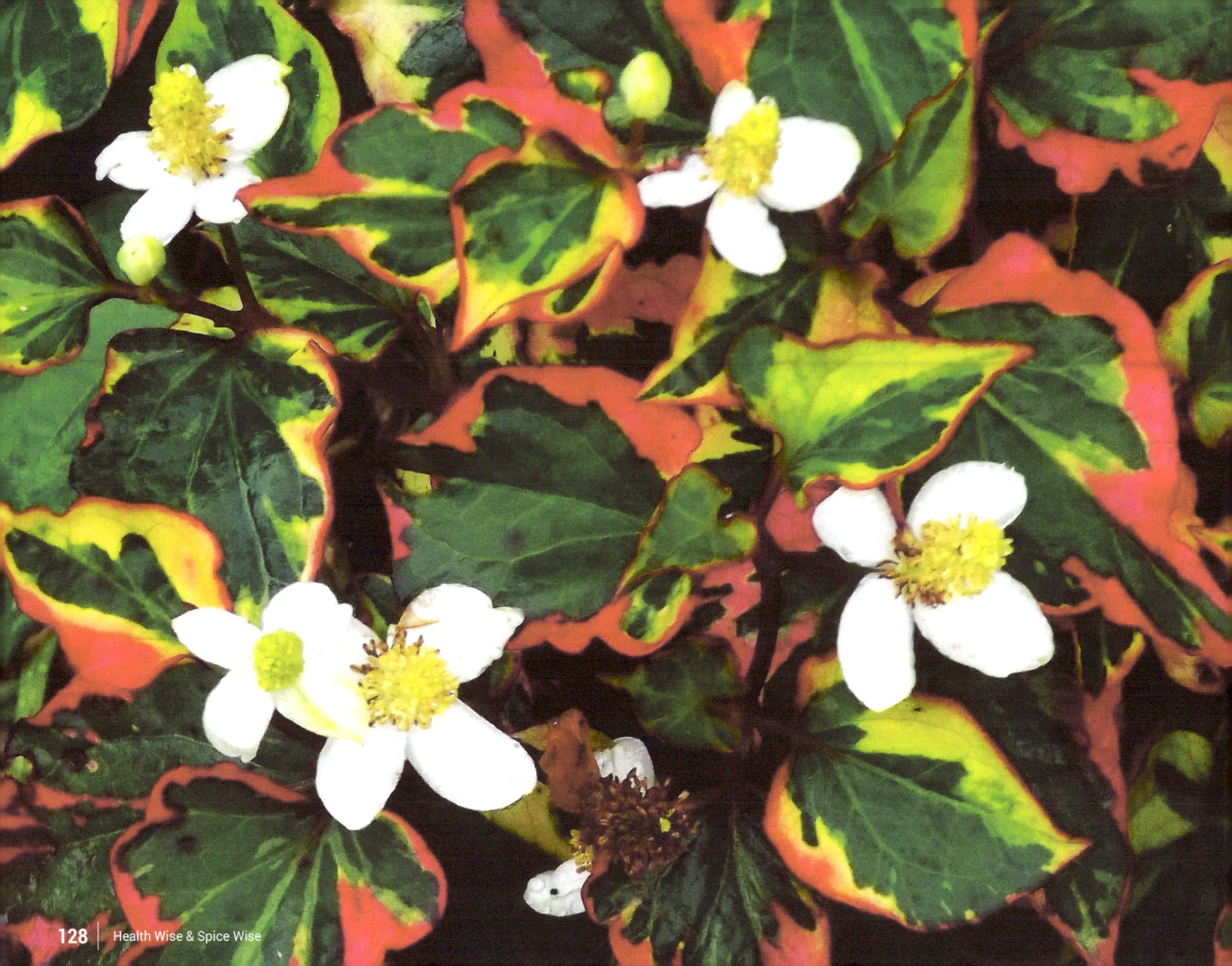

CHAMELEON PLANT (HOUTTUYNIA CORDATA)

Chameleon plant, scientifically known as Houttuynia cordata, is an aromatic herb used as a spice in various Asian cuisines. Also called fish mint, fish leaf, rainbow plant, or Chinese lizard tail, this plant has a distinctive culinary profile that makes it particularly valued in specific regional cooking traditions.

BOTANICAL BACKGROUND

Chameleon plant is a herbaceous perennial native to Southeast Asia that grows 0.6-1 meter tall. It's a flowering plant in the Lizard's Tail family that spreads via rhizomes and thrives in moist, shady locations. The plant produces heart-shaped leaves and has variegated foliage that gives it ornamental appeal.

FLAVOR PROFILE

The most distinctive characteristic of chameleon plant is its unique "fishy" flavor and aroma. The leaves have been described as tasting like fishy cilantro, with a pungent, somewhat acquired taste that not everyone enjoys. When cooked, the plant can impart a fish-like flavor to vegetarian dishes that would otherwise require fish stock, making it valuable for creating umami-rich plant-based meals.

CULINARY USES

REGIONAL APPLICATIONS

Chameleon plant is particularly prominent in Manipuri cuisine from northeastern India, where both the leaves and fresh rhizomes are used extensively. This regional cooking style incorporates many aromatic leaves and fermented fish flavors, making it quite distinct from mainstream Indian cuisine and more similar to Southeast Asian cooking.

COOKING METHODS

The tender leaves and flowers can be consumed in multiple ways:

- Raw in salads and on sandwiches
- Added to soups, stews, and curry dishes
- Used in stir-fries
- Fried in batter as a type of pakora or fritter
- Julienned over noodle salads
- Incorporated into fish meals and other protein dishes
- Ground into powder for seasoning

USAGE CONSIDERATIONS

The strong, distinctive flavor of chameleon plant means it works best in cuisines that already incorporate bold, pungent flavors. It pairs well with fermented ingredients and other strongly flavored herbs and spices. The plant's ability to add fish-like umami makes it especially valuable in vegetarian cooking where depth of flavor is desired.

The leaves are typically used fresh, though they can be dried for later use. The rhizomes are also edible and provide a different flavor profile than the leaves, offering additional culinary versatility.

CINNAMON (CINNAMOMUM ZEYLANICUM)

BOTANICAL BACKGROUND

- Evergreen tree, family Lauraceae.
- Native to Sri Lanka & S. India; grown in tropics.
- Grows 10–15 m; bark dried into quills.
- Inner bark & leaves aromatic.
- "True cinnamon," distinct from cassia.

COMMON CULINARY APPLICATIONS

- Ground or sticks in sweet & savory dishes.
- Key in desserts, baked goods, puddings.
- Used in curries, stews, rice, mulled drinks.
- Added to teas, coffees, liqueurs.
- Flavor: warm, sweet, woody, mildly spicy.

TYPES / VARIETIES

- Ceylon (C. zeylanicum) – delicate, sweet.
- Cassia (C. cassia) – strong, spicy, common.
- Saigon (C. loureiroi) – very aromatic.
- Indonesian (C. burmannii) – mild, economical.

CULINARY

desserts, breads, curries, rice, chai, garam masala, mulled drinks.

HEALTH

antioxidant, anti-inflammatory; aids digestion, relieves nausea; may regulate sugar & cholesterol; supports colds & respiratory health; antimicrobial, oral care.

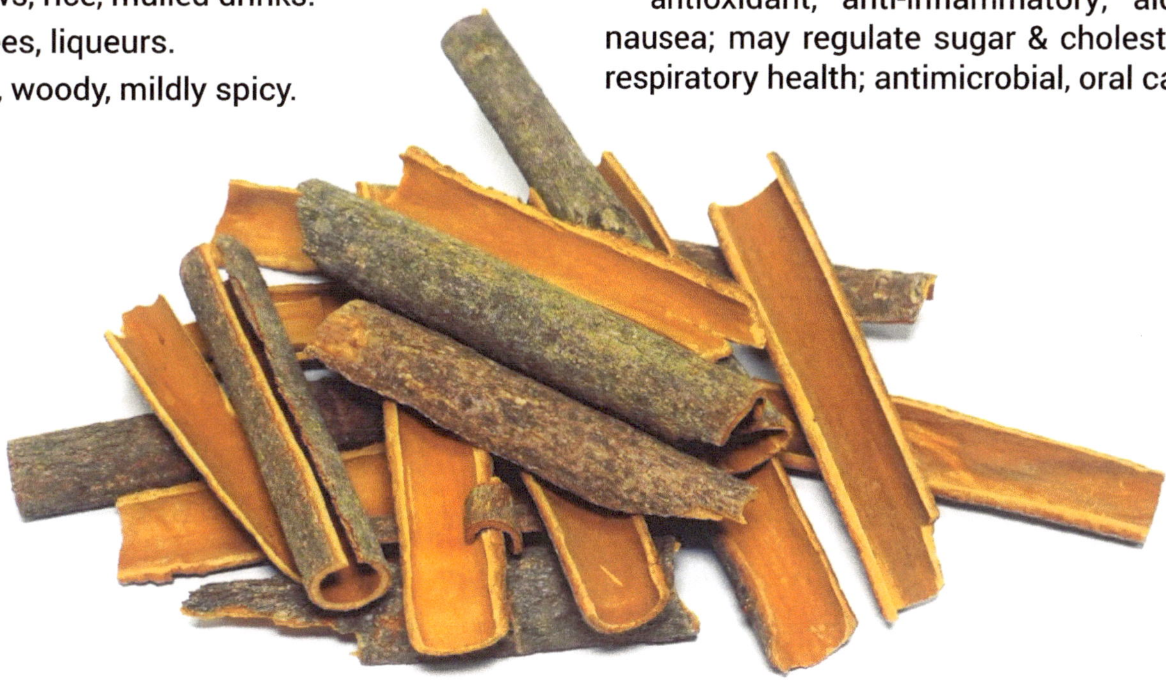

CLOVES (SYZYGIUM AROMATICUM)

BOTANICAL BACKGROUND

- Evergreen tree, family Myrtaceae.
- Native to the Maluku Islands (Indonesia); cultivated in tropical regions worldwide.
- Grows 10–12 m tall with glossy green leaves and small red flower buds.
- Flower buds harvested before blooming and dried into clove spice.
- Known for strong, sweet, and pungent aroma due to eugenol content.

COMMON CULINARY APPLICATIONS

- Whole or ground in spice blends (garam masala, pumpkin spice, chai masala).
- Used in baked goods, desserts, and sweet pastries.
- Flavoring for meats, stews, sauces, and pickles.
- Infused in teas, mulled wines, and hot beverages.
- Adds warm, sweet, aromatic, slightly bitter flavor.

TYPES / VARIETIES

- Indonesian Cloves – most common, strong aroma and flavor.
- Madagascan Cloves – large, high oil content, very aromatic.
- Zanzibar Cloves – slightly milder, used in East African cuisine.
- Sri Lankan Cloves – high-quality spice, strong, pungent aroma.

CULINARY

used whole in savory dishes, ground in sweets, teas, spice blends, marinades, and beverages.

HEALTH

rich in antioxidants and eugenol; may support oral health, digestion, and immunity; traditionally used for toothaches, respiratory relief, and anti-inflammatory purposes; may aid blood sugar regulation and improve circulation.

Coconut is an incredibly versatile ingredient with numerous culinary and non-culinary applications. Here's a comprehensive overview of the various uses of coconut in cooking and beyond:

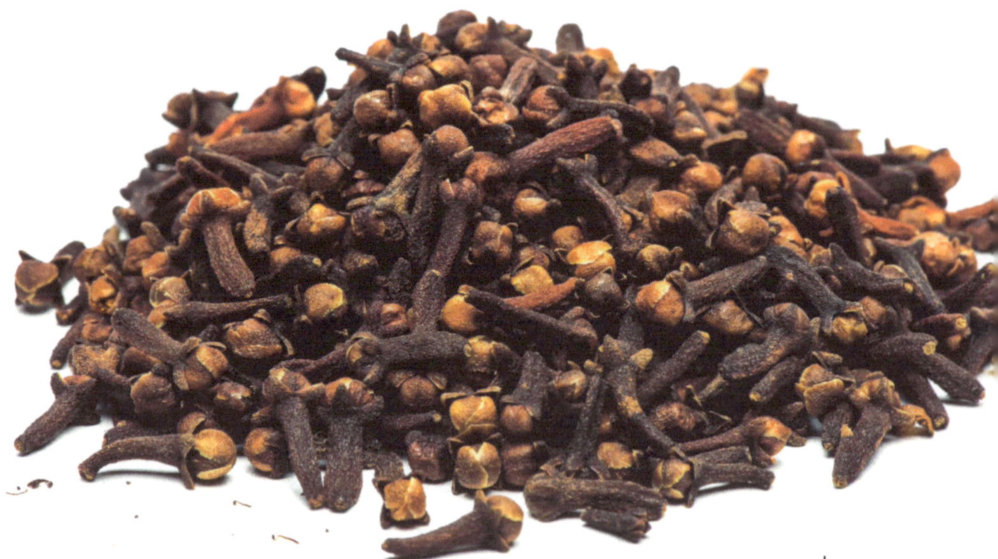

COCONUT (COCOS NUCIFERA)

FORMS USED IN COOKING

Coconut Milk and Cream - Coconut milk is extracted from grated coconut meat mixed with water. It's a cornerstone of many cuisines, particularly in Southeast Asian, Caribbean, and Indian cooking. The milk enhances savory curries, stews, and soups, providing a smooth, velvety texture. It also works beautifully in sweet applications, serving as a base for desserts like Thai coconut custard or Brazilian coconut brigadeiros. Coconut cream, which is thicker and richer than coconut milk, can replace heavy cream in most recipes, offering similar richness with a subtle coconut flavor.

FRESH COCONUT MEAT

The white, fleshy part of the coconut offers rich texture and mild sweetness. Fresh coconut meat can be eaten as a snack, added to fruit salads for tropical flavor, or blended into smoothies for a creamy, nutritious boost. It can be grated or shredded and sprinkled over fruit bowls, yogurt, or smoothie bowls for added texture and flavor.

DESICCATED COCONUT

This dried, shredded coconut is ideal for baking applications. Its moisture-absorbing properties make it perfect for adding texture and subtle coconut flavor to cookies, cakes, and bars. It's the main ingredient in coconut macaroons and is commonly used in various baked goods.

COCONUT OIL

Coconut oil has a nut-like quality with some sweetness and is commonly used in baked goods, pastries, and sautés. It can be used for sautéing, frying, or baking, and adds a distinct flavor to meals. Movie theater chains sometimes use it to pop popcorn. It serves as an excellent replacement for solid fats in various recipes.

SAVORY APPLICATIONS

Curries and Stews - Coconut milk and cream are essential in many curry preparations, providing richness and balancing spicy flavors. They create smooth, luxurious textures in stews and braised dishes.

SOUPS

Coconut milk adds depth and creaminess to soups without dairy, making it popular in both traditional recipes and modern plant-based cooking.

RICE DISHES

Coconut milk can be used to cook rice, creating aromatic and flavorful side dishes that pair well with spicy or bold-flavored main courses.

MARINADES AND SAUCES

Coconut milk serves as an excellent base for marinades, particularly for grilled meats and seafood, and can be incorporated into various sauces.

SWEET APPLICATIONS

Desserts - Coconut is used in countless dessert preparations, from puddings and custards to ice creams and frozen treats. It provides natural sweetness and tropical flavor.

BAKING

Shredded coconut, coconut flour, and coconut oil are popular in baking, offering texture, flavor, and moisture to cakes, cookies, and pastries.

FROSTINGS AND FILLINGS

Coconut cream and coconut milk can be whipped and used in frostings and fillings, adding tropical twist to traditional desserts.

SPECIALTY COCONUT PRODUCTS

Coconut Vinegar - Made from coconut water or coconut sap, coconut vinegar serves as a natural alternative to synthetic vinegar. It's used in pickles, salad dressings, and sauces as both a flavoring and preserving ingredient. It's high in vitamins and minerals including calcium, phosphorus, iron, and sodium.

COCONUT WATER

The clear liquid inside young coconuts is consumed as a refreshing beverage and can be used in cocktails, smoothies, and as a base for marinades.

COCONUT SUGAR

Made from coconut palm sap, this natural sweetener can replace regular sugar in recipes, offering a lower glycemic index and subtle caramel flavor.

COCONUT FLOUR

A gluten-free flour alternative made from dried coconut meat, popular in paleo and gluten-free baking.

REGIONAL CUISINE APPLICATIONS

Southeast Asian Cuisine - Coconut milk is fundamental in Thai, Malaysian, and Indonesian cooking, appearing in curries, soups like tom kha gai, and desserts.

CARIBBEAN COOKING

Coconut features prominently in Caribbean cuisine, from rice and peas to coconut-based desserts and beverages.

INDIAN CUISINE

Fresh coconut, coconut milk, and coconut oil are extensively used in South Indian cooking, particularly in Kerala cuisine.

PACIFIC ISLAND COOKING

Coconut is a staple ingredient throughout Pacific island cuisines, used in both savory and sweet preparations.

MODERN CULINARY TRENDS

Plant-Based Cooking - Coconut products serve as excellent dairy alternatives in vegan and plant-based cooking, providing richness and flavor without animal products.

GLUTEN-FREE BAKING

Coconut flour and coconut-based products are popular in gluten-free baking applications.

HEALTH-CONSCIOUS COOKING

Various coconut products are embraced in paleo, keto, and other health-focused dietary approaches.

The versatility of coconut makes it invaluable in both traditional and modern cooking, offering options for every meal from breakfast smoothies to elaborate dinner curries and decadent desserts.

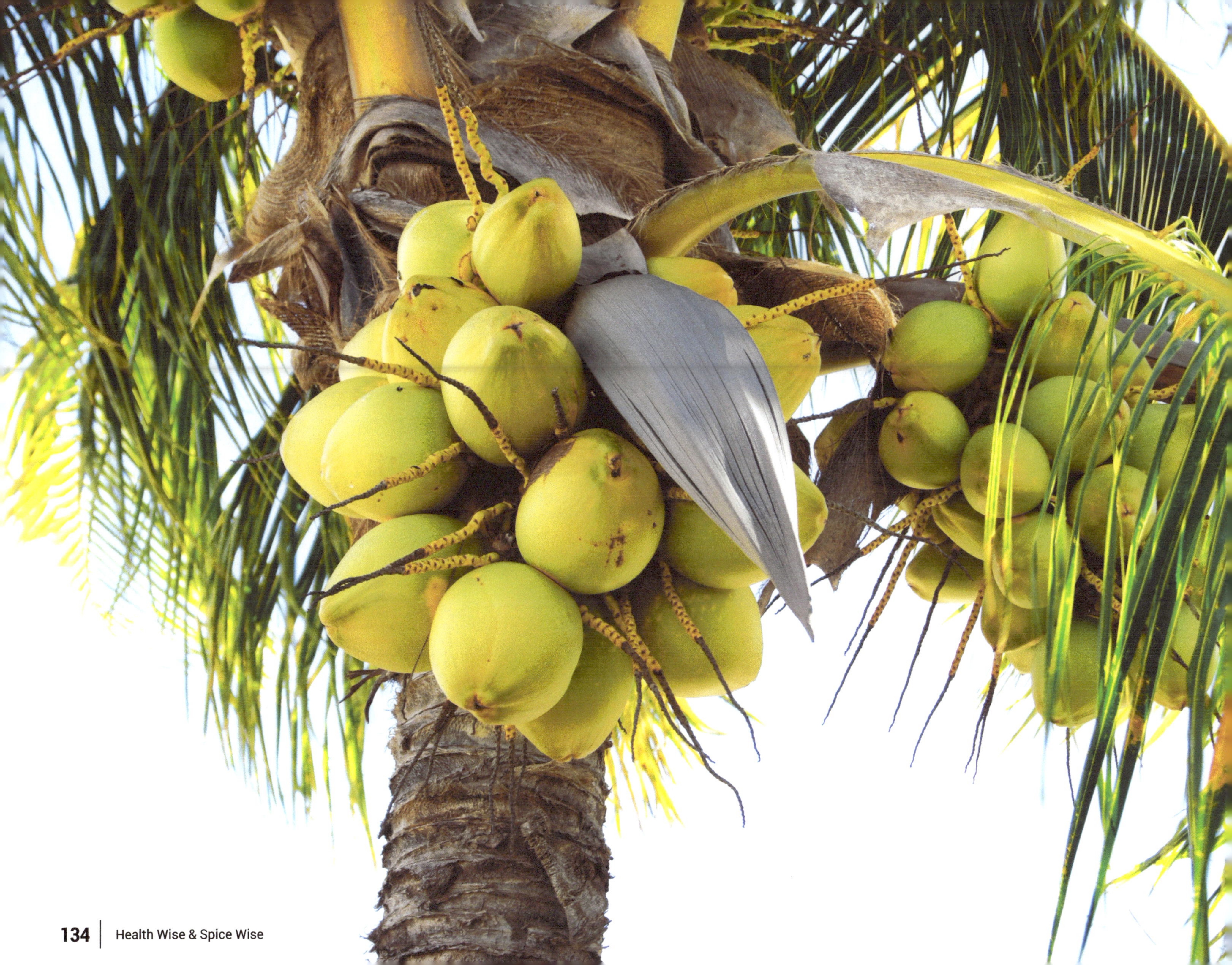

CORIANDER (CORIANDRUM SATIVUM)

Has many properties, including antioxidant, antibacterial, and anti-inflammatory properties. Coriander is also a source of vitamins, minerals, and essential oils.

ANTIOXIDANT PROPERTIES

- Coriander contains phenolics, such as caffeic acid, protocatechuic acid, and glycitin, which give it antioxidant properties
- Coriander's antioxidant properties may help protect against neurodegenerative diseases, cancer, and metabolic syndrome

ANTIBACTERIAL PROPERTIES

- Coriander essential oil may have antibacterial effects
- Coriander's essential oils may have antifungal properties

ANTI-INFLAMMATORY PROPERTIES

- Coriander's natural anti-inflammatory properties may help reduce inflammation and arthritis symptoms

NUTRITIONAL PROPERTIES

- Coriander leaves are rich in vitamins A, C, and K, and contain moderate amounts of minerals
- Coriander seeds contain dietary fiber, calcium, selenium, iron, magnesium, and manganese
- Other properties Coriander may help lower blood pressure and Coriander may help lower blood sugar.
- Coriander is a popular spice used in cooking around the world.

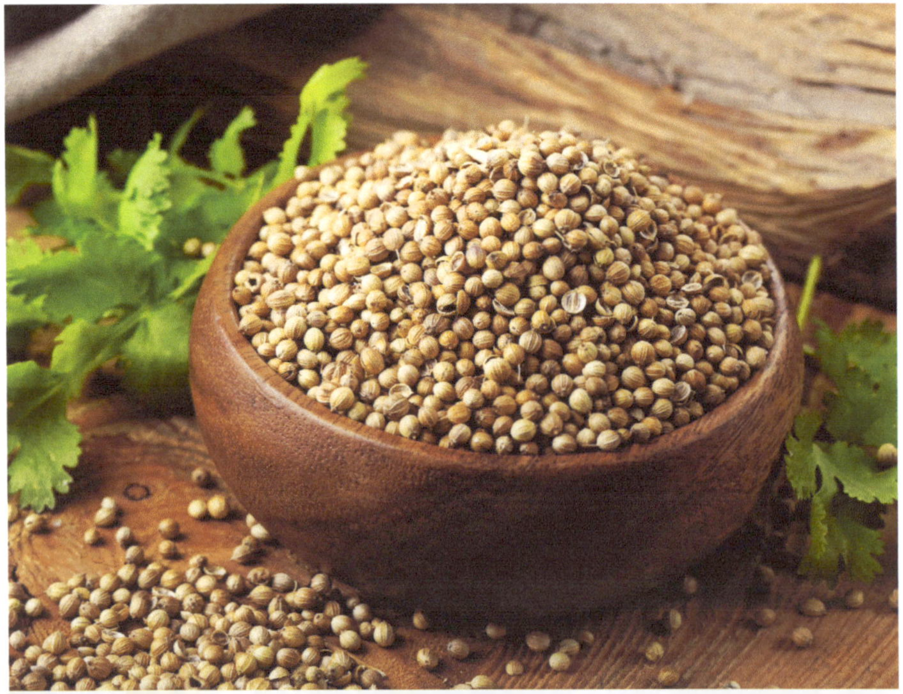

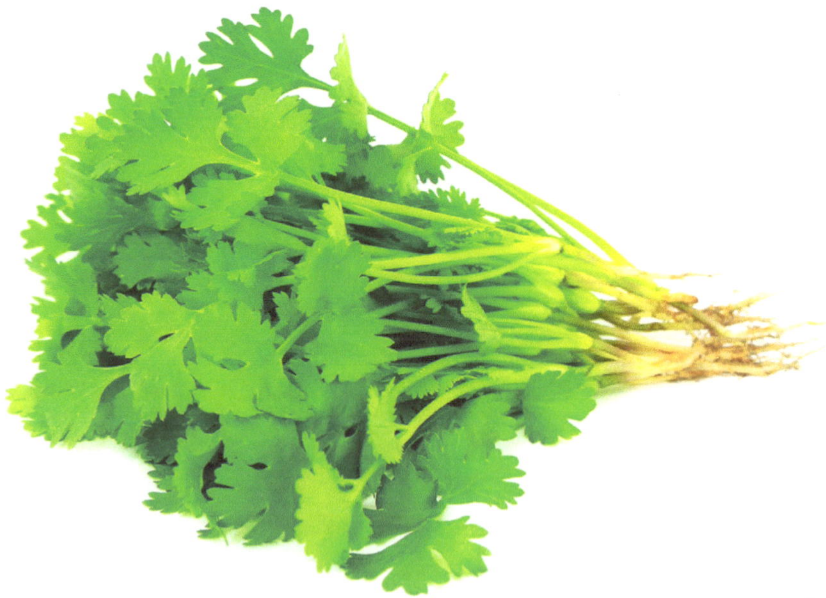

CUBEB PEPPER (PIPER CUBEBA)

Ashanti pepper (uziza, edo pepper, guinea cubeb) (Piper guineense)

BOTANICAL BACKGROUND

- Piper guineense, family Piperaceae; climbing perennial vine.
- Native to West Africa; produces small, wrinkled, dark green to black berries.
- Leaves are aromatic; fruits are dried and used as spice.
- Known as Ashanti pepper, uziza, edo pepper, or Guinea cubeb.

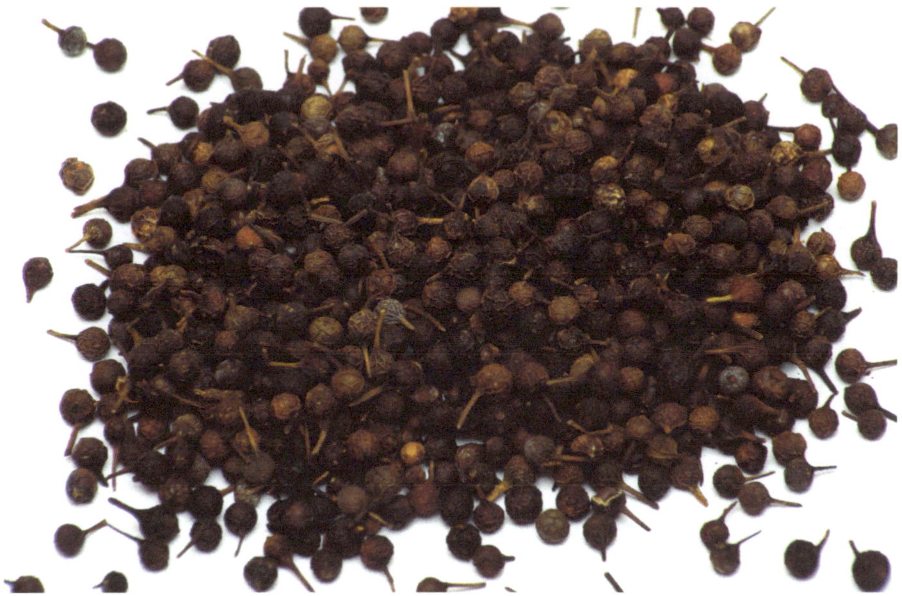

COMMON CULINARY APPLICATIONS

- Adds pungent, slightly bitter, and peppery flavor to soups and stews.
- Used in traditional West African dishes, especially vegetable and meat soups.
- Leaves sometimes used fresh for seasoning.

TYPES / VARIETIES

- Whole dried berries – used ground or whole in cooking.
- Ground spice – powdered for convenience in soups and sauces.
- Fresh leaves – aromatic, used in local soups and sauces.

CULINARY USES

- Seasoning for soups, stews, and sauces.
- Ground or crushed into spice blends for meats, fish, and vegetables.
- Leaves used fresh in traditional soups for aroma and flavor.

HEALTH BENEFITS

- Contains antioxidants; may support immunity and reduce oxidative stress.
- Traditionally used to aid digestion and relieve gastrointestinal discomfort.
- Exhibits antimicrobial and anti-inflammatory properties.
- May help regulate blood pressure and support respiratory health.

CUMIN (CUMINUM CYMINUM)

BOTANICAL BACKGROUND

- Cumin is a slender annual herb native to the eastern Mediterranean and parts of Egypt.
- The plant reaches 30-50 cm tall, with small white or pink flowers.
- Seeds are elongated, brownish, and emit a warm, earthy, and slightly bitter aroma.

COMMON CULINARY APPLICATIONS

- Cumin is a foundational spice in Middle Eastern, Indian, Mexican, and North African cuisines.
- Used extensively in curry powders, chili blends, and spice rubs.

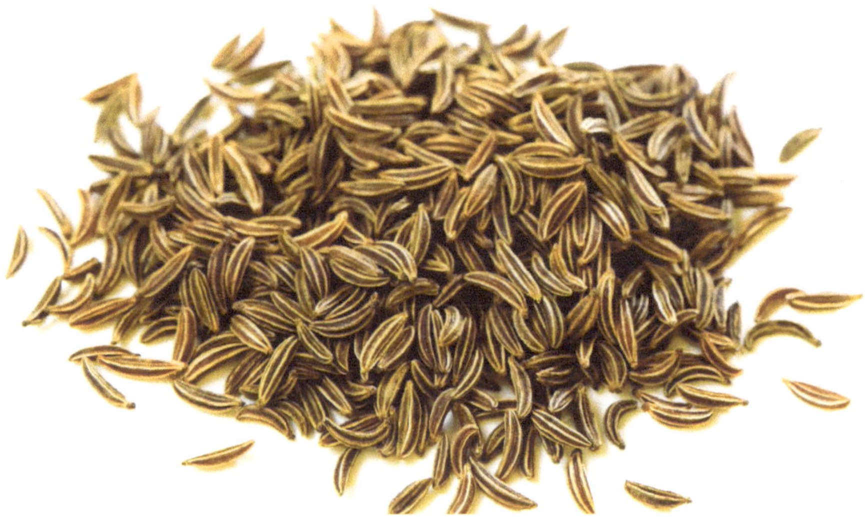

TYPES / VARIETIES

- Several cultivars exist, differing in seed size, color, and essential oil content.
- White and black cumin are different species, with distinct flavors.

CULINARY USES

- Seeds are often dry roasted to intensify flavor before grinding.
- Integral in soups, stews, meat dishes, rice, and vegetable preparations.
- Key spice in blends like ras el hanout, baharat, and garam masala.

HEALTH BENEFITS

- Stimulates digestion and reduces bloating.
- Antioxidant and antimicrobial effects promote overall health.
- Some evidence suggests immune system and blood sugar regulation support.

CULINARY USES

- Enhances soups, stews, and lentil dishes.

"Cumin awakens the digestive fire and nourishes the body's vitality." — **Dr. Sara Malik**

CURRY LEAF (MURRAYA KOENIGII)

BOTANICAL BACKGROUND

- Evergreen shrub/tree, family Rutaceae.
- Native to India and Sri Lanka; cultivated in tropical regions.
- Grows 4–6 m tall; pinnate, aromatic leaves.
- Small white flowers;produces black berries with seeds.
- Valued for culinary and traditional medicinal uses.

COMMON CULINARY APPLICATIONS

- Used fresh or lightly sautéed in Indian and Sri Lankan cooking.
- Flavoring for curries, dals, chutneys, soups, and rice dishes.
- Tempered in oil with mustard seeds, garlic, or chili for aroma.
- Enhances soups, stews, and vegetable dishes.
- Adds aromatic, slightly citrusy, and savory flavor.

TYPES / VARIETIES

- Murraya koenigii var. koenigii – common culinary type.
- Murraya koenigii var. zeylanica – Sri Lankan variety, stronger aroma.
- Dwarf cultivars – suitable for pots and home gardens; culinary use.
- Hybrid selections – selected for leaf size and aroma.

CULINARY

- fresh or fried leaves in curries, soups, chutneys, rice, and spice blends.
- Used in pickling cucumbers, carrots, and other vegetables.
- Sprinkled on bread, salads, and roasted vegetables.

HEALTH BENEFITS

- Rich in antioxidants and essential oils.
- Supports digestion; relieves bloating and gas.
- May have antimicrobial and anti-inflammatory properties.
- Traditionally used for respiratory issues and menstrual discomfort.
- rich in antioxidants, vitamins A, C, and minerals; aids digestion; supports liver and heart health; may have anti-diabetic and anti-inflammatory properties; traditionally used for hair and skin care.

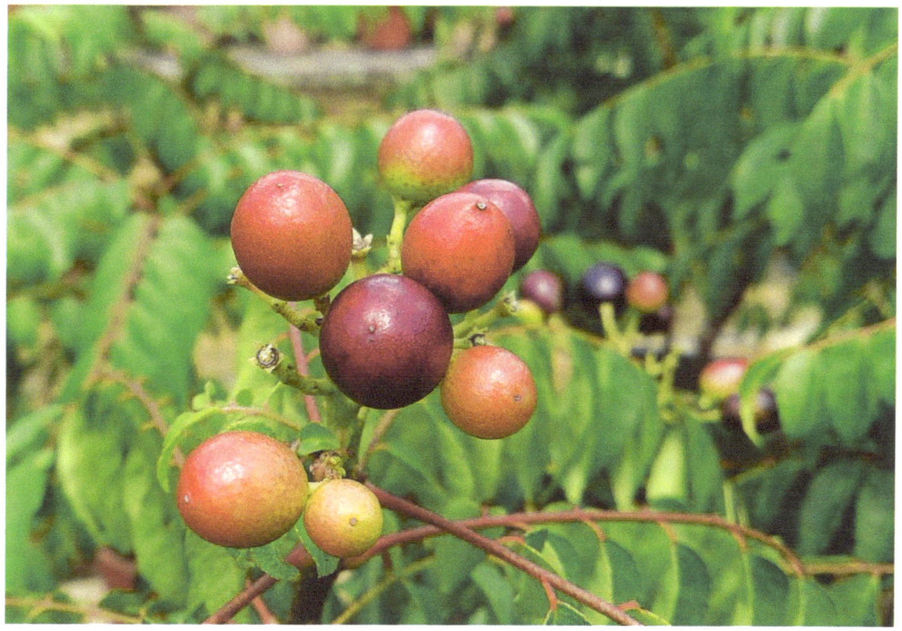

DILL SEED (ANETHUM GRAVEOLENS)

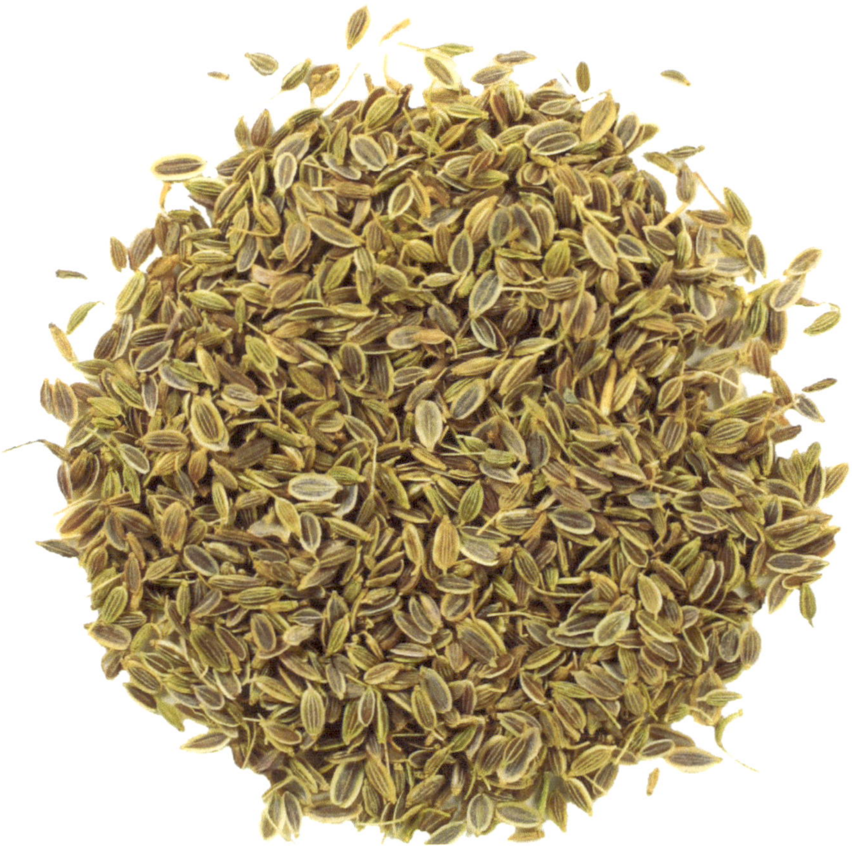

BOTANICAL BACKGROUND

- Seeds of Anethum graveolens, family Apiaceae.
- Native to the Mediterranean and West Asia; cultivated worldwide.
- Annual herb with feathery leaves and yellow umbrella-shaped flowers.
- Seeds are small, oval, brownish, aromatic, and harvested from umbels.

COMMON CULINARY APPLICATIONS

- Flavoring in soups, stews, pickles, and sauces.
- Added to bread, pastries, and vegetable dishes.
- Used in spice blends and for seasoning fish and poultry.

TYPES / VARIETIES

- Common Dill – standard culinary variety with mild aroma.
- Bouquet Dill – primarily grown for fresh leaves; seeds also usable.
- Fernleaf Dill – ornamental and culinary; delicate flavor.

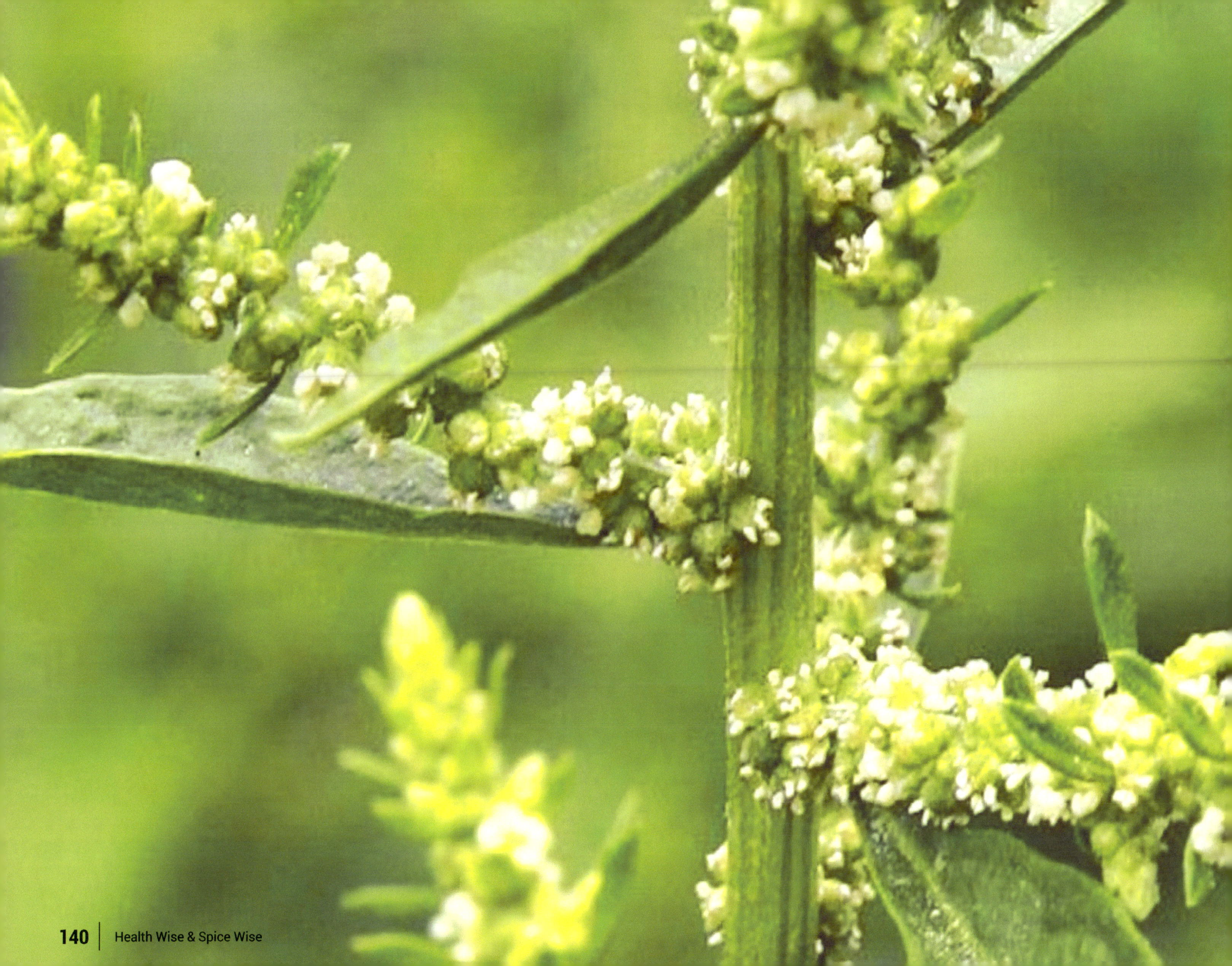

EPAZOTE (CHENOPODIUM AMBROSIOIDES)

Epazote (Dysphania ambrosioides), also known as Mexican tea, wormseed, or goosefoot, is a distinctive herb that plays a crucial role in traditional Mexican cuisine. This pungent leafy herb has become synonymous with authentic Mexican cooking, particularly for its unique pairing with bean dishes.

BOTANICAL BACKGROUND AND CHARACTERISTICS

Epazote is an annual herb native to Central and South America. The name comes from the Nahuatl language, combining Aztec words meaning "skunk" and "sweat," which aptly describes its distinctive aroma. The herb has a petroleum-like, pungent odor that might initially seem off-putting to those unfamiliar with it.

FLAVOR PROFILE

Despite its strong smell, epazote transforms dramatically when cooked. The herb has a complex flavor that's difficult to describe - it's been characterized as gasoline-like, earthy, and intensely aromatic. When heated, these harsh notes mellow into something uniquely savory that enhances rather than overwhelms dishes.

PRIMARY CULINARY USES

Bean Dishes - Epazote's most famous application is in bean cookery, where it serves a dual purpose. Beyond adding its distinctive flavor, epazote contains compounds that help break down proteins in beans that typically cause intestinal gas. This makes it not just a flavoring agent but a digestive aid, which is why it's considered essential in traditional pot beans (frijoles de olla).

COOKING METHODS AND TIMING

Epazote is a delicate herb that should be added near the end of cooking to preserve its flavor and aromatic properties. Overcooking can cause the herb to become bitter and lose its distinctive characteristics. Fresh epazote is preferred when available, though dried versions can be substituted.

AVAILABILITY AND FORMS

Epazote is available both fresh and dried. Fresh epazote offers the most vibrant flavor and is preferred for most applications. The dried form works well in longer-cooking dishes where the herb will have time to rehydrate and release its flavors.

CULTURAL SIGNIFICANCE

In Mexican cuisine, epazote represents more than just an ingredient - it's a cultural marker of authenticity. Many traditional cooks consider dishes like black beans incomplete without epazote, and its presence often distinguishes home-style Mexican cooking from restaurant adaptations.

SUBSTITUTION CONSIDERATIONS

There is no direct substitute for epazote's unique combination of flavor and functional properties. While some cooks might suggest oregano or other herbs as alternatives, none can replicate epazote's distinctive taste or its gas-reducing properties in bean dishes.

FENNEL (FOENICULUM VULGARE)

Has many properties, including antioxidant, anti-inflammatory, and digestive health benefits. Fennel is also a good source of nutrients like potassium, calcium, magnesium, and iron.

ANTIOXIDANT PROPERTIES

- Fennel contains antioxidants like chlorogenic acid, quercetin, Rosmarinic acid, and apigenin.
- Antioxidants can help reduce the risk of chronic diseases like cancer and heart disease.

ANTI-INFLAMMATORY PROPERTIES

- Fennel has anti-inflammatory properties.
- Fennel can help relieve bloating, stomachache, colic, and flatulence.

DIGESTIVE HEALTH BENEFITS

- Fennel can help with digestive disorders like bloating, stomach ache, colic, and flatulence.
- Fennel tea can help with heartburn, loss of appetite, and colic in infants.

OTHER PROPERTIES

- Fennel has antispasmodic properties.
- Fennel has diuretic properties.
- Fennel has expectorant and antitussive properties.
- Fennel has galactogogue properties, which can increase breast milk production.
- Fennel has carminative properties, which can help reduce infant colic.

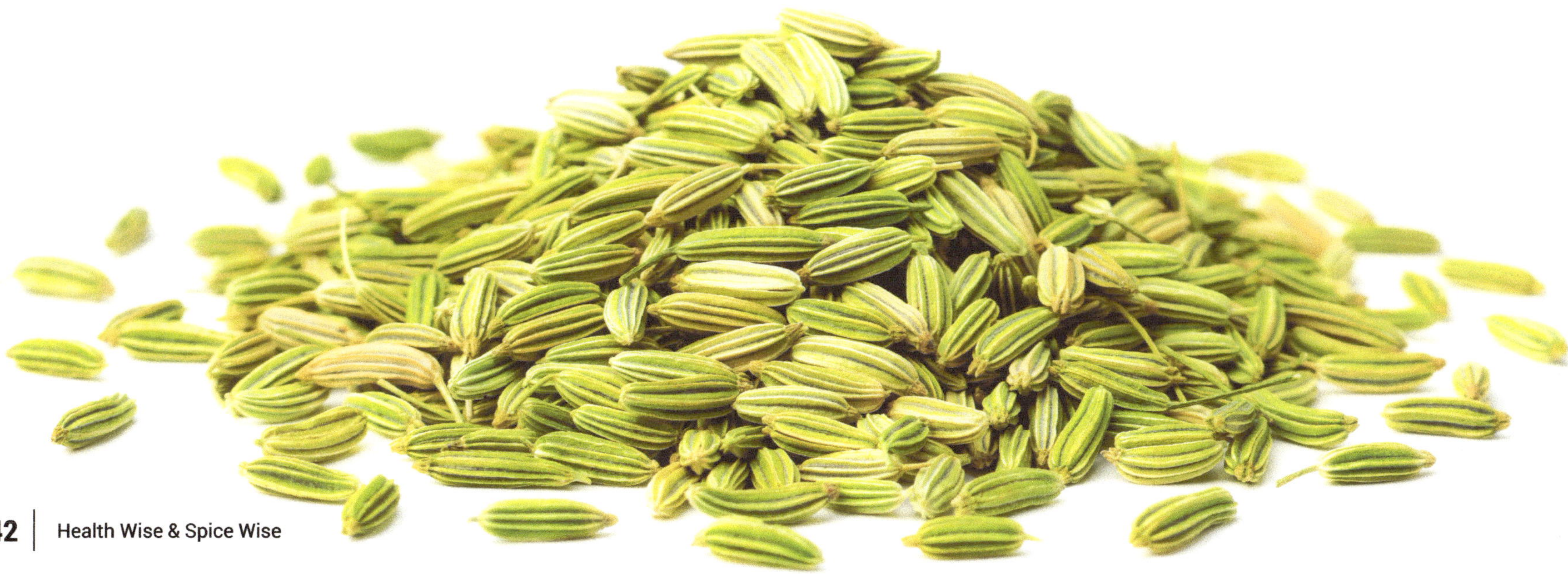

FENUGREEK (TRIGONELLA FOENUM-GRAECUM)

TRIGONELLAFOENUM-GRAECUM

Fenugreek is a legume with many health benefits. It has antioxidant, anti-inflammatory, and anti-diabetic properties. Fenugreek is also used as a spice and in food products.

HEALTH BENEFITS

- Anti-diabetic: Fenugreek can help improve blood sugar control and diabetes.
- Anti-inflammatory: Fenugreek can help reduce inflammation.
- Antioxidant: Fenugreek can help reduce oxidative stress.
- Anti-carcinogenic: Fenugreek may have anti-cancer properties.
- Anti-cholesterolemic: Fenugreek can help lower cholesterol levels.
- Antimicrobial: Fenugreek can help fight bacteria and fungi.
- Hepatoprotective: Fenugreek can help protect the liver.
- Galactogogue: Fenugreek can help increase breast milk production.

OTHER USES

- Fenugreek is used as a flavor enhancer in many cuisines.
- Fenugreek is used as a food stabilizer, adhesive, and emulsifying agent.
- Fenugreek is used in the development of healthy baked goods and extruded products.

TOXICITY

Some studies have shown that fenugreek can have serious toxicological side effects, including anti-fertility and abortifacient effects.

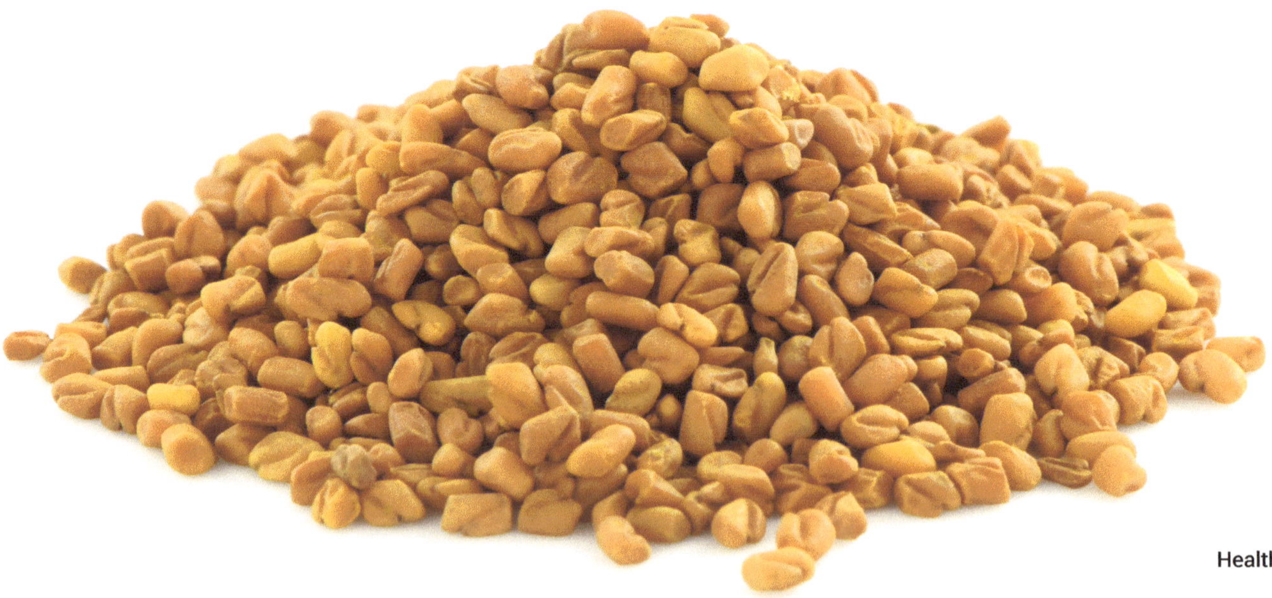

FILÈ (SASSAFRAS) (SASSAFRAS ALBIDUM)

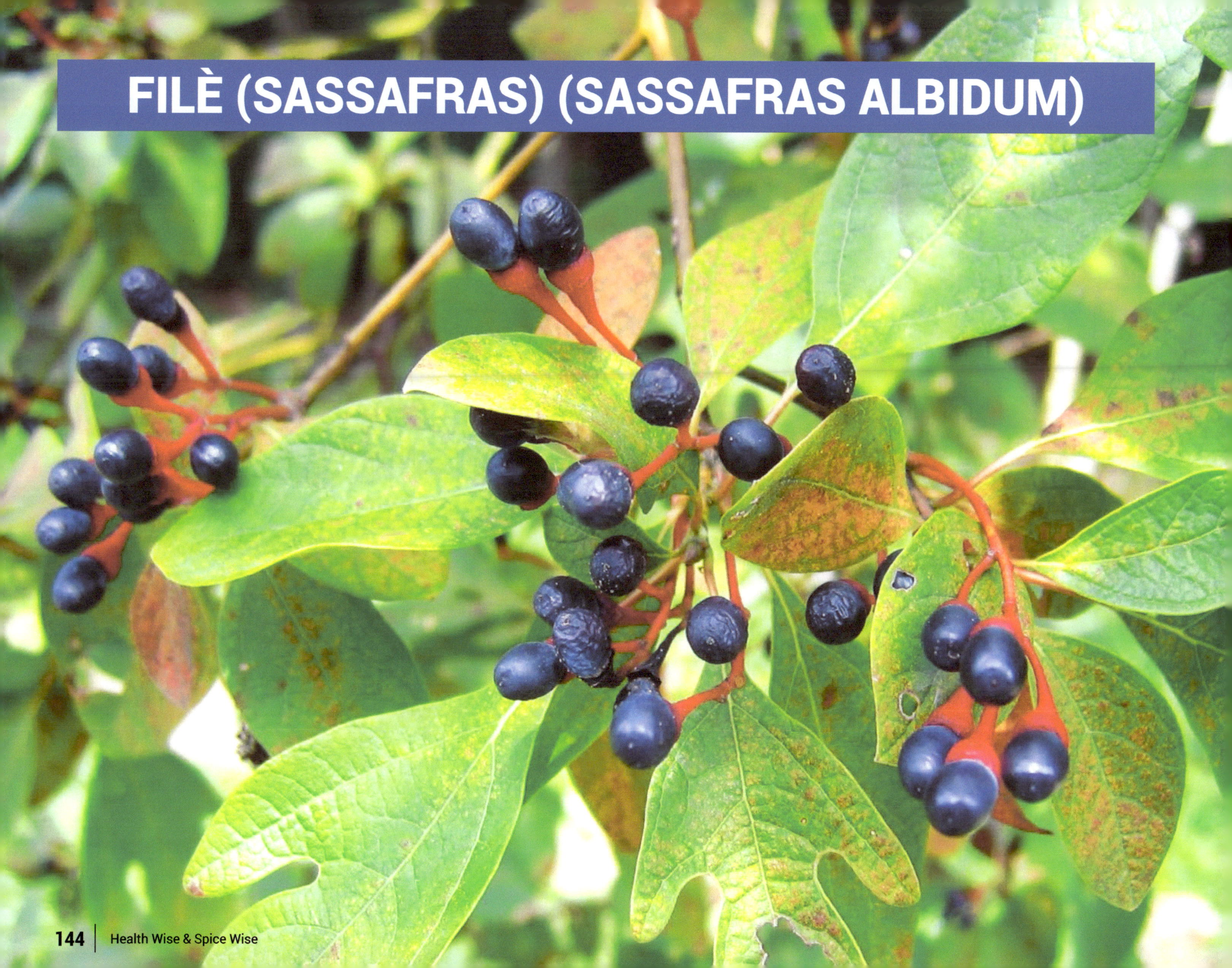

CULINARY USES

- Filé Powder (the most important modern use): The dried and ground leaves of sassafras, known as filé powder, are a key ingredient in Creole and Cajun cooking, especially in gumbo. The powder adds a unique flavor and thickening quality that elevates these traditional dishes.
- The leaves, which are used to make filé powder, contain significantly lower amounts of safrole and are generally considered safe for consumption. Filé powder continues to be a popular ingredient in culinary applications.
- Root Beer & Teas: This tree and its composite parts have been used in foods ranging from root beer and salads to sassafras root tea and flavoring agents in Creole cuisine.
- The dried root bark, steeped to a tea that was served with milk and sugar, made a popular drink called "saloop," offered at almost every street corner in England up through the early 1900s (per Mother Earth News)
- Modern Safe Use: Today, safrole-free sassafras teas are a way to enjoy its aromatic qualities without health concerns. For culinary enthusiasts, filé powder made from dried leaves is an excellent addition to soups and stews, offering a unique flavor and texture. (Ref: LongLifeNutri)

TRADITIONAL HEALTH BENEFITS

- Sassafras has been used medicinally in many ways, including to strengthen immunity, prevent cancer, detoxify the body, relieve pain, increase energy, alleviate inflammation, treat kidney ailments, purify the blood, and treat malaria, scurvy, rheumatoid arthritis, gonorrhea, herpes, shingles, and measles. (Ref: Herbsociety)

OTHER NOTED TRADITIONAL USES INCLUDE:

- Rheumatism and gout relief – a trusted remedy for thousands of years in various parts of the world. Inflammation affects the body in many ways, which means this impressive plant can also help improve gastrointestinal processes and the symptoms of arthritis, as well as headaches. (Ref: Organic Facts)
- Topical skin applications – applying a poultice of sassafras leaves to affected areas can reduce inflammation or discoloration from boils, sores, and rashes. The presence of tannic acid and a unique compound called Sassafridis believed to provide these benefits. (Ref: Organic Facts)
- Native Americans used infusions made from its root bark as a remedy to treat fevers, diarrhea, and rheumatism. (Ref: Memorial Sloan Kettering Cancer Center)

IMPORTANT SAFETY WARNING

- Sassafras contains safrole, a volatile oil which has been classified as a likely carcinogen to humans, and has been banned as a food additive by the FDA. It caused liver cancer in laboratory animals, and the risk of developing cancer increases with the amount consumed and duration of consumption. (Ref: Memorial Sloan Kettering Cancer Center)
- One cup of tea made with 2.5 grams of sassafras contains about 200 mg of safrole – approximately 4.5 times the dose that researchers think is poisonous. So in 1976, the US FDA ruled that sassafras could no longer be sold as sassafras tea. (Ref: WebMD)

FINGERROOT (BOESENBERGIA PANDURATA)

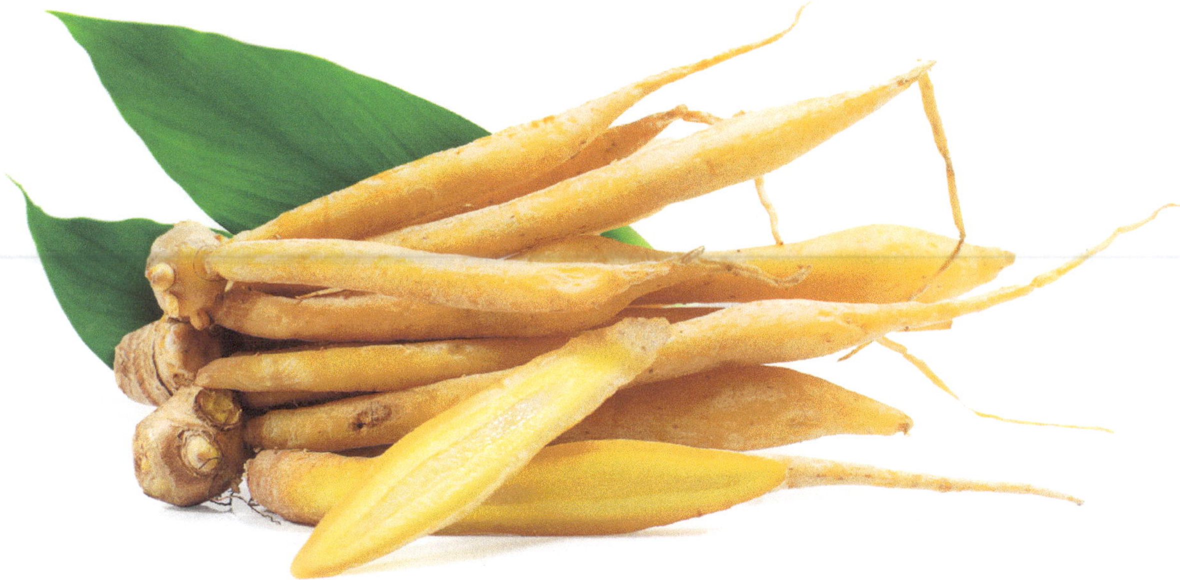

Also known by its Thai name krachai, Chinese keys, Chinese ginger, or lesser galangal, is a distinctive culinary and medicinal herb belonging to the ginger family (Zingiberaceae). Native to Southeast Asia, particularly from southern Yunnan Province in China to west Malaysia, this unique rhizome has earned its common name from its characteristic finger-like appearance.

BOTANICAL CHARACTERISTICS AND NAMES

The plant gets its English name "fingerroot" because the rhizome resembles fingers growing from a central piece. In various Southeast Asian cultures, it's known by different names: krachai in Thai, temu kunci in Indonesian (where "kunci" means "key," referring to the shape), and k'jeay in Khmer. The alternative name "Chinese keys" is commonly used in Singapore.

PHYSICAL DESCRIPTION

Fingerroot produces broad, light green leaves that grow upright, averaging 7 to 12 centimeters in width and 25 to 50 centimeters in length. The underground rhizome develops the characteristic finger-like projections that give the plant its distinctive appearance and name.

FLAVOR PROFILE

Fingerroot has a complex flavor that distinguishes it from other members of the ginger family. It's described as milder and sweeter than regular ginger, with a subtle peppery quality and earthy undertones. The taste is less sharp than ginger but more aromatic than galangal, offering a unique middle ground between these related spices.

PRIMARY CULINARY USES

- **Thai Cuisine** - Fingerroot is most prominently used in Thai cooking, where it's considered an essential ingredient. It appears in various traditional dishes including:
- **Fish Curries** - Particularly valuable in fish-based curry preparations where it complements the seafood without overwhelming delicate flavors

- **Jungle Curry** - A spicy northern Thai curry that doesn't contain coconut milk, where krachai adds depth and complexity
- **Kanom Jeen Nam Ya** - A famous southern Thai dish featuring fermented rice noodles with a spiced fish curry sauce
- **Hot and Spicy Spaghetti** - A Thai-Western fusion dish combining krachai with holy basil and chilies over pasta
- **Fish Soups** - Often paired with kaffir lime leaves to create aromatic broths.

SOUTHEAST ASIAN APPLICATIONS

- **Beyond Thai cuisine, fingerroot appears in** - Indonesian Cooking: Used as a spice and in the production of tempeh (fermented soybean cake)
- Vietnamese Cuisine: Occasionally found in markets but less commonly used than in Thai cooking
- **Malaysian Dishes** - Used in various traditional preparations Cooking Methods and Techniques
- **Fingerroot can be used in multiple ways** - Fresh rhizomes sliced or chopped for curries and stir-fries
- Young rhizomes eaten raw as vegetables
- Dried and ground into powder for seasoning
- Added to soups and broths for aromatic depth
- Used in vegetable stews and main dishes

COMPLEMENTARY INGREDIENTS

Fingerroot pairs exceptionally well with:

- Garlic and chili peppers
- Lemongrass and galangal
- Kaffir lime leaves
- Fish sauce and coconut milk
- Holy basil and other Thai herbs

AVAILABILITY AND FORMS

In Western countries, fingerroot is typically found pickled or frozen in Asian markets, as fresh fingerroot has a limited shelf life and doesn't travel well. It's available in several forms:

- Fresh rhizomes (when available in specialty Asian markets)
- Frozen fingerroot pieces
- Pickled fingerroot
- Dried fingerroot powder
- Live plants for home cultivation

MEDICINAL PROPERTIES

Beyond its culinary uses, fingerroot has been used traditionally in herbal medicine. Research has shown it contains beneficial compounds including alkaloids, essential oils, flavonoids, and phenolics. It's particularly rich in boesenbergin and has demonstrated anti-allergic, antibacterial, anticancer, anti-inflammatory, antioxidant, and antiulcer activities.

STORAGE AND HANDLING

Fresh fingerroot should be stored in the refrigerator and used relatively quickly due to its perishable nature. Frozen fingerroot can be used directly in cooking without thawing. The dried powder form has a much longer shelf life and provides convenience for regular use.

Fingerroot represents one of those uniquely Southeast Asian ingredients that adds an irreplaceable dimension to traditional dishes, particularly in Thai cuisine where it's considered indispensable for achieving authentic flavors in many regional specialties.

GARDEN CRESS (LEPIDIUM SATIVUM)

Has many properties, including nutritional value, medicinal properties, and use in cooking.

NUTRITIONAL VALUE

- **Seeds :** Contain protein, essential fatty acids, and minerals like calcium, iron, potassium, and phosphorus
- **Leaves :** Contain minerals like calcium, iron, magnesium, and zinc
- **Raw :** Contains vitamins A, C, and K, as well as dietary minerals

MEDICINAL PROPERTIES

- **Anti-inflammatory :** Contains bioactive compounds like gallic acid, caffeic acid, and protocatechuic acid
- **Antioxidant :** Contains bioactive compounds like gallic acid, caffeic acid, and protocatechuic acid
- **Anti-hypertensive :** Contains bioactive compounds like gallic acid, caffeic acid, and protocatechuic acid
- **Anti-diabetic :** Contains bioactive compounds and fiber that can help reduce blood sugar levels
- **Laxative :** Can help treat constipation
- **Anti-anemic :** Contains calcium and can help boost hemoglobin levels
- **Hepatoprotective :** Can help protect the liver
- **Immunomodulatory :** Can help strengthen the immune system

OTHER PROPERTIES

- Can help with hormonal balance and menstrual cycles
- Can help with bone strength
- Can help with milk production in breastfeeding mothers

Garden cress has been used for medicinal and culinary purposes for centuries.

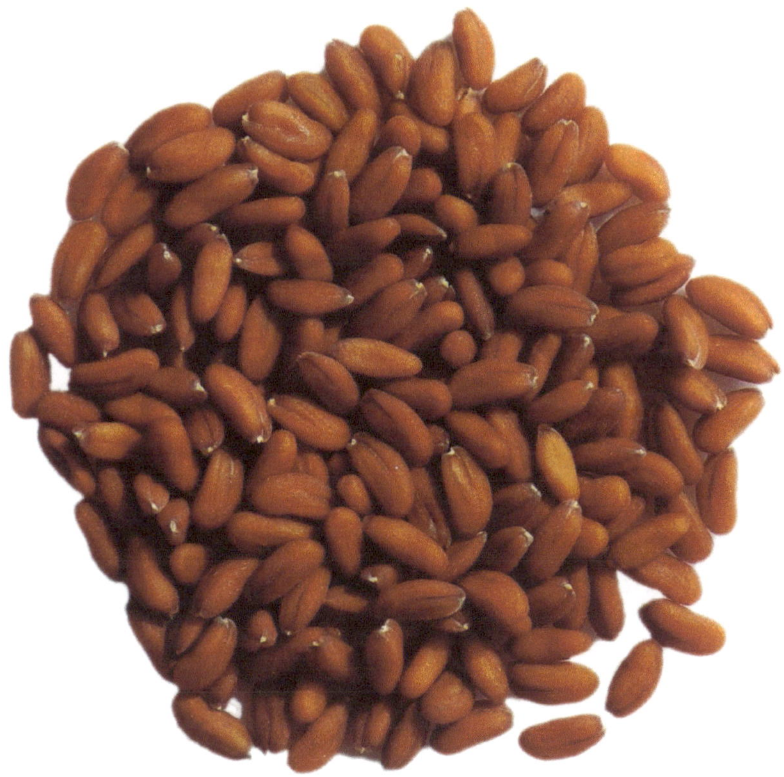

GARLIC (ALLIUM SATIVUM)

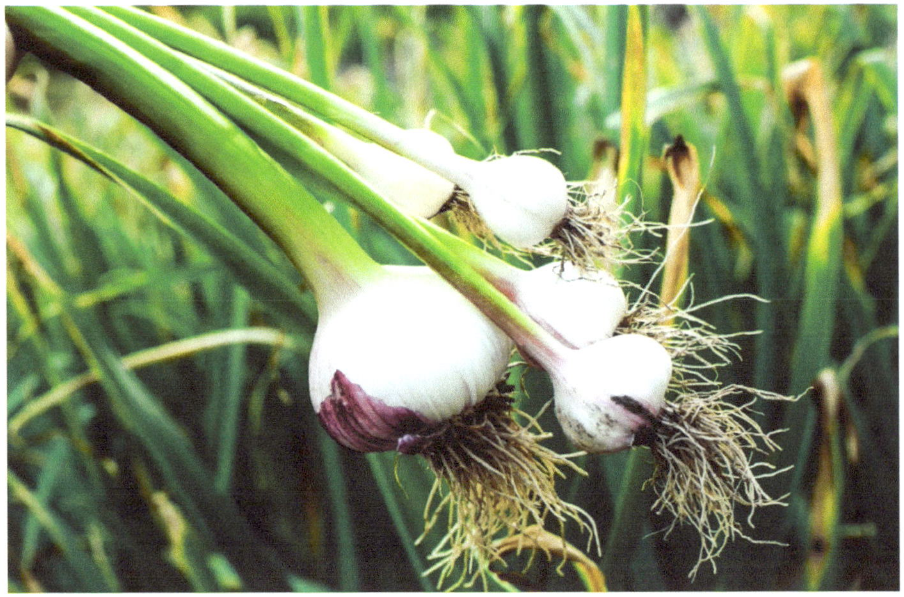

BOTANICAL BACKGROUND

- Bulbous perennial, family Amaryllidaceae.
- Native to Central Asia; widely cultivated.
- Bulbs with cloves; flat leaves; umbels of flowers.
- Pungent aroma from allicin.

COMMON CULINARY APPLICATIONS

- Used raw, sautéed, roasted, or fried.
- Added to sauces, soups, stews, stir-fries, curries, meats, seafood.
- Used in pickles, dips, dressings.

TYPES / VARIETIES

- Softneck – mild, long storage.
- Hardneck – strong, with flower stalks.
- Elephant Garlic – mild, large cloves.
- Purple Stripe/Rocambole – aromatic.

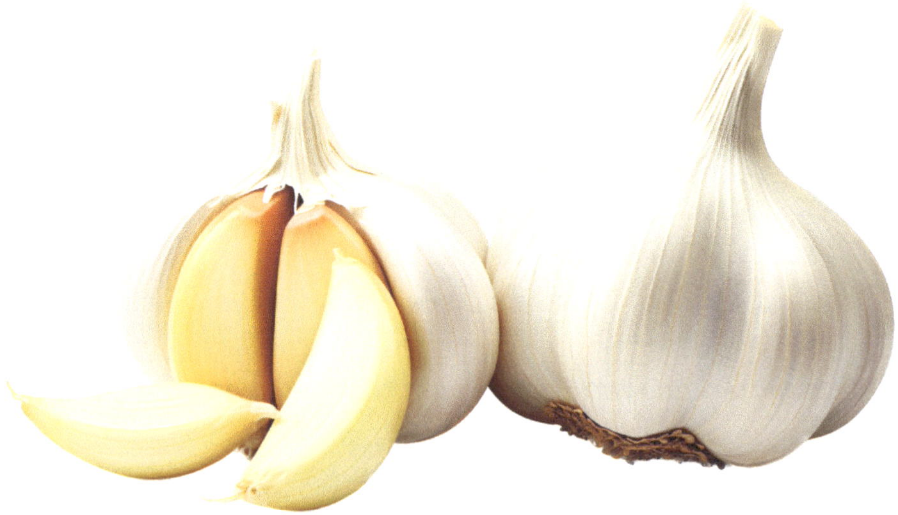

CULINARY USES

- Enhances savory dishes and spice blends.
- Roasted or sautéed for mellow taste.
- Minced/crushed for marinades, sauces, dips.

HEALTH BENEFITS

- Rich in antioxidants; supports immunity.
- Allicin may reduce blood pressure, cholesterol.
- Antimicrobial and anti-inflammatory.

GINGER (ZINGIGER OFFICINALE)

Ginger (Zingiber officinale) is a widely used spice known for its distinct flavor and numerous health benefits. Here are some of its key properties and health benefits:

NUTRITIONAL CONTENT

- **Gingerol :** The primary active compound responsible for its pungent flavor and medicinal properties.
- **Vitamins and Minerals :** Contains vitamins B3 and B6, as well as minerals like magnesium, potassium, copper, and manganese.
- **Antioxidants :** High in antioxidants, which help protect cells from oxidative stress and damage.

HEALTH BENEFITS

- **Digestive Health :** Aids in digestion, alleviates nausea, and reduces symptoms of indigestion and bloating.
- **Anti-inflammatory :** Reduces inflammation and can help alleviate conditions like arthritis and muscle pain.
- **Pain Relief :** Known for its analgesic properties, providing relief from headaches, menstrual pain, and joint pain.
- **Immune System Boost :** Strengthens the immune system and helps fight off infections.
- **Anti-nausea :** Effective in reducing nausea, including motion sickness, morning sickness, and chemotherapy-induced nausea.
- **Cardiovascular Health :** Supports heart health by reducing blood pressure, improving circulation, and lowering cholesterol levels.
- **Antimicrobial Properties :** Has antibacterial and antiviral properties that help fight infections.
- **Weight Management :** Enhances metabolism and promotes fat burning, aiding in weight management.

USAGE

- **Culinary Uses :** Ginger is used to flavor a wide variety of dishes, including stir-fries, soups, sauces, and desserts. It can be used fresh, dried, powdered, or as an oil or juice.
- **Medicinal Uses :** Consumed as a tea, supplement, or essential oil for its health benefits.
- **Aromatherapy :** Ginger essential oil is used in aromatherapy for its warming and invigorating effects.

Ginger is a versatile spice that not only adds a zesty kick to your meals but also offers numerous health benefits.

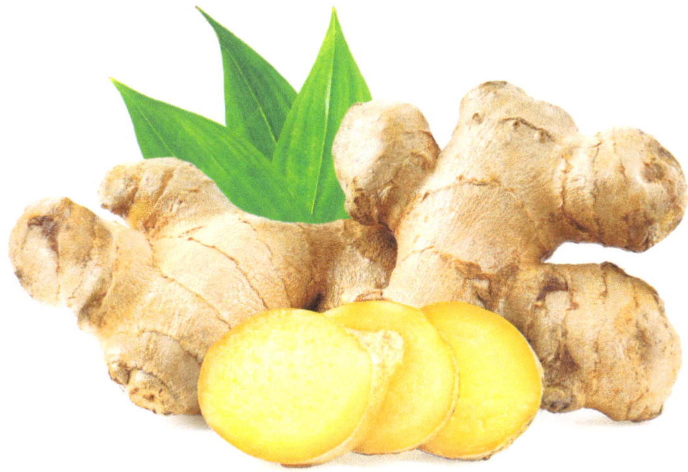

GRAINS OF PARADISE (MELEGUETA PEPPER) (AFRAMOMUM MELEGUETA)

BOTANICAL BACKGROUND

- Aframomum melegueta, family Zingiberaceae; perennial herb native to West Africa.
- Produces small, reddish-brown seeds known as grains of paradise or melegueta pepper.
- Seeds are aromatic, pungent, and slightly citrusy; used as a spice.

COMMON CULINARY APPLICATIONS

- Adds warm, peppery, and citrusy flavor to soups, stews, and sauces.
- Used in West African traditional dishes, seasonings, and spice blends.
- Sometimes used in beverages, pickling, and marinades.

TYPES / VARIETIES

- Whole seeds – dried for grinding when needed.
- Ground spice – convenient for cooking and seasoning.
- Rarely, used in extracted oils for flavoring.

CULINARY USES

- Seasoning for soups, stews, and sauces.
- Ground into spice blends for meats, fish, and vegetables.
- Used in beverages or as a pepper substitute in cooking.

HEALTH BENEFITS

- Rich in antioxidants; supports immune function.
- Traditionally used to aid digestion and relieve bloating.
- Exhibits antimicrobial and anti-inflammatory properties.
- May help stimulate appetite and enhance metabolism.

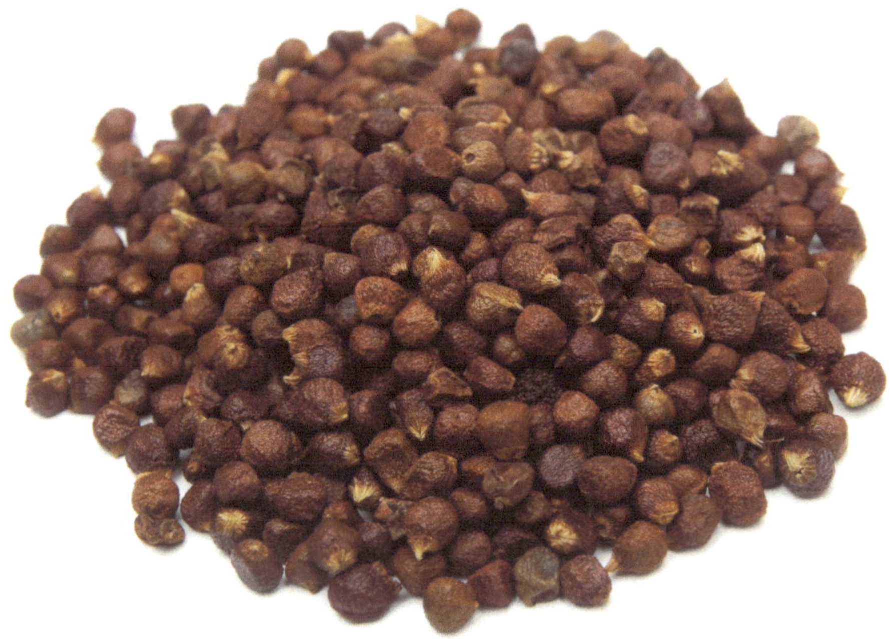

GREATER GALANGA (ALPINIA GALANGA)

Greater galangal (Alpinia galanga), also known as Thai ginger or simply galangal, is an aromatic rhizome closely related to ginger and turmeric that plays a fundamental role in Southeast Asian cuisine. Native to Java and South and Southeast Asia, this distinctive spice has been cultivated and traded for centuries.

NAMES AND REGIONAL VARIATIONS

Greater galangal is known by various names across different cultures. In Thai, it's called kha, in Javanese it's laos, and in Sundanese it's laja. Other regional names include romdeng in Cambodia, pa de kaw in Myanmar, nankyō in Japan, and hóng dòu kòu in Mandarin Chinese. In South Asian languages, it's known as pedda dumprashtamu in Telugu and pae-reeya-ra-thai in Tamil.

FLAVOR PROFILE AND CHARACTERISTICS

Greater galangal has a distinctive flavor that differs significantly from its ginger cousin. It's more peppery and earthy than ginger, with a sharp, pine-like aroma and a slightly medicinal quality. The flavor is complex, offering citrusy, spicy, and slightly floral notes with a lingering warmth that doesn't have ginger's heat.

PRIMARY CULINARY USES

SOUTHEAST ASIAN CUISINE

Greater galangal is essential in numerous traditional dishes across Southeast Asia:

Thai Cooking : Galangal is a cornerstone ingredient in Thai cuisine, particularly in curry pastes where it provides depth and complexity. It's indispensable in popular soups like tom yum (hot and sour soup) and tom kha gai (chicken and coconut milk soup).

Indonesian Cuisine : Used extensively in dishes like soto and opor, galangal adds aromatic depth to these traditional preparations.

Cambodian Cooking : An essential component in kroeung, the foundational spice paste used throughout Cambodian cuisine.

Vietnamese Applications : Particularly prominent in Huế cuisine, where it's used in dishes like tré and other regional specialties.

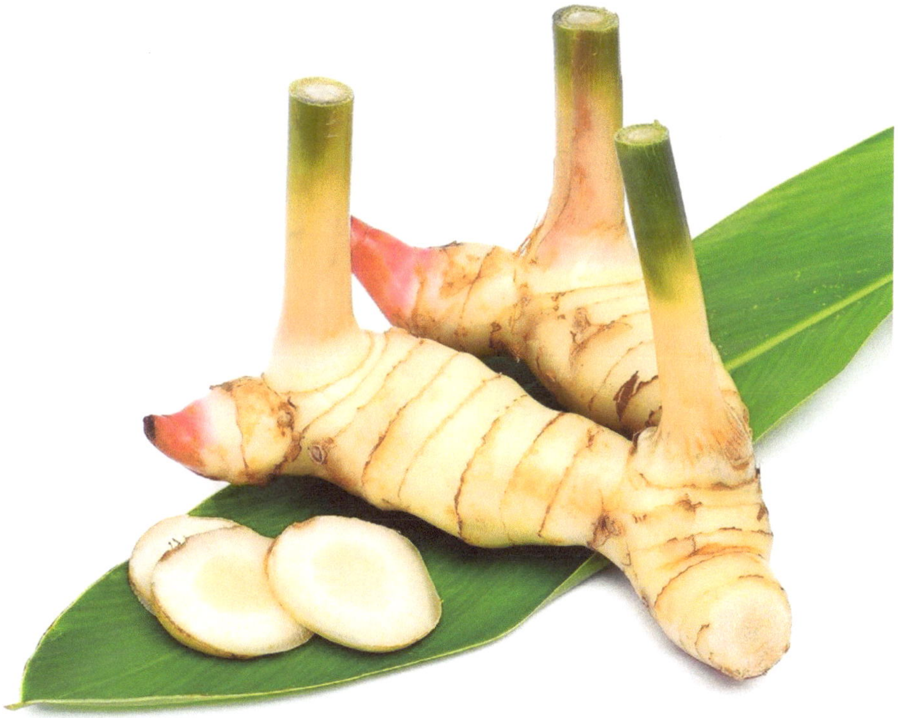

COOKING METHODS AND APPLICATIONS

Greater galangal can be used in several forms and preparation methods:

Fresh Form : Fresh galangal rhizome is preferred when available, offering the most vibrant flavor and aroma. It can be sliced, minced, or pounded into curry pastes.

Dried and Powdered : Dried galangal provides convenience and longer storage life, making it widely available globally.

Young Parts : The sprouts and young flowers are consumed as vegetables or used as spicing agents in various dishes.

Essential Oil : Extracted from the rhizome for flavoring applications in foods and beverages.

COMPLEMENTARY INGREDIENTS AND PAIRINGS

Galangal pairs exceptionally well with:

- Coconut milk in curries and soups
- Lemongrass and kaffir lime leaves
- Chili peppers and garlic
- Fish sauce and tamarind
- Shallots and ginger
- Thai basil and cilantro

COMMERCIAL AND INDUSTRIAL USES

Beyond home cooking, greater galangal serves as a flavoring agent in various commercial applications including sausages, spicy condiments, and herbal teas. It's also used in the development of functional foods and nutraceutical formulations.

PREPARATION AND STORAGE

Fresh galangal should be peeled before use, similar to ginger. It can be grated, sliced thin, or pounded in a mortar and pestle for curry pastes. Fresh rhizomes store well in the refrigerator and can be frozen for longer storage. The dried form requires soaking before use in some applications.

MEDICINAL AND HEALTH APPLICATIONS

Traditionally, greater galangal has been used for various health purposes including:

- Digestive aid and appetite stimulation
- Mouth hygiene and oral health
- Detoxification properties
- Anti-inflammatory applications

The rhizome contains beneficial compounds that have demonstrated potential health benefits in traditional medicine systems.

SUBSTITUTION GUIDELINES

While ginger is sometimes suggested as a substitute, it cannot replicate galangal's unique flavor profile. Lesser galangal (Alpinia officinarum) is closer in taste but still distinct. For authentic Southeast Asian dishes, particularly Thai curries and soups, there's no adequate substitute for greater galangal's distinctive contribution to the flavor profile.

Greater galangal represents one of the most important aromatic ingredients in Southeast Asian cooking, providing irreplaceable depth and complexity that defines the authentic taste of many traditional dishes from the region.

HYSSOP (HYSSOPUS OFFICINALIS)

Hyssop (Hyssopus officinalis) is a small herbaceous plant from the mint family, widely known for its medicinal properties and use in cooking. Here are some notable properties and health benefits:

NUTRITIONAL CONTENT

- **Essential Oils :** Hyssop contains essential oils such as pinocamphone, isopinocamphone, and beta-pinene.
- **Vitamins and Minerals :** Rich in vitamins A and C, and minerals like calcium, iron, and potassium.

HEALTH BENEFITS

- **Respiratory Health :** Hyssop is often used to treat respiratory issues like coughs, colds, and bronchitis due to its expectorant properties.
- **Digestive Aid :** Helps to relieve digestive problems like gas, bloating, and indigestion.
- **Anti-inflammatory :** Known for its ability to reduce inflammation and alleviate pain.
- **Antimicrobial Properties :** Has antiseptic and antimicrobial properties that help in fighting infections.
- **Boosts Immune System :** Strengthens the immune system due to its rich nutrient content.
- **Mental Clarity :** Believed to have mild stimulating effects that improve mental clarity and concentration.
- **Wound Healing :** Topically used for its wound-healing properties, it helps in cleaning and healing cuts and bruises.

USAGE

- **Culinary Uses :** Hyssop leaves and flowers are used to flavor salads, soups, stews, and meat dishes.
- **Medicinal Uses :** Can be consumed as a tea, tincture, or essential oil for its health benefits.
- **Aromatherapy :** Hyssop essential oil is used in aromatherapy for its uplifting and invigorating scent.

Hyssop has been valued for centuries for its wide range of applications in traditional medicine and culinary practices. Have you ever tried using hyssop in your cooking or as a remedy?

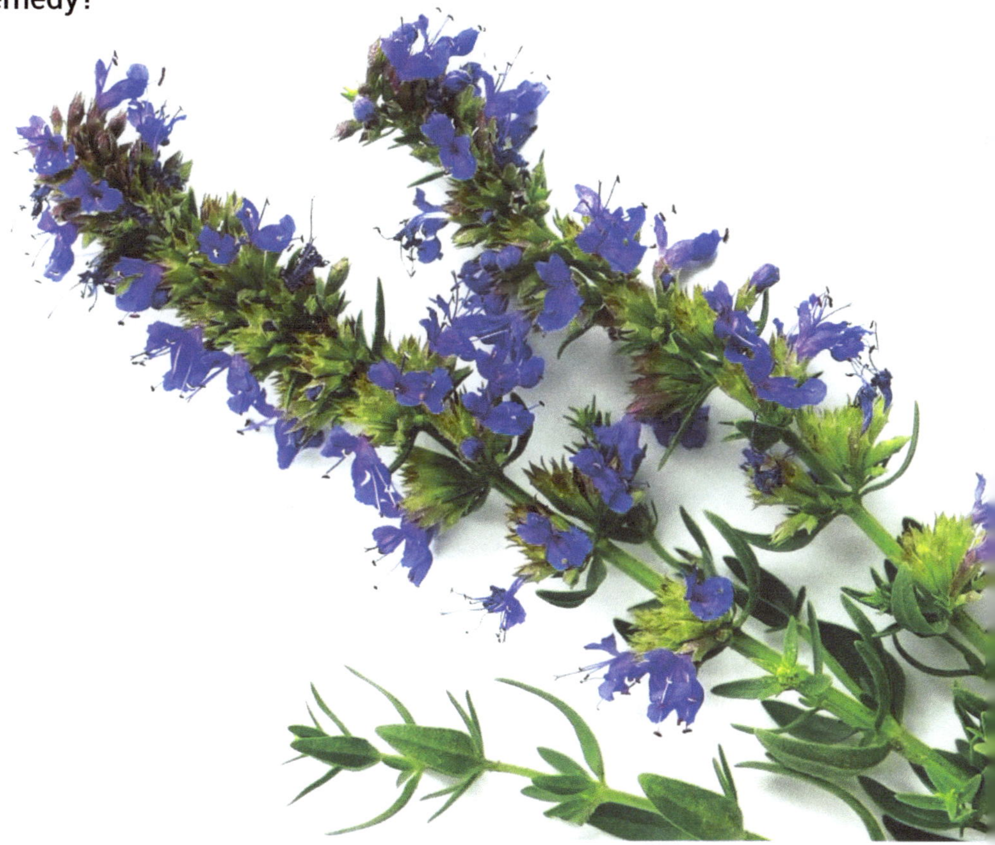

INDIAN BAY LEAF (CINNAMOMUM TAMALA)

BOTANICAL BACKGROUND

- Evergreen tree, family Lauraceae.
- Native to India, Nepal, Bhutan; cultivated in tropical/ subtropical regions.
- Grows 10–15 m tall; aromatic lance-shaped leaves.
- Small greenish-white flowers;produces small dark berries.
- Known as "tej patta"; used in culinary and medicinal traditions.

COMMON CULINARY APPLICATIONS

- Whole leaves in curries, biryanis, dals, and stews.
- Added to rice, soups, and slow-cooked meats for aroma.
- Tempered in oil with spices to release flavor.
- Infused in sauces, pickles, and marinades.
- Provides warm, sweet, cinnamon-like, slightly clove aroma.

TYPES / VARIETIES

- C. tamala var. tamala – most common culinary type.
- C. tamala var. indica – Indian subcontinent variety, aromatic leaves.
- Wild Himalayan types – stronger aroma; used in traditional medicine.
- Cultivated hybrids – larger leaves, higher aromatic oil content.
- Culinary
- Leaves - whole or crushed in curries, rice dishes, stews, sauces, spice blends.

HEALTH BENEFITS

Antioxidants and essential oils; aids digestion, reduces bloating, supports respiratory health; traditional oral hygiene and anti-inflammatory uses; may help regulate blood sugar.

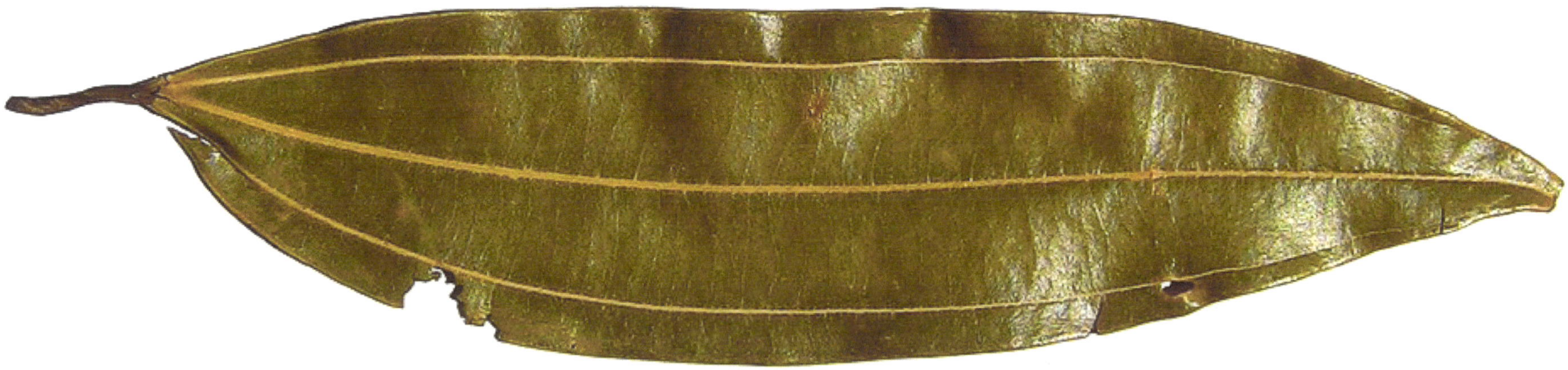

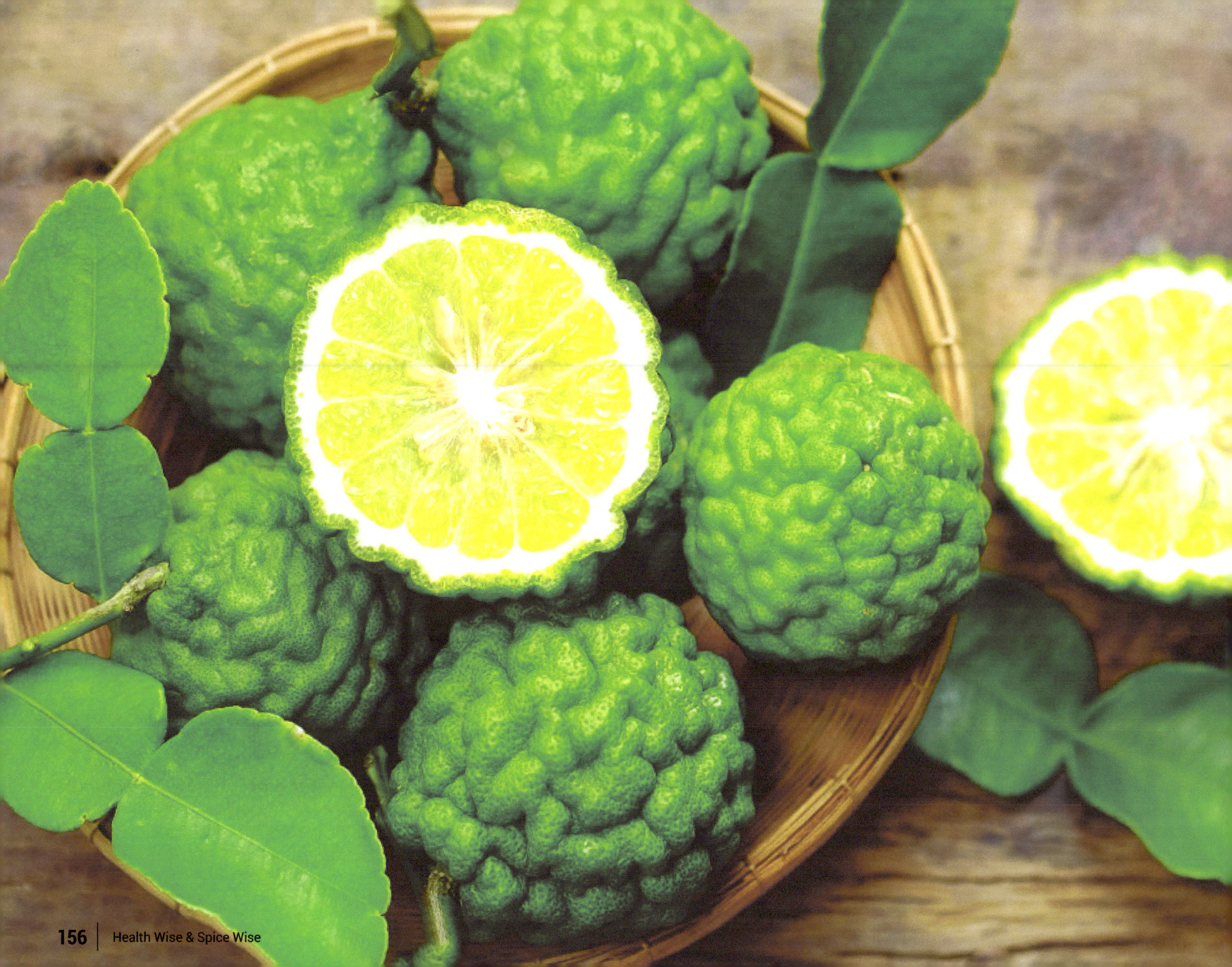

KAFFIR LIME (CITRUS HYSTRIX)

Kaffir lime, (Citrus hystrix), is a distinctive citrus fruit whose leaves are one of the most essential ingredients in Southeast Asian cuisine. This aromatic herb has gained international recognition for its unique culinary properties and intense fragrance.

Botanical Characteristics and Identification

The makrut lime tree produces leaves with a highly distinctive appearance. The leaves have a unique double-leaf hourglass shape that looks like two pointed oval leaves connected at their tips. This characteristic formation makes them easily recognizable and distinguishes them from other citrus leaves.

AROMA AND FLAVOR PROFILE

Makrut lime leaves possess an intensely citrus fragrance that's released when the leaves are crushed or cut. The flavor is more pungent and aromatic than regular lime, with a complex profile that includes bright citrus notes combined with floral and slightly pine-like undertones. Each leaf is very strong in flavor, so only a few are needed to make a significant impact on a dish.

PRIMARY CULINARY USES

THAI CUISINE

Makrut lime leaves are integral to Thai cooking and are considered crucial ingredients in many famous Thai dishes. They're essential in tom yum goong (spicy shrimp soup), tom kha gai (chicken coconut soup), and panang curry. The leaves add a distinctive aromatic quality that's fundamental to authentic Thai flavors.

SOUTHEAST ASIAN APPLICATIONS

Beyond Thai cuisine, the leaves are commonly used in Lao soups, curries, and other Southeast Asian dishes. They're particularly valued in Malaysian and Indonesian cooking for their ability to add depth and complexity to curries and stews.

Cooking Methods and Techniques

Makrut lime leaves can be used in several ways:

Whole Leaves : Most commonly added whole to curries during the later stages of cooking, then removed before serving (similar to bay leaves). They infuse the dish with flavor without being eaten.

Finely Sliced : When cut lengthwise on either side of the tough middle vein and then sliced thinly or chopped finely, the leaves can be added to salads, sambals, stir-fries, and even used to flavor condiments like mayonnaise.

In Pastes and Marinades : The leaves can be blended into curry pastes and marinades to infuse other ingredients with their pungent flavors.

Aromatic Enhancement : Fresh leaves can be bruised or torn to release their intense aroma during cooking.

THE FRUIT VS. THE LEAVES

While the leaves are prized for cooking, the fruit itself has limited culinary use. The juice is very bitter and isn't typically used in cooking. However, the rind emits an intense citrus fragrance and can be used for aromatic purposes. The fruit's bumpy, brain-like appearance makes it easily identifiable.

LAVENDER (LAVANDULA ANGUSTIFOLIA)

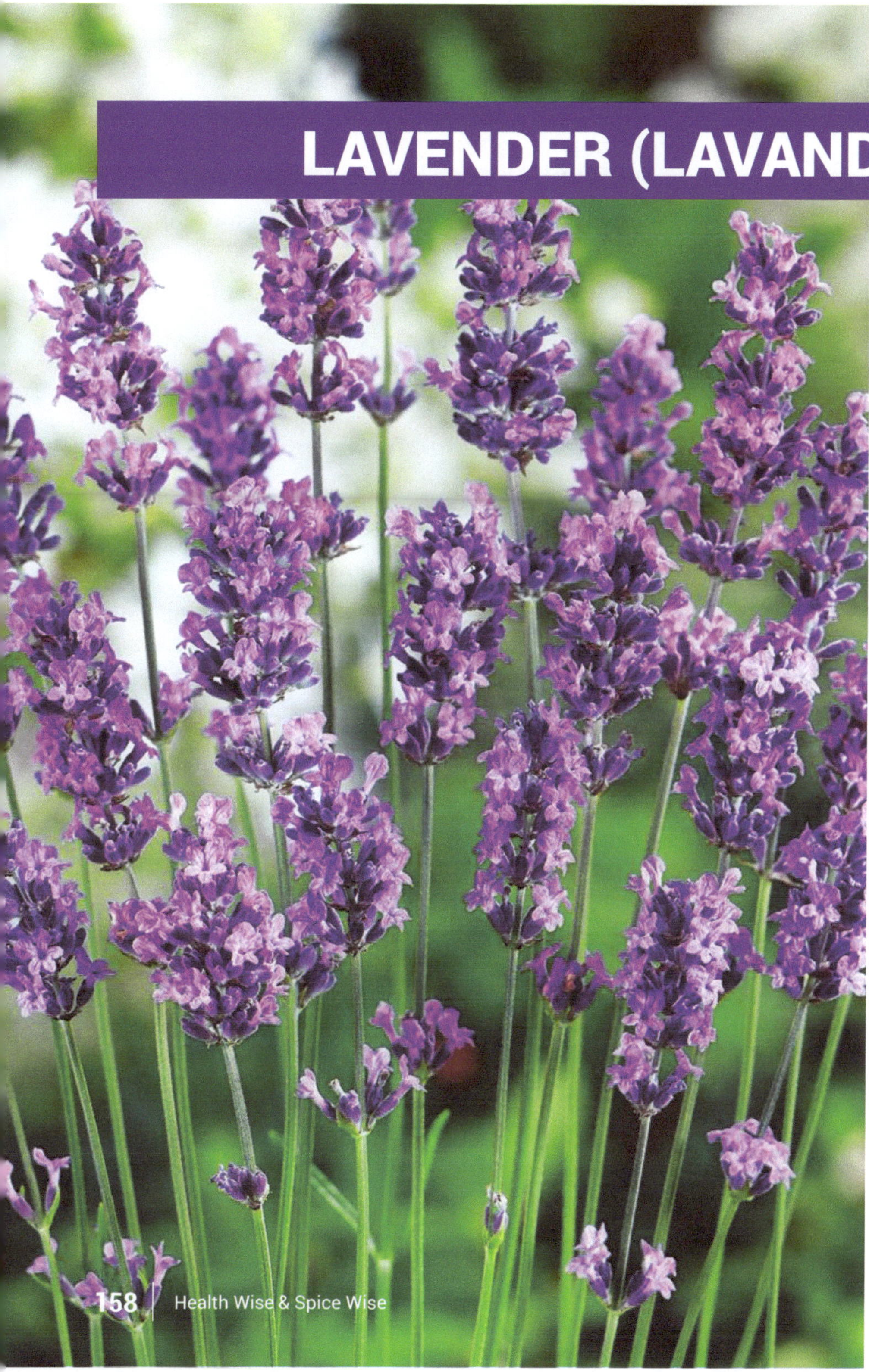

Lavender (Lavandulaangustifolia) is one of the most versatile herbs with applications spanning culinary, medicinal, aromatherapy, and craft uses. This fragrant Mediterranean herb offers numerous benefits and applications beyond its beautiful purple flowers.

CULINARY APPLICATIONS

Flavor Profile and Parts Used

- Lavender has a pungent floral flavor and aroma with subtle notes of herbaceousness, earthiness, and mint. The flower buds, leaves, and stems can be used fresh or dried in dishes ranging from sweet floral desserts to heartier meat dishes. The best time to harvest is when flower stalks are full of buds about to open, as opened flowers become bitter and overly floral.

SWEET APPLICATIONS

Lavender excels in dessert preparations including:

- Baked Goods: Added to cake batter, frosting, cookies, and bread for a unique floral twist
- Desserts: Crème brûlée, ice cream, and custards benefit from lavender's aromatic qualities
- Sugar and Syrups: Lavender-infused sugar (made by burying buds in sugar for a week) and simple syrups for beverages
- Beverages: Teas, lemonades, iced teas, and cocktails

SAVORY APPLICATIONS

Lavender works particularly well in savory dishes where it can:

- Cut through rich and fatty foods, lifting overall flavor
- Enhance lamb dishes with its aromatic qualities
- Be included in herb blends with rosemary, oregano, thyme, and sage for meat rubs
- Add depth to marinades and sauces for roasted vegetables
- Enhance pizza dough with 1-2 teaspoons per recipe

USAGE GUIDELINES

When using lavender in cooking, remember that dried lavender is more potent than fresh. Use 1/3 the quantity of dried flowers compared to fresh - if a recipe calls for 3 teaspoons fresh lavender, use only 1 teaspoon dried.

NON-CULINARY USES

Aromatherapy and Wellness

Lavender is renowned for its calming and relaxation properties:

- Essential Oils: Created by steeping lavender buds in carrier oils like olive or coconut oil
- Sleep Aid: Lavender sachets placed under pillows or in bedrooms
- Stress Relief: Used in aromatherapy for inducing relaxation
- Therapeutic Properties: Traditional uses include treating burns, insect bites, and spasms

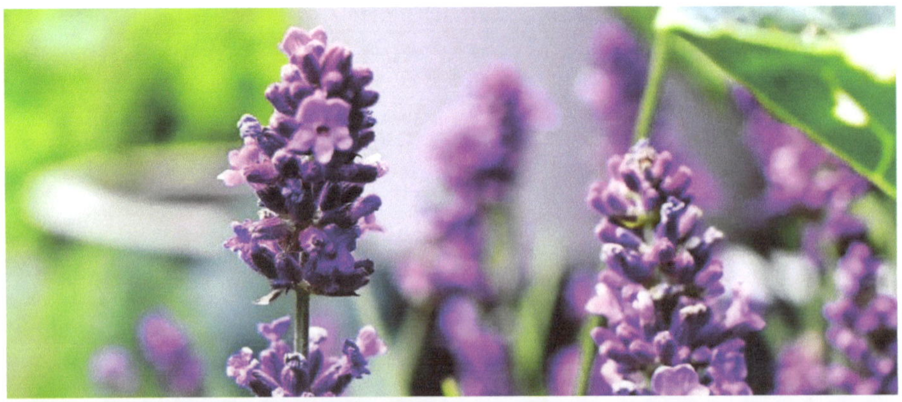

HOME AND HOUSEHOLD USES

Lavender serves numerous domestic purposes:

- **Natural Fragrance :** Dried lavender buds used in potpourri and room fresheners
- **Scented Sachets :** Placed in wardrobes and drawers to naturally scent clothing
- **Cleaning Products :** Added to homemade soaps and cleaning solutions
- **Bath Products :** Used in bath salts and bath oils for relaxation

CRAFT AND DECORATIVE APPLICATIONS

Lavender's visual appeal makes it popular in crafts:

- Floral Arrangements: Both fresh and dried lavender in bouquets and centerpieces
- **Wreaths :** Dried lavender incorporated into decorative wreaths
- **Natural Confetti :** Dried flower petals used for special occasions
- **DIY Projects :** Including lavender playdough for sensory activities

BEAUTY AND PERSONAL CARE

Lavender appears in numerous beauty applications:

- **Skin Care :** Added to lotions, creams, and facial products
- **Hair Care :** Used in shampoos and hair treatments
- **Natural Perfumes :** Essential oil used in fragrance blends

English Lavender (Lavandula angustifolia) is the preferred variety for culinary applications due to its sweet, delicate flavor. Other varieties like French lavender may be too strong or camphor-like for food use.

LEMON GRASS (CYMBOPOGON CITRATUS)

- **Scientific Name** : Cymbopogon citratus (main culinary variety)
- **Family :** Poaceae (grass family)
- **Common names :** Lemongrass, fever grass, citronella grass (though citronella is a different Cymbopogon species)
- **Native to :** South and Southeast Asia
- **Appearance :** Tall perennial grass with long, slender green leaves and a bulbous base resembling a green onion stalk.

CULINARY USES

Lemongrass is widely used in Asian cuisine, particularly Thai, Vietnamese, Malaysian, and Indian dishes.

- Flavor: Fresh, lemony, slightly sweet with earthy undertones.
- Used in: Soups (like Tom Yum), curries, teas, marinades, and herbal infusions.
- Edible parts: The tender white lower stalk is most often used for cooking.
- Form available: Fresh stalks, dried, powdered, or as essential oil.

MEDICINAL AND HEALTH BENEFITS

Lemongrass has long been used in Ayurvedic and traditional medicine for its therapeutic properties.

KEY BENEFITS:

- Antimicrobial & Antifungal: Helps fight bacteria, fungi, and yeast infections.
- Antioxidant: Contains citral and flavonoids that protect cells from oxidative damage.
- Anti-inflammatory: Reduces swelling and inflammation.
- Digestive aid: Relieves bloating, constipation, and stomach cramps.
- Relaxant: Lemongrass tea has mild sedative effects — aids sleep and reduces anxiety.
- Detoxification: Promotes urination and helps flush out toxins.
- Insect repellent: Lemongrass oil (rich in citronellal) repels mosquitoes naturally.

ACTIVE COMPOUNDS

- Citral (geranial + neral) – main aromatic compound responsible for lemon scent and antibacterial effect.
- Myrcene, limonene, and citronellal – contribute to fragrance and medicinal activity.
- Flavonoids and phenolic compounds – provide antioxidant and anti-inflammatory effects.

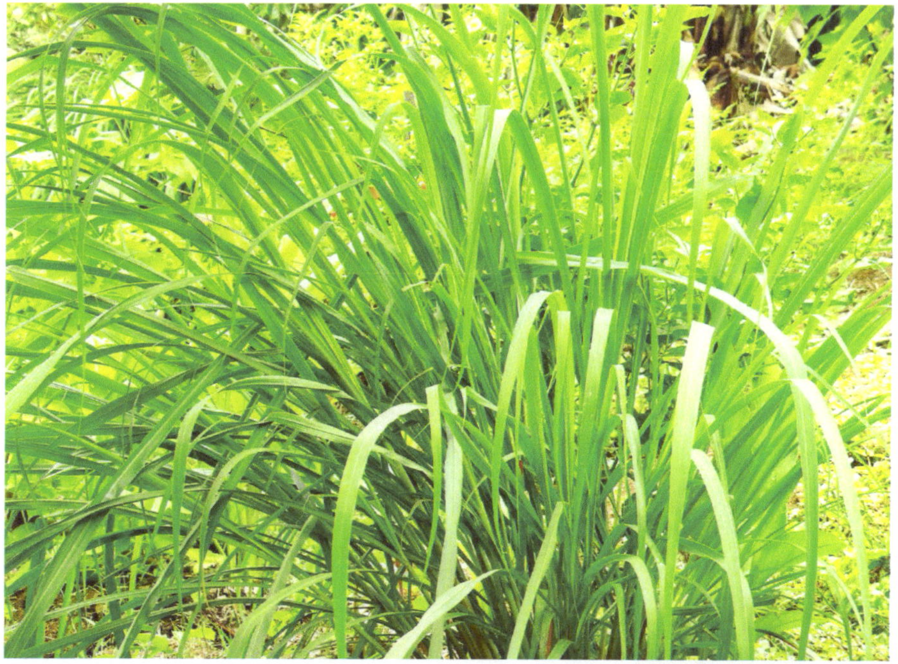

LEMON VERBENA (LIPPIA CITRIODORA)

- Scientific Name : Aloysia citrodora (formerly Lippia citriodora)
- Family : Verbenaceae
- Common names: Lemon verbena, Louisa, Lemon beebrush
- Native to : South America (Argentina, Chile, Peru)
- Appearance : Woody shrub, 1–3 m tall, with elongated, pointed green leaves that release a strong lemon scent when crushed.

CULINARY USES

Lemon verbena is prized for its intense, clean lemon fragrance often stronger and more floral than lemongrass or lemon balm.

USED IN

- Teas and infusions (hot or iced herbal tea)
- Desserts: Custards, sorbets, cakes, and jellies
- Savory dishes: Poultry, fish, marinades, and vinaigrettes
- Flavoring: Used to scent sugars, syrups, and liqueurs

FORMS AVAILABLE

- Fresh leaves, dried leaves, or essential oil (for aromatherapy or perfumery—not for ingestion).

MEDICINAL AND HEALTH BENEFITS

- In both European herbalism and South American folk medicine, Lemon Verbena is valued for its calming, digestive, and antioxidant effects.

KEY BENEFITS

- Digestive aid: Relieves indigestion, gas, bloating, and cramps.
- Calming & sleep-promoting: Mild sedative—helps reduce anxiety, insomnia, and stress.
- Anti-inflammatory: Eases joint pain and muscle soreness.
- Antioxidant: Protects cells from oxidative stress.
- Immune support: May boost the immune system due to its polyphenols.
- Metabolic support: Some studies show mild lipid-lowering effects.
- Mild antipyretic: Traditionally used to help lower fever.

ACTIVE COMPOUNDS

- Citral (neral + geranial) – lemon scent, antimicrobial
- Verbascoside (acteoside) – antioxidant, anti-inflammatory
- Luteolin and apigenin derivatives – flavonoids with calming properties
- Geraniol, limonene, cineol – aromatic compounds contributing to fragrance and biological activity.

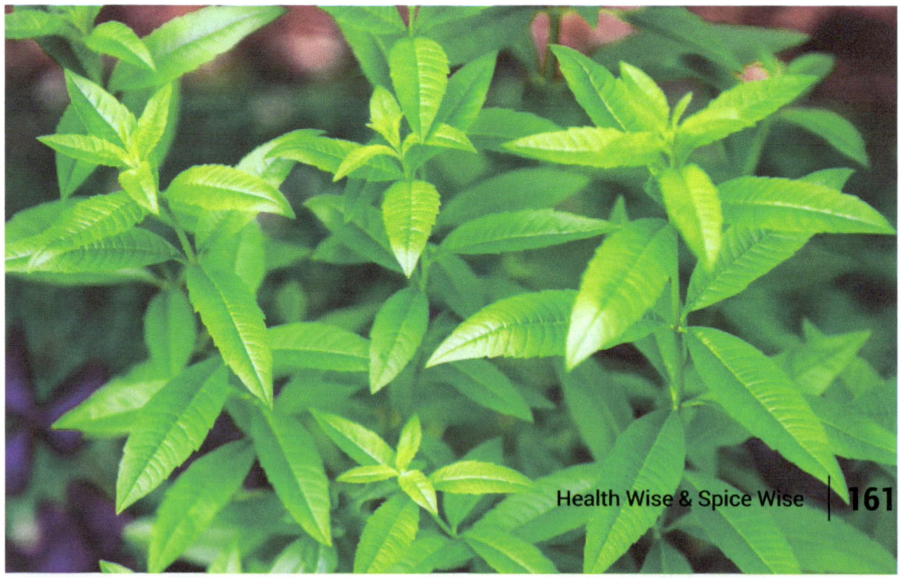

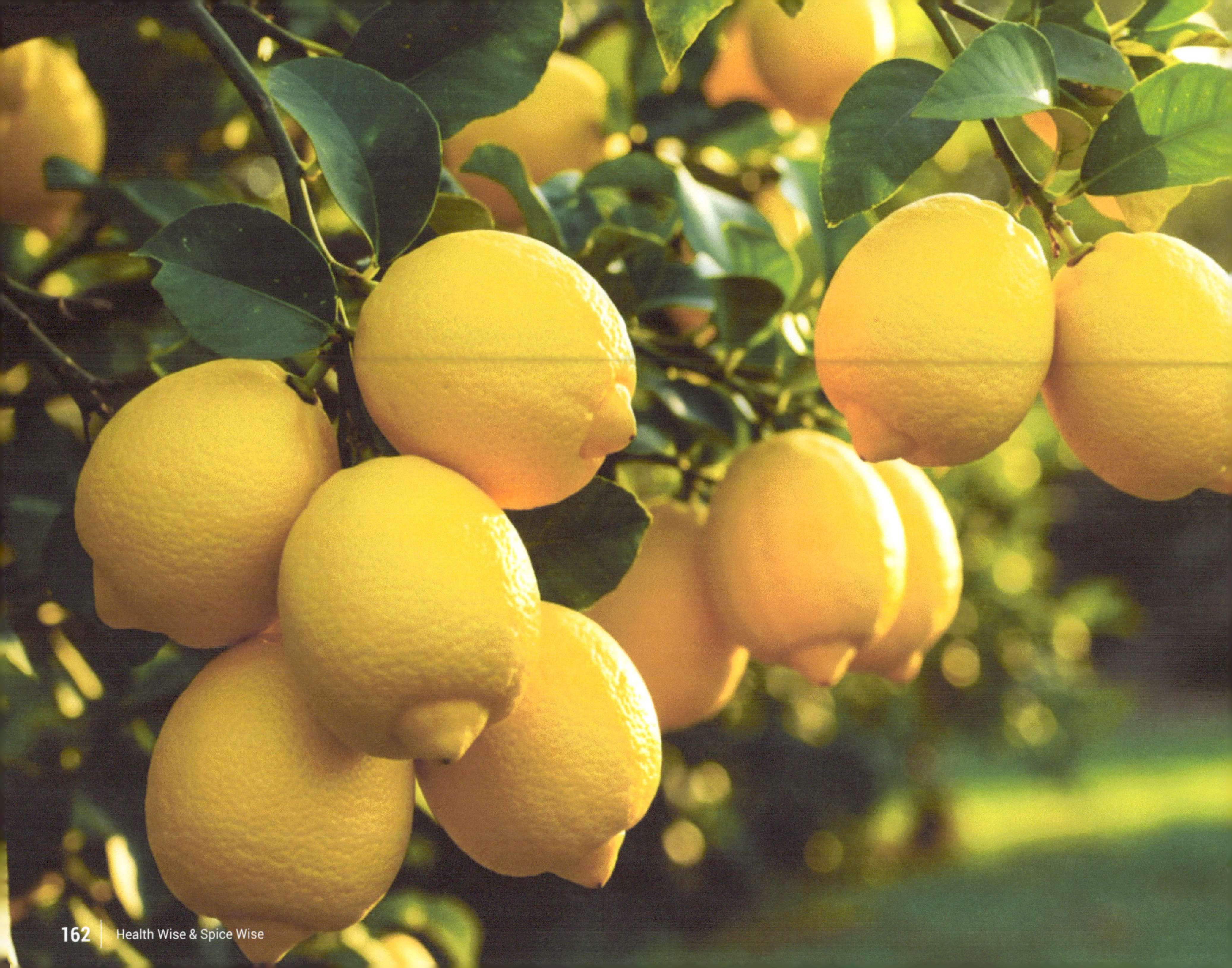

LEMON (CITRUS LIMON)

BOTANICAL OVERVIEW

- Scientific name:Citrus limon
- Family: Rutaceae (citrus family)
- Common names: Lemon, Nimbu (India), Citronnier (French)
- Origin: Believed to have originated in Northeast India and Northern Burma; later spread through the Mediterranean.
- Appearance: Small evergreen tree (3–6 meters) with glossy green leaves, fragrant white-purple flowers, and bright yellow oval fruits.

CULINARY USES

Lemon is one of the world's most widely used citrus fruits, valued for its sharp flavor, fragrance, and acidity.

COMMON CULINARY APPLICATIONS

- Juice: For drinks, dressings, marinades, and preservation.
- Zest (peel): Used in baking, desserts, and flavoring.
- Whole fruit: Used for pickles, marmalades, and preserved lemons.
- Leaves (in some cuisines): Used for subtle lemon aroma in teas or broths.

POPULAR DISHES & USES

- Lemon tea, lemonade, lemon rice, lemon chicken, lemon tart, and countless sauces and salad dressings.

MEDICINAL AND HEALTH BENEFITS

Lemon has been a cornerstone of both traditional and modern natural medicine due to its vitamin-rich, cleansing, and antimicrobial properties.

KEY BENEFITS

- Rich in Vitamin C: Strengthens immunity and helps fight colds and infections.
- Antioxidant: Neutralizes free radicals and supports skin and heart health.
- Detoxifying: Supports liver function and helps flush out toxins.
- Oral Health: Acidic nature helps whiten teeth and fight bacteria (but excessive direct use can erode enamel).
- Mood Booster: The aroma has uplifting, stress-reducing effects.
- Aids Digestion: Lemon water stimulates gastric juices and bile production.
- Weight Management: Warm lemon water in the morning can aid metabolism.
- Skin Benefits: Helps lighten dark spots, fight acne, and promote collagen synthesis.

ACTIVE COMPOUNDS

- Citric acid: Key acid providing tangy taste and aiding detoxification.
- Vitamin C (ascorbic acid): Powerful antioxidant and immune booster.
- Flavonoids (hesperidin, diosmin, eriocitrin): Anti-inflammatory and antioxidant.
- Limonene: Found in peel; has antibacterial, antifungal, and anticancer properties.
- Pectin: Soluble fiber that supports gut health and lowers cholesterol.

LESSER GALANGA (KAEMPFERIA GALANGA)

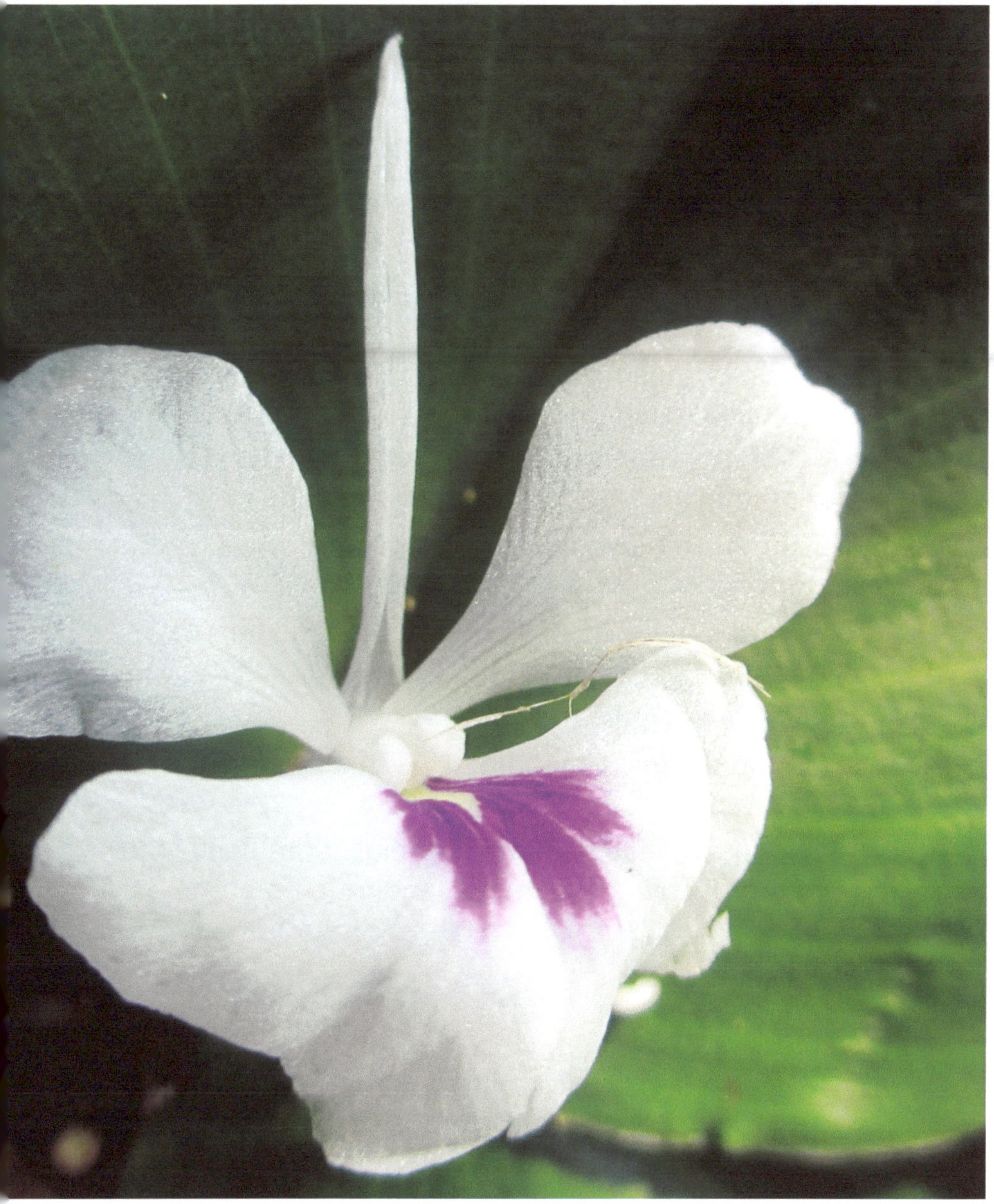

BOTANICAL OVERVIEW

- Scientific name: Alpinia officinarum&Kaempferia galanga
- Family: Zingiberaceae (Ginger family)
- Common names: Lesser galangal, Galanga, Kulanjan (India), Kha khae (Thailand), Galangal root
- Related species: Alpinia galanga (Greater Galangal) – similar but milder in flavor and larger in rhizome size
- Native to: Southern China (Hainan), and widely cultivated in India, Southeast Asia, and Indonesia

APPEARANCE

- Perennial herb, 1–1.5 m tall
- Narrow lance-shaped leaves (20–30 cm long)
- Flowers are white with red streaks
- Rhizomes are reddish-brown, aromatic, and fibrous with a spicy flavor

CULINARY USES

Lesser galangal is a traditional Asian spice valued for its warm, peppery, slightly pine-like aroma and sharp taste.

USED IN

- Indian, Thai, and Indonesian cuisine
- Curries, soups, meat dishes, and herbal teas
- Spice blends: An ingredient in some curry powders and Thai pastes
- Liqueurs: Flavoring for European herbal liqueurs like Benedictine and Chartreuse

FLAVOR PROFILE

Aromatic, spicy, slightly sweet, and more pungent than ginger with hints of pine, citrus, and pepper.

MEDICINAL AND HEALTH BENEFITS

Lesser galangal has been used for centuries in Ayurveda, Unani, and Traditional Chinese Medicine (TCM) for its warming, digestive, and antimicrobial properties.

KEY BENEFITS

- Digestive aid: Stimulates appetite, relieves indigestion, nausea, and gas.
- Antimicrobial: Effective against bacteria, fungi, and parasites.
- Anti-inflammatory: Helps with arthritis and joint pain.
- Cardiovascular support: Improves circulation and may help regulate cholesterol.
- Respiratory relief: Used in cough, bronchitis, and sore throat preparations.
- Cognitive and energy booster: Mild stimulant; historically used to enhance vitality.
- Antioxidant: Protects cells from oxidative damage.
- Metabolic support: Traditionally used in obesity and metabolic sluggishness.

ACTIVE COMPOUNDS

- Galangin : Flavonoid with strong antioxidant, anti-inflammatory, and antimicrobial effects.
- Alpinia & Kaempferide : Bioactive compounds with antibacterial and hepatoprotective properties.
- Cineole, Eugenol, and Pinene : Contribute to aroma and respiratory benefits.
- Tannins & Resins: Aid in digestion and wound healing.

People with acid reflux or ulcers should use with caution due to its pungency.

BENEFITS

Aids digestion, eases cough and sore throat, and boosts energy.

- Comparison: Lesser Galangal vs. Ginger vs. Greater Galangal
- Feature Lesser Galangal (Alpinia officinarum) Greater Galangal (Alpinia galanga) Ginger (Zingiber officinale)
- Flavor Sharp, peppery, pine-like Mild, citrusy, sweet Warm, spicy, mild
- Color (rhizome) Reddish-brown Pale yellow Light brown
- Texture Hard and fibrous Softer Moist and fibrous
- Primary use Medicinal, spice Culinary (Thai cuisine) Universal culinary spice
- Active compound Galangin Galangol Gingerol

Medicinal focus Digestive, antimicrobial, stimulant Anti-inflammatory, stomachic Antiemetic, anti-inflammatory.

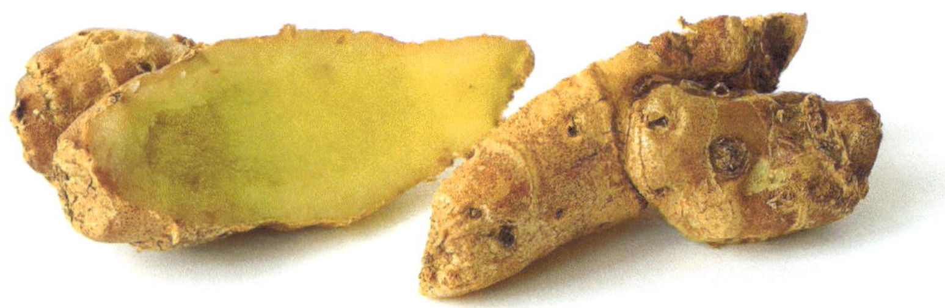

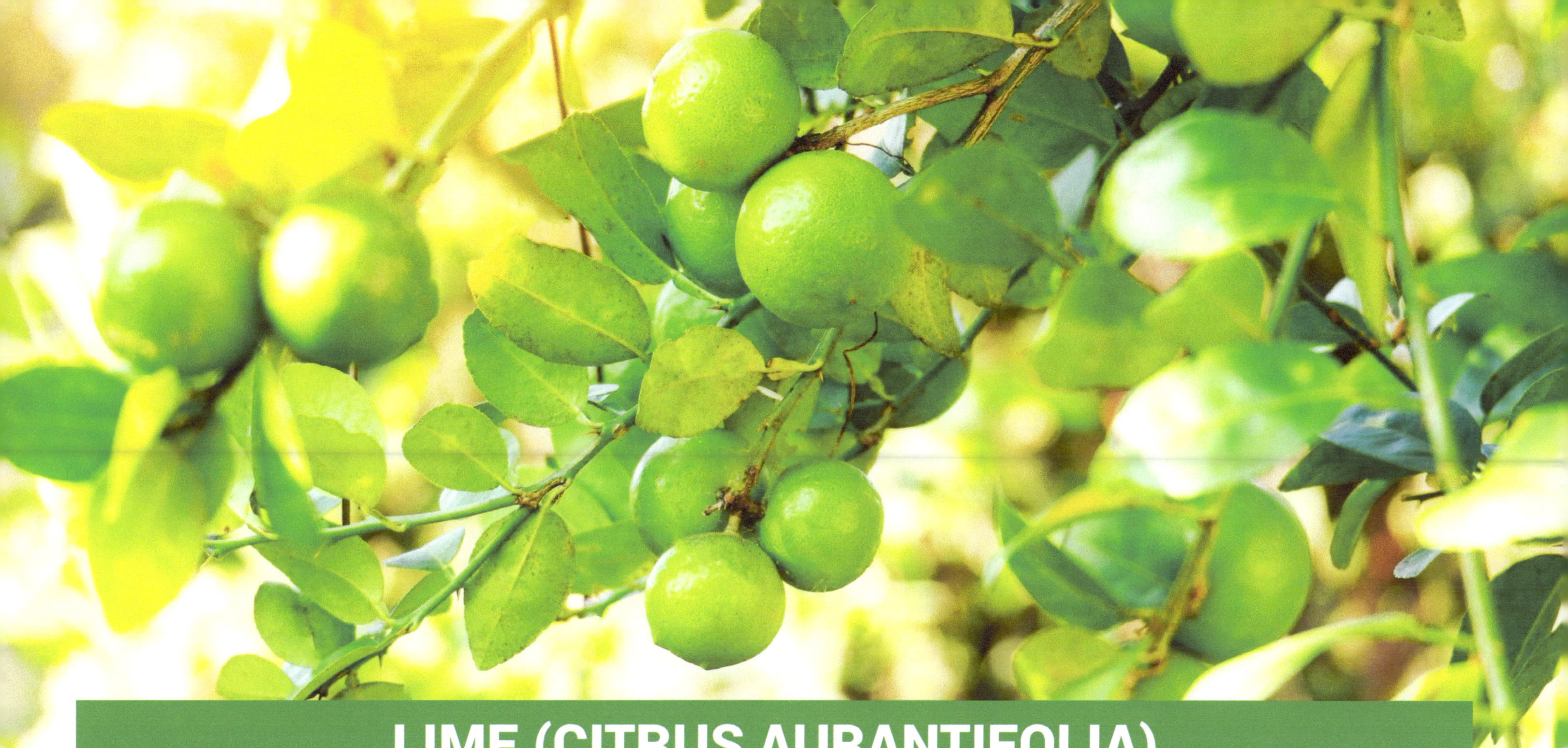

LIME (CITRUS AURANTIFOLIA)

LEMON OVERVIEW

BOTANICAL INFORMATION

- Scientific name: Citrus limon
- Family: Rutaceae (Citrus family)
- Origin: Likely from northern India and Myanmar; later cultivated widely in the Mediterranean and Americas.
- Type: Small evergreen tree (3–6 m) with glossy leaves and fragrant white-purple flowers.
- Fruit: Oval, bright yellow when mature, with a thick rind and juicy acidic pulp.

CULINARY USES

- Used in beverages, desserts, marinades, sauces, and salads.
- Lemon juice: Adds acidity and freshness to dishes.
- Zest (outer peel): Used in baking and flavoring.
- Preserved lemons: Common in Middle Eastern and North

African cuisine.

- Drinks: Lemonade, lemon tea, lemon water.

MEDICINAL & HEALTH BENEFITS

- Vitamin C powerhouse: Strengthens immunity and supports collagen production.
- Digestive support: Stimulates bile flow and aids digestion.
- Skin health: Brightens complexion, helps acne and pigmentation (topically diluted).
- Cardiovascular health: Flavonoids support heart and vessel function.
- Respiratory relief: Soothes throat and helps break down mucus.
- Detoxifying effect: Mild diuretic and liver tonic.

ACTIVE COMPOUNDS

- Citric acid – provides acidity, aids metabolism.
- Limonene – aromatic compound with antimicrobial properties.
- Vitamin C (ascorbic acid) – antioxidant.
- Flavonoids: Hesperidin, diosmin, eriocitrin.

LIME OVERVIEW

BOTANICAL INFORMATION

- Scientific names:
- Citrus aurantiifolia — Key lime (smaller, more acidic)
- Citrus latifolia — Persian or Tahiti lime (larger, milder, seedless)
- Family: Rutaceae
- Origin: Southeast Asia, later cultivated in tropical and subtropical regions worldwide.
- Type: Small thorny tree or shrub (2–4 m tall).
- Fruit: Round or oval, green when fresh, turns yellow when overripe, with thin smooth rind.

CULINARY USES

- Essential in Indian, Thai, Mexican, Caribbean, and Middle Eastern cuisines.
- Juice: Used for drinks, chutneys, curries, and marinades.
- Zest: Adds intense citrus aroma to dishes and baked goods.
- Beverages: Lime soda, mojito, lime water, and traditional nimbu pani (Indian limeade).

MEDICINAL & HEALTH BENEFITS

- Rich in Vitamin C: Boosts immunity, fights infections.
- Detox & digestion: Enhances digestion and liver function.
- Antibacterial & antiviral: Lime oil and juice inhibit pathogen growth.
- Mood enhancer: Lime aroma reduces fatigue and enhances alertness.
- Skin care: Lime extracts in cosmetics help exfoliation and acne control.
- Antioxidant: Prevents oxidative stress and supports tissue repair.

ACTIVE COMPOUNDS

- Citric acid
- Vitamin C (ascorbic acid)
- Limonene and linalool
- Flavonoids: Naringin, hesperidin, eriocitrin
- Coumarins: Contribute to aroma and antimicrobial effect.

CULTIVATION NOTES (BOTH LEMON AND LIME)		
FEATURE	**LEMON**	**LIME**
Climate	Subtropical to Mediterranean	Tropical to subtropical
Temperature range	25–35 °C	20–30 °C
Soil	Well-drained sandy loam, pH 5.5–7.0	Similar, slightly more tolerant of alkalinity
Propagation	Grafting or budding	Grafting or air layering
Fruiting time	2–3 years (grafted plants)	2–3 years
Major producers	India, Italy, USA, Spain, Mexico	India, Mexico, Brazil, Thailand

ESSENTIAL OIL		
PROPERTY	**LEMON OIL**	**LIME OIL**
Extraction	Cold pressing of peel	Cold pressing or steam distillation
Aroma	Bright, fresh, sweet-citrus	Sharp, tangy, slightly bitter
Key Compounds	Limonene, citral	Limonene, beta-pinene
Uses	Skin care, cleaning, aromatherapy	Perfumery, cleaning, mood uplifting
Precautions	Photosensitive	Photosensitive

PRECAUTIONS (BOTH)

- Highly acidic — can erode tooth enamel if used excessively.
- Lemon and lime oils are photosensitive — avoid sunlight after topical use.
- Overuse may cause stomach acidity or irritation in sensitive individuals.

COMPARISON : LEMON VS. LIME		
PROPERTY	LEMON OIL	LIME OIL
Feature	Lemon (Citrus limon)	Lime (Citrus aurantiifolia / latifolia)
Fruit Color	Bright yellow when ripe	Green (turns yellow when ripe)
Shape	Oval or oblong	Round or slightly oval
Taste	Tart but slightly sweet	More acidic and bitter
Aroma	Fresh, floral-citrus	Sharp, tangy-citrus
Juice Content	Higher volume, milder acidity	Less juice, stronger acidity
Vitamin C (per 100 g)	~53 mg	~29 mg
Main Compound	Citric acid, limonene	Citric acid, limonene, naringin
Best For	Baking, desserts, sauces, detox drinks	Savory dishes, cocktails, chutneys
Oil Extraction	Cold-pressed peel	Cold-pressed or steam-distilled peel
Major Producers	India, USA, Italy, Spain	India, Mexico, Brazil, Thailand
pH (juice)	2.2-2.4	2.0-2.2
Shelf Life (fruit)	Longer	Shorter (spoils faster)
Medicinal Focus	Immune and skin health	Digestion and liver support
Color in Cuisine	Brightens visually	Adds tang without color

IN SHORT

- Lemon = milder, sweeter acidity, more Vitamin C, ideal for desserts and drinks.
- Lime = sharper, stronger tang, more aromatic bitterness, ideal for savory dishes and tropical beverages. Both are rich in antioxidants, vitamin C, and cleansing properties, making them valuable in both culinary and medicinal use.

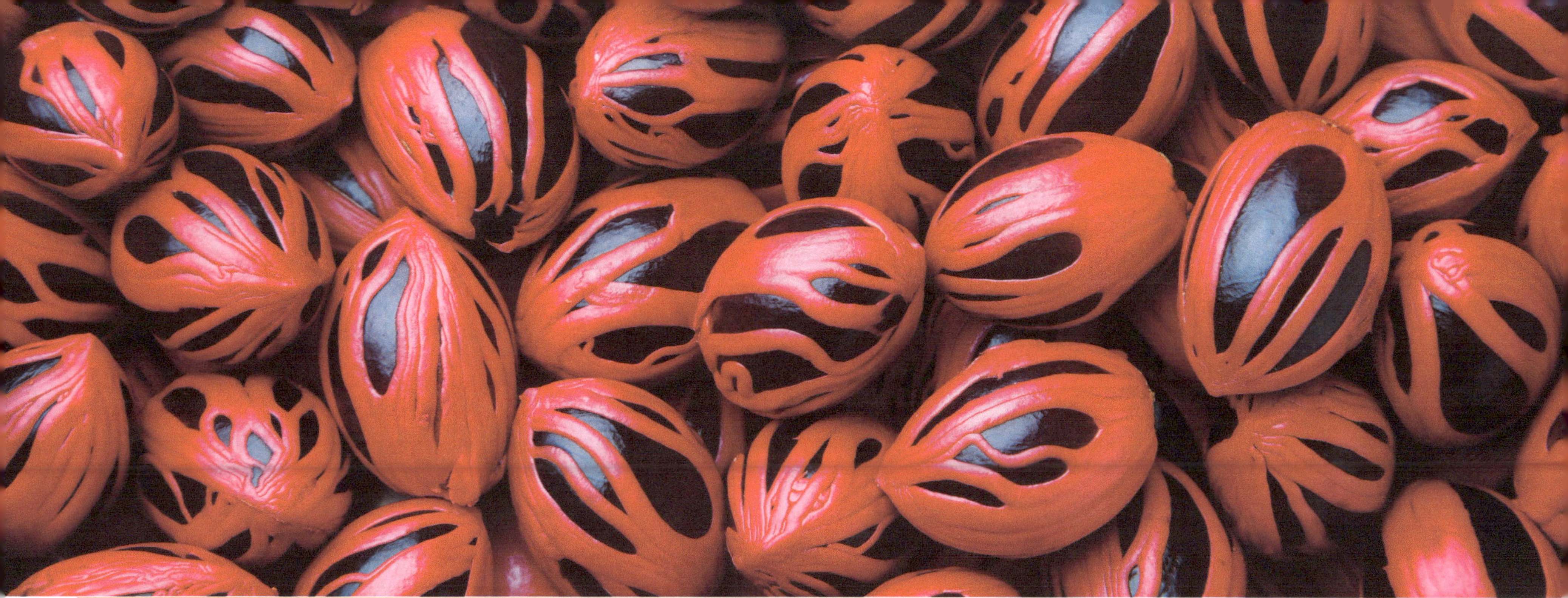

NUTMEG AND MACE (MYRISTICA FRAGRANS)

Nutmeg (Myristica fragrans) is a popular spice made from the seed of the nutmeg tree. It is known for its warm, sweet, and slightly spicy flavor. Here are some key properties and health benefits of nutmeg:

NUTRITIONAL CONTENT

- Essential Oils: Contains essential oils such as myristicin, elemicin, eugenol, and safrole.
- Vitamins and Minerals: Rich in vitamins A, C, and E, as well as minerals like calcium, iron, magnesium, and manganese.
- Antioxidants: High in antioxidants, which help protect against oxidative stress and damage.

HEALTH BENEFITS

- Digestive Health: Aids in digestion, relieves stomach cramps, and reduces bloating.
- Pain Relief: Has analgesic properties that help alleviate pain, including headaches and joint pain.
- Anti-inflammatory: Reduces inflammation and can help alleviate conditions like arthritis.
- Sleep Aid: Known to promote relaxation and improve sleep quality due to its mild sedative effects.
- Antimicrobial Properties: Has antibacterial and antifungal properties that help fight infections.

- Oral Health: Used in dental care products for its ability to freshen breath and combat oral bacteria.
- Cognitive Health: Enhances cognitive function and may help protect against neurodegenerative diseases.
- Detoxification: Helps detoxify the liver and kidneys, promoting overall health.

USAGE

- Culinary Uses: Nutmeg is used to flavor a variety of dishes, including desserts, beverages, sauces, and spice blends. It is a key ingredient in dishes like eggnog, mulled wine, and pumpkin pie.
- Medicinal Uses: Can be consumed as a tea, supplement, or essential oil for its health benefits.
- Aromatherapy: Nutmeg essential oil is used in aromatherapy for its warming and calming effects.

Mace

- When ripe, it splits open to reveal a hard brown nutmeg seed surrounded by a bright red lacy covering — this red aril is mace.
- Once dried, mace turns yellowish-orange or light brown, becoming brittle and aromatic.
- So:
- Mace = the dried outer aril (covering) of the nutmeg seed.
- Nutmeg = the dried kernel inside.

CULINARY USES

- Mace has a warm, aromatic, slightly sweet, and more delicate flavor than nutmeg.
- It's widely used in both sweet and savory dishes.

COMMON USES

- In Indian cuisine: Garam masala, biryanis, kormas, pickles.
- In Western cuisine: Cakes, pastries, doughnuts, puddings, sauces, sausages, soups.
- In European cooking: Adds aroma to béchamel sauce, stews, and spice blends.
- Beverages: Used in mulled wine, hot chocolate, and spiced teas.

FLAVOR PROFILE:

- Warm, sweet-spicy, with notes of cinnamon and pepper — subtler and more refined than nutmeg.

MEDICINAL AND HEALTH BENEFITS

Mace shares many of nutmeg's therapeutic properties but is milder and less likely to irritate digestion.

KEY BENEFITS:

- Digestive aid: Stimulates appetite, relieves nausea, indigestion, and gas.
- Nervine tonic: Calming and mildly sedative; reduces stress and anxiety.
- Anti-inflammatory: Helps with joint pain and muscle soreness.
- Antibacterial & antifungal: Prevents microbial infections.
- Circulatory booster: Improves blood flow and heart function.
- Detoxification: Supports liver health.
- Cognitive support: Enhances alertness in small doses.
- Metabolic & sexual tonic: Traditionally used as an aphrodisiac and energy booster in Ayurveda and Unani medicine.

LONG PEPPER (PIPER LONGUM)

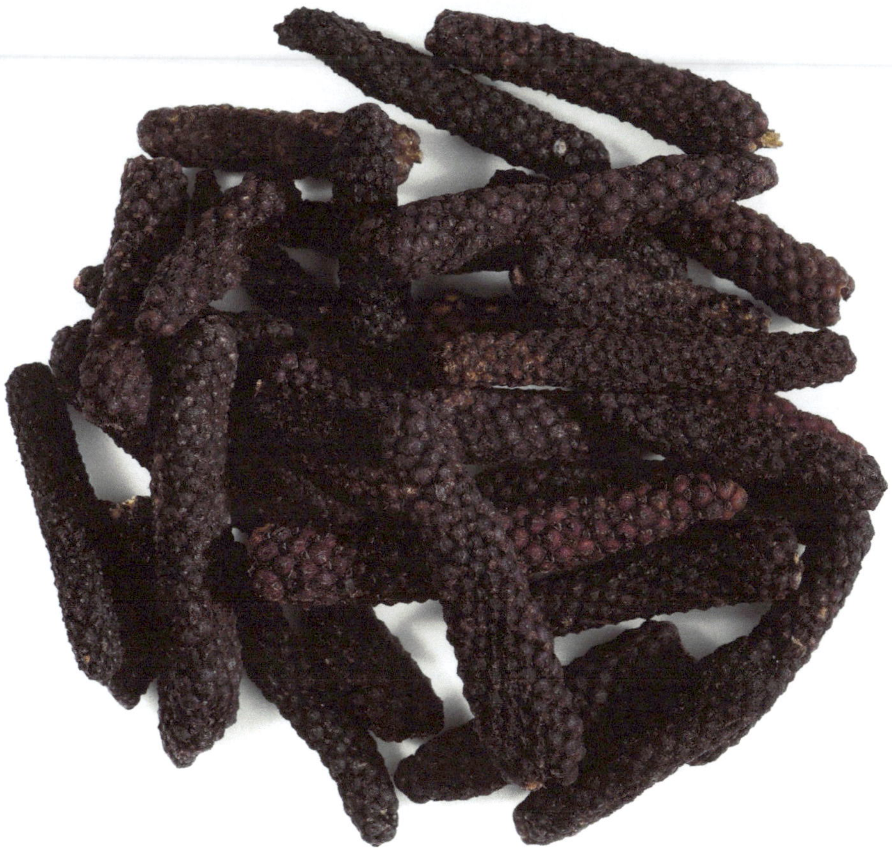

BOTANICAL BACKGROUND

- Perennial climbing vine, family Piperaceae.
- Native to India, Indonesia, and tropical Asia.
- Produces elongated, cylindrical spikes of tiny berries.
- Grows 2–5 m; prefers humid, tropical climates.
- Known as "pippali"; used in culinary, medicinal, and traditional Ayurveda.

COMMON CULINARY APPLICATIONS

- Ground or whole in curries, stews, and soups.
- Flavoring for meat dishes, pickles, and sauces.
- Used in spice blends and traditional garam masala.
- Adds warm, pungent, slightly sweet, and complex heat.

TYPES / VARIETIES

- Indian Long Pepper (Piper longum var. longum) – most common culinary type.
- Indonesian Long Pepper (Piper longum var. piperinum) – slightly milder, aromatic.
- Wild Himalayan types – smaller spikes, stronger flavor.
- Cultivated hybrids – selected for larger spikes and higher pungency.

CULINARY

- whole or ground in curries, rice dishes, stews, sauces, spice blends.

HEALTH

supports digestion, relieves bloating and flatulence; traditionally used for respiratory health (coughs, colds, asthma); antimicrobial and anti-inflammatory properties; may stimulate appetite and metabolism.

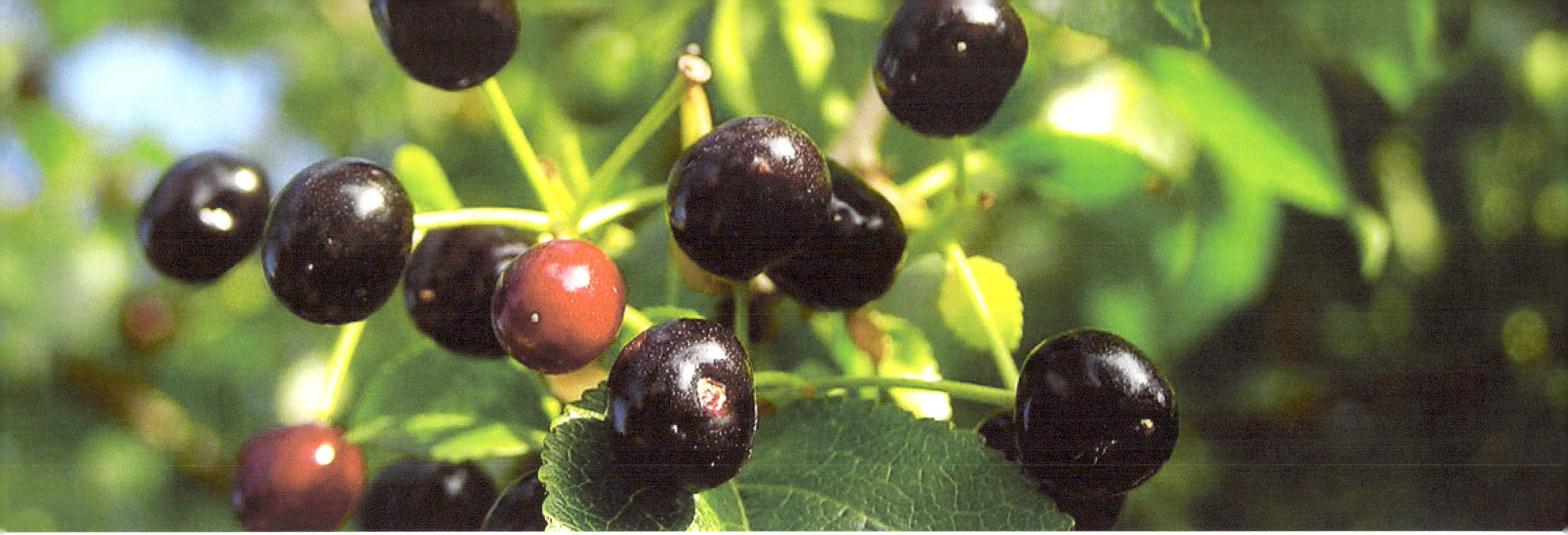

MAHALEB CHERRY (PRUNUS MAHALEB)

Mahlab kernels come from the seeds of the Prunus mahaleb, otherwise known as St. Lucie, a kind of wild cherry plant.

PRUNUSMAHALEB

- Has many properties, including pharmaceutical, cosmetic, and culinary uses.

PHARMACEUTICAL PROPERTIES

- Anti-oxidant and anti-bacterial Mahaleb seed extract has been shown to treat kidney stones and respiratory tract infections.

ANTI-INFLAMMATORY

- The bark, wood, and seeds of the Mahaleb cherry contain coumarin, which has anti-inflammatory properties.

COUMARINS

- Coumarins are anti-inflammatory compounds that may help fight diseases like asthma, Alzheimer's, and heart disease.

COSMETIC PROPERTIES

- Dye: Mahaleb can be used as a dye.

CULINARY PROPERTIES

- Flavor: Mahaleb seeds have a special taste and odor and are often used in bakeries, mostlyused in Middle Eastern and European baked goods.
- Spice: Mahaleb can be used as a spice in festive bakes.
- Sprinkle: Mahaleb can be sprinkled on sauteed vegetables, creamy soups, rice, and dishes with carrots or pumpkin.

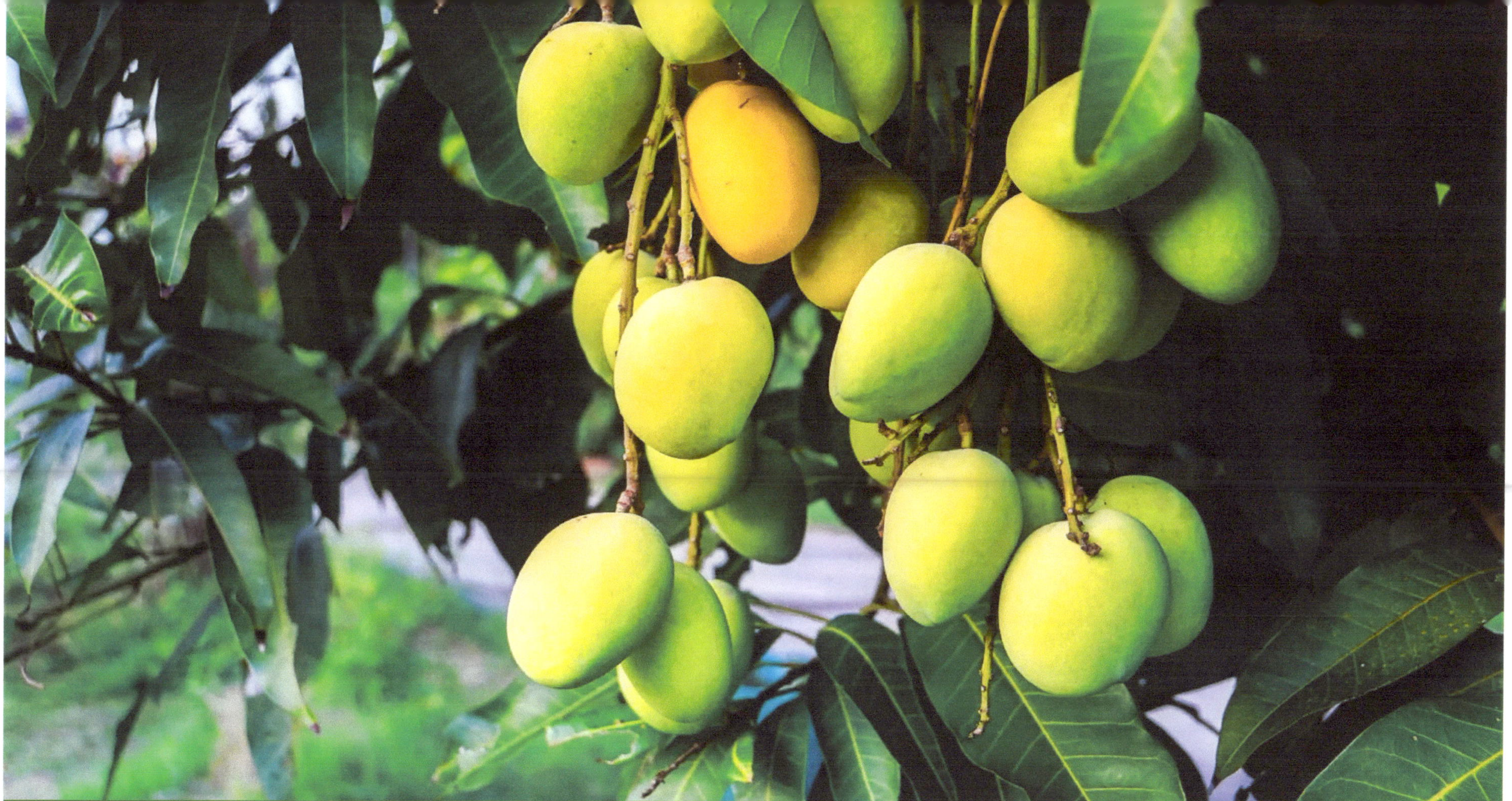

MANGO (MANGIFERA INDICA)

CULTIVATION & GROWTH

- Thrives in tropical and subtropical climates with a distinct dry season to trigger flowering.
- Requires full sun, deep well-drained soil, and warm temperatures (24–27°C / 75–80°F optimal).
- Sensitive to frost — even brief cold spells can damage young trees.
- Grown commercially across India, China, Thailand, Mexico, Indonesia, Pakistan, and Brazil.
- India is the world's largest producer, accounting for nearly 40% of global mango output.
- Over 500 named varieties exist worldwide, including Alphonso, Dasheri, Kesar, Ataulfo, Tommy Atkins, and Kent.

CULINARY

- Eaten fresh as a dessert fruit – one of the most beloved fruits globally.
- Used in juices, smoothies, lassis, sorbets, ice creams, and jams.
- Unripe (green) mangoes are used extensively in pickles (achar), chutneys, and raw salads (e.g., green mango salad in Southeast Asia).
- Amchur (dried mango powder) is a tangy spice widely used in Indian cooking.
- Used in sauces, marinades, salsas, and desserts across tropical cuisines.
- Mango pulp is processed into juices, nectars, and concentratesfor global export.

MEDICINAL & TRADITIONAL USES:

- Leaves, bark, seeds, and fruit are all used in Ayurvedic and traditional medicine.
- Rich in mangiferin, a natural antioxidant with anti-inflammatory and antiviral properties.
- Traditionally used to manage diabetes, digestive disorders, and skin conditions.
- Mango leaf tea is used in some cultures to help regulate blood sugar levels.
- Seed kernel oil (mango butter) is used in cosmetics and skincare for its moisturizing properties.

NON-CULINARY

- Mango wood is used in furniture, flooring, and musical instruments.
- Mango butter, extracted from the seed, is used in lotions, soaps, and hair products.
- Leaves are used in Hindu and Buddhist rituals – strung at doorways during festivals and auspicious ceremonies.

NUTRITIONAL PROFILE (RIPE FRUIT, PER 100G)

Mango is a nutritional powerhouse

- Vitamin C: 36 mg (about 40% of daily value)
- Vitamin A / Beta-carotene: High – responsible for the deep orange color
- Folate (Vitamin B9): Important for cell health
- Potassium: Supports heart and muscle function
- Dietary Fiber: Aids digestion
- Polyphenols: Including mangiferin, quercetin, and gallic acid – powerful antioxidants.
- Low in fat and sodium

CULTURAL & HISTORICAL SIGNIFICANCE

- Revered as the National Fruit of India, Pakistan, and the Philippines.
- The paisley pattern, iconic in textiles worldwide, is derived from the shape of the mango.
- Mentioned in ancient Sanskrit texts, Buddhist literature, and the Ramayana and Mahabharata – mango groves were places of meditation and royal gifting.
- Emperor Akbar is said to have planted a grove of 100,000 mango trees, known as the Lakhi Bagh, in the 16th century.
- The word "mango" derives from the Tamil word māngāi, which passed into Portuguese as manga during the spice trade era.
- Mango leaves and fruits are central to festivals like Ugadi, Vishu, and Gudi Padwa across South and Southeast Asia.

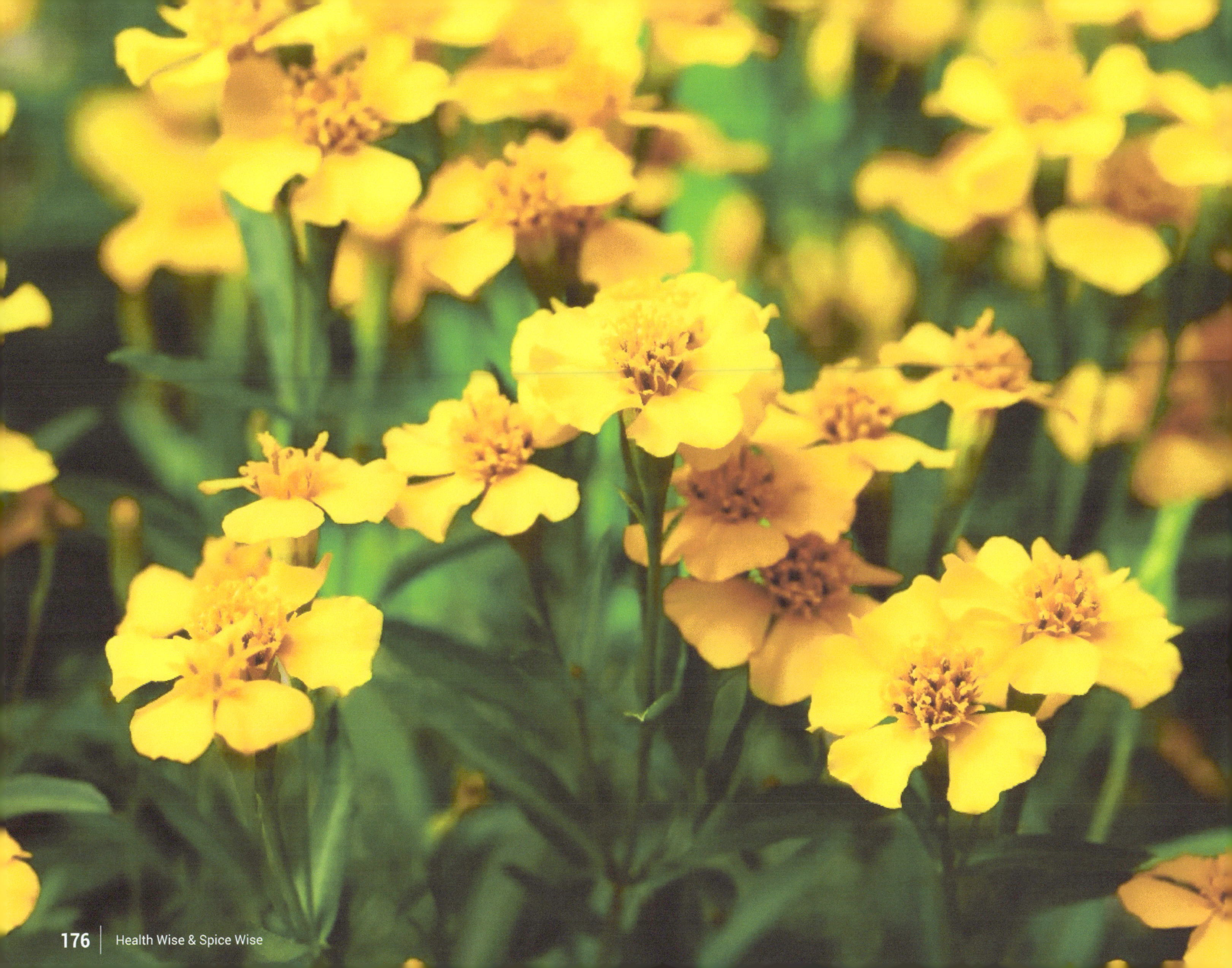

MEXICAN TARRAGON (TAGETES LUCIDA)

It is native to Mexico and Central America, where it has been used for centuries in culinary, medicinal, and ritual contexts. Despite its name and flavor similarities, it is not related to French Tarragon (Artemisia dracunculus) but is instead a member of the marigold genus.

CULINARY USES

- The leaves carry a strong anise/tarragon-like flavor with sweet, slightly spicy undertones – making it an excellent substitute for French Tarragon in hot climates.
- Used fresh or dried to flavor fish, chicken, eggs, salads, soups, and sauces.
- Popular in vinaigrettes and herb butters.
- Flowers are edible and make a beautiful garnish.
- Widely used in Mexican cuisine – especially to flavor a traditional hot drink called té de pericón (pericón tea).
- Pairs well with tomatoes, citrus, corn, and beans.
- Used to make anise-flavored liqueurs and beverages in Mexico.
- Can be used to infuse vinegars and oils, much like French tarragon.

MEDICINAL & TRADITIONAL USES:

- One of the most important sacred and medicinal herbs of the Aztec civilization.
- The Aztecs called it yauhtli and used it in offerings to Tlaloc, the rain god, as well as in purification rituals and religious ceremonies.
- Traditionally used to treat digestive complaints – bloating, indigestion, colic, and stomach cramps.
- Used as a febrifuge (fever reducer) and to relieve headaches and colds.
- Applied topically for skin conditions and as an insect repellent.
- Contains compounds including estragole, anethole, and methyleugenol – responsible for its anise scent and various bioactive properties.
- Historically used in Mesoamerican ritual medicine – burned as incense and mixed into ritual drinks to induce altered states during ceremonies.
- Modern research suggests potential anti-inflammatory, antimicrobial, and antifungal properties.

NUTRITIONAL & PHYTOCHEMICAL PROFILE

- Key compounds found in Mexican Tarragon include:
  - **Estragole (methyl chavicol)** : The primary essential oil component, responsible for the anise flavor
  - **Anethole** : Also found in anise and fennel; anti-inflammatory properties
  - **Quercetin and other flavonoids** : Antioxidants
  - **Tannins** : Astringent, antimicrobial properties
  - **Methyleugenol** : Aromatic compound with reported sedative and analgesic effects.

MARJORAM (MAJORANA HORTENSIS)

BOTANICAL BACKGROUND

- Perennial herb, family Lamiaceae.
- Native to the Mediterranean region; widely cultivated worldwide.
- Aromatic, bushy plant with small oval leaves and tiny white or pink flowers.
- Known for sweet, mild, slightly citrusy aroma.

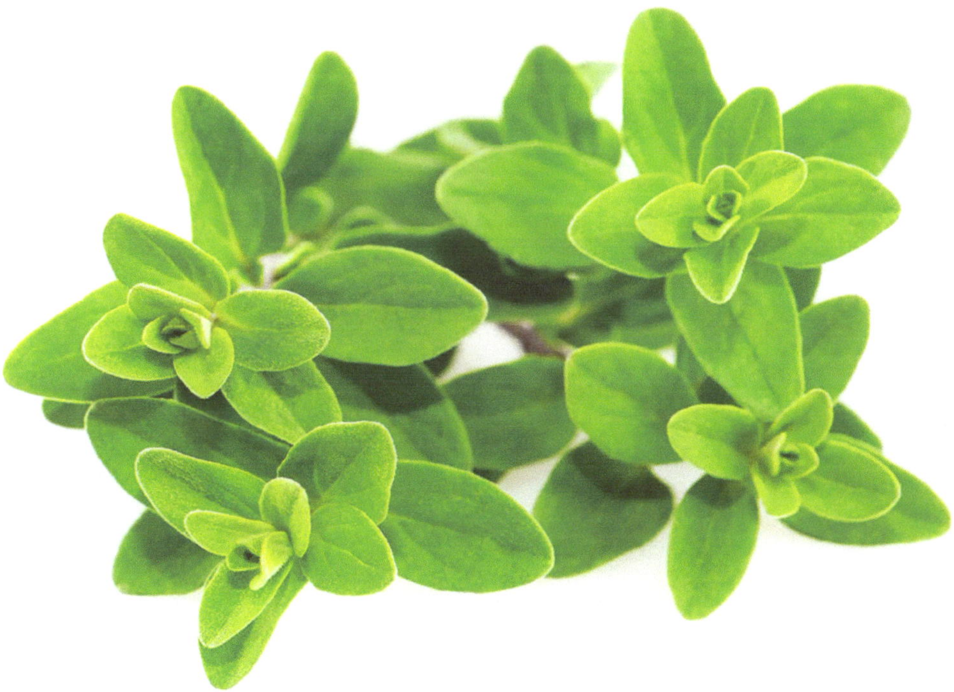

COMMON CULINARY APPLICATIONS

- Added fresh or dried to soups, stews, sauces, and salad dressings.
- Used in meat, poultry, and vegetable dishes.
- Included in spice blends, marinades, and herb mixes like herbes de Provence.

TYPES / VARIETIES

- Sweet Marjoram – mild, commonly used in cooking.
- Wild Marjoram (Oregano) – stronger flavor, sometimes used interchangeably with oregano.
- Compact Marjoram – ornamental and culinary use.

CULINARY USES

- Enhances soups, stews, sauces, and gravies.
- Added to roasted meats, vegetables, and pasta dishes.
- Used in herb blends, dressings, and marinades.

HEALTH BENEFITS

- Rich in antioxidants; supports digestion and immunity.
- Possesses antimicrobial and anti-inflammatory properties.
- Traditionally used for respiratory issues, stress relief, and mild pain.
- May improve circulation and promote heart health.

MYRTLE (MYRTUS COMMUNIS)

Myrtle (Myrtus communis) is a flowering plant with many properties, including antibacterial, anti-inflammatory, and antioxidant properties. Myrtle has been used for cooking and healing for thousands of years.

PROPERTIES

- Antibacterial: Myrtle contains chemicals that may help fight bacteria and fungus
- Anti-inflammatory: Myrtle has anti-inflammatory properties that may help reduce swelling
- Antiseptic: Myrtle has antiseptic properties that may help with respiratory tract ailments, colds, and bronchitis
- Astringent: Myrtle has astringent properties that may help with acne, oily skin, and tight pores
- Stress management: Myrtle may help with stress management and anxiety relief

USES

- Skin health: Myrtle may help with acne, oily skin, and tight pores
- Food flavoring: The dried flowers, fruits, and leaves of myrtle can be used to flavor food
- Bay leaf substitute: The leaves of myrtle can be used as a substitute for bay leaves
- Meat flavoring: The wood of myrtle can be used to flavor meats
- Symbol of love and beauty: Myrtle is often used in bouquets for weddings and special occasions to symbolize love, beauty, and loyalty

SAFETY

- Myrtle essential oil is considered safe, but caution is advised when pregnant or breastfeeding

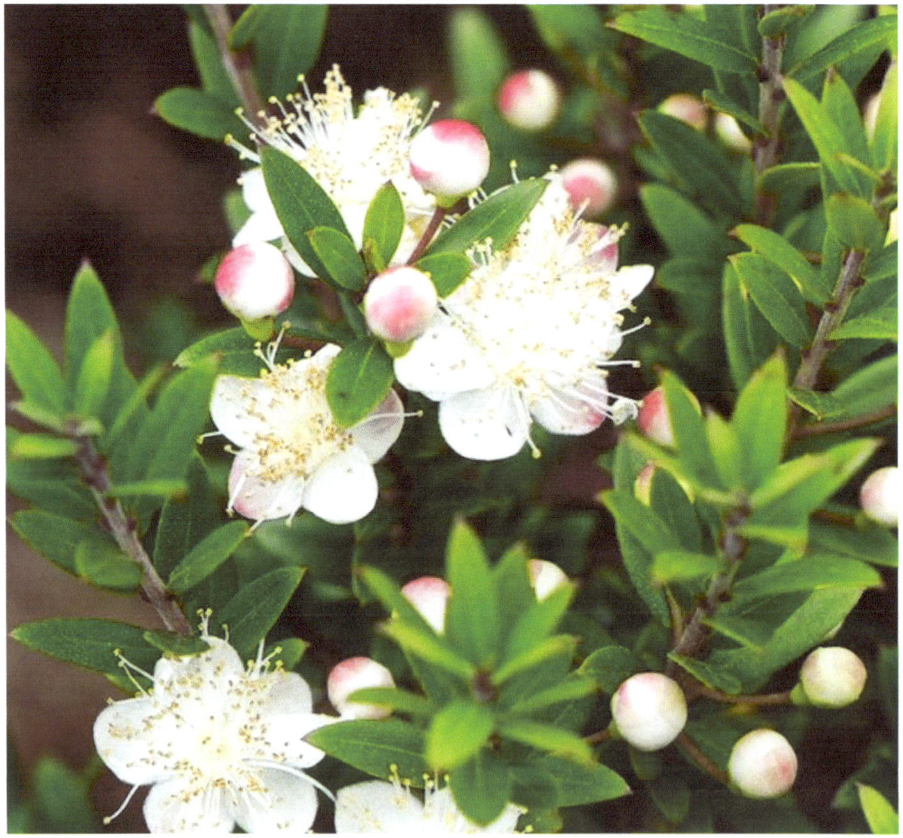

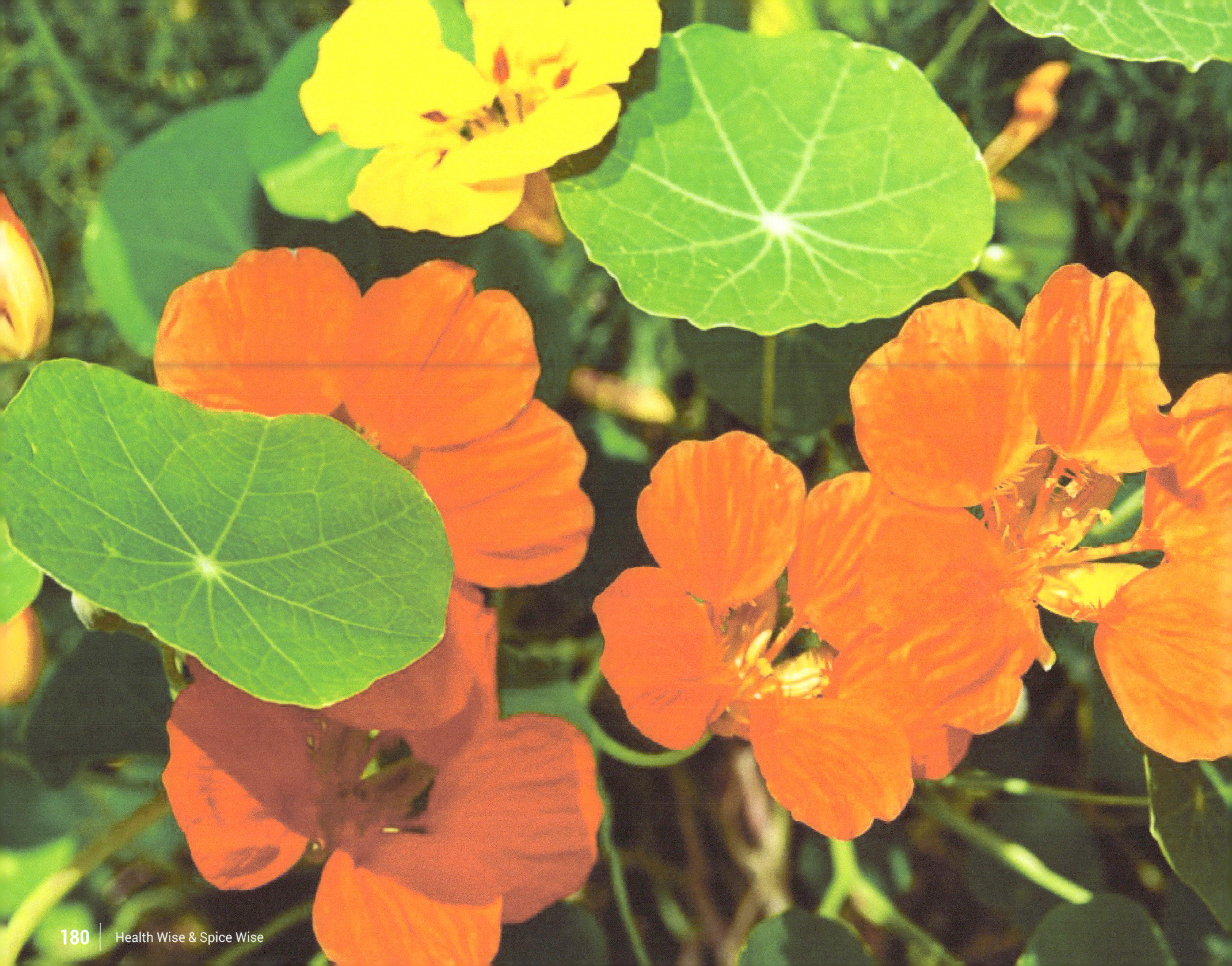

NASTURTIUM (TROPAEOLUM MAJUS)

CULINARY USES:

- One of the most versatile edible ornamental plants is edible: flowers, leaves, stems, and seeds.
- Flowers: Have a sweet, mildly peppery, slightly spicy flavor; used fresh in salads, as garnishes, and to decorate cakes and desserts.
- Leaves: Peppery, similar to watercress; used in salads, sandwiches, pestos, and wraps.
- Seeds (unripe): Pickled in vinegar to make a caper substitute — known as "poor man's capers"; a popular practice since the 17th century in Europe.
- Stems: Tender young stems are edible, with a similar flavor to the leaves.
- Commonly used in gourmet and farm-to-table cuisine for its vibrant color and peppery bite.
- The whole plant is rich in Vitamin C — historically used by sailors to prevent scurvy.
- Pairs well with cheese, eggs, smoked salmon, avocado, and citrus.

MEDICINAL & TRADITIONAL USES:

- Used extensively in South American traditional medicine by indigenous Andean cultures long before European contact.
- The plant contains glucotropaeolin, a glucosinolate that breaks down into benzyl isothiocyanate — the compound responsible for its peppery heat and potent antimicrobial properties.
- Traditionally used to treat respiratory infections, coughs, bronchitis, and urinary tract infections.
- Has demonstrated antibiotic activity — studied as a natural alternative to synthetic antibiotics for respiratory and urinary infections.
- Used topically for wound healing, scalp health, and hair growth stimulation.
- The juice of the leaves has been applied as a mild antiseptic.
- Used in European herbal medicine since the 17th century as a blood purifier and immune tonic.

NUTRITIONAL & PHYTOCHEMICAL PROFILE

- Nasturtium is surprisingly nutritious:
  - Vitamin C: Very high — leaves and flowers are excellent sources
  - Vitamin A / Lutein & Zeaxanthin: Important for eye health
  - Iron, Calcium, and Phosphorus: Present in useful amounts
  - Glucotropaeolin: A glucosinolate with antimicrobial and anticancer research interest
  - Benzyl isothiocyanate: Potent natural antibiotic compound
  - Flavonoids and carotenoids: Antioxidants responsible for the vivid flower colors
  - Quercetin and Kaempferol: Anti-inflammatory flavonoids

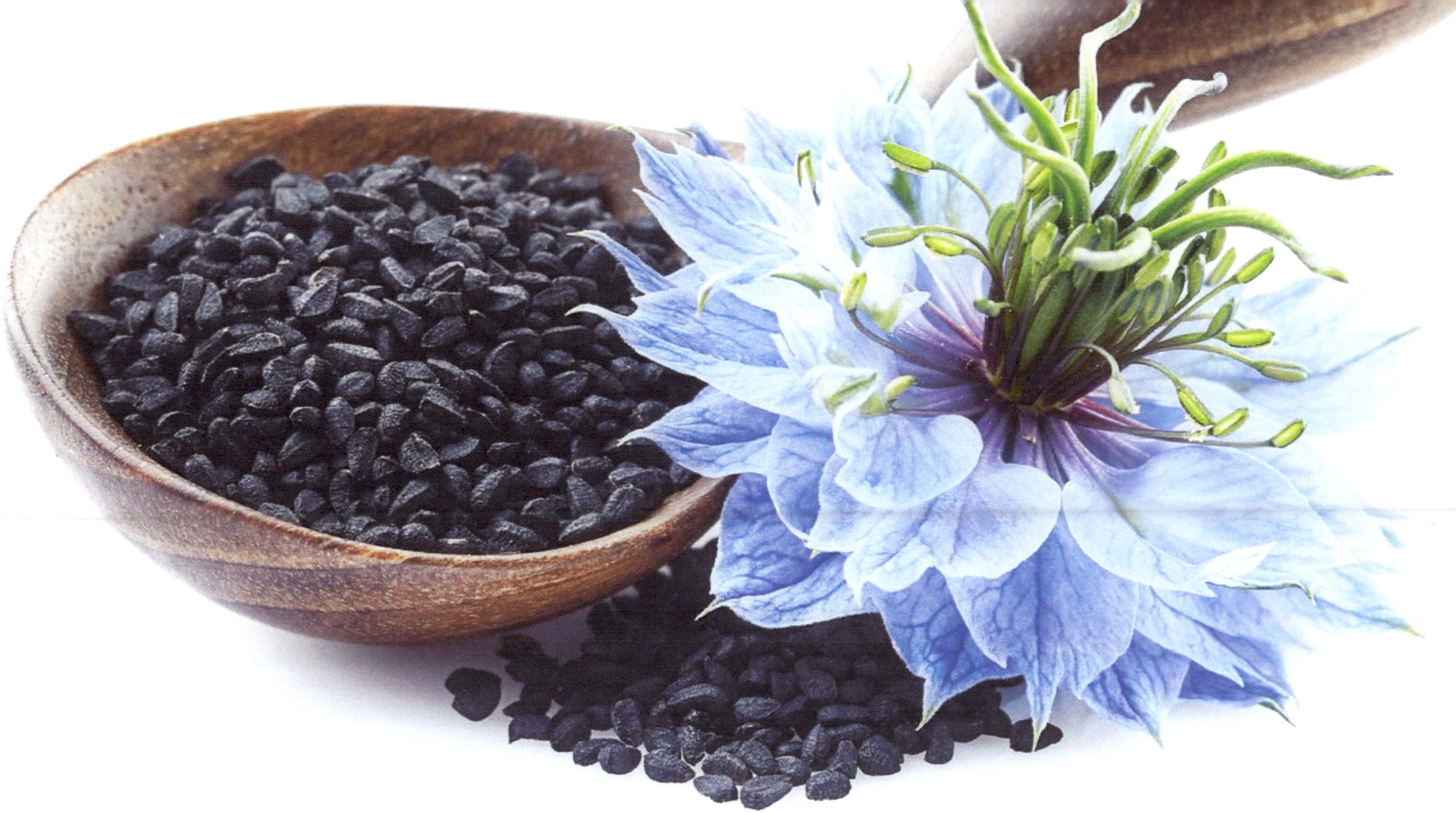

NIGELLA (NIGELLA SATIVA)

Common names include Black seed, Black Cumin, Black Caraway etc.

NIGELLA SATIVA (CULINARY)

- Leaves: Finely divided, feathery, thread-like — giving a delicate, lacy appearance.
- Flowers: Pale blue-white or whitish, five-petaled, with a somewhat star-like shape; delicate and elegant.
- Seed pods: Inflated, balloon-like capsules that split open to release small, angular, jet-black seeds with a rough, matte surface.
- Seeds: Tiny, about 2–3 mm, three-cornered, intensely black — the most commercially important part of the plant.

CULINARY USES

- The seeds of Nigella sativa have a complex, warm, slightly bitter, peppery flavor with notes of onion, oregano, and black pepper.
- Widely used in South Asian, Middle Eastern, North African, and Eastern European cuisines.
- Sprinkled on naan bread, flatbreads, and bagels — a defining flavor of many traditional breads.
- Used in Indian spice blends — notably PanchPhoron (Bengali five-spice), where it is a key ingredient.
- Added to pickles, chutneys, curries, lentil dishes, and vegetable stir-fries.
- Used to flavor cheeses in some Eastern European and Middle Eastern traditions.
- Common in Egyptian and Turkish spice markets.
- Seeds can be lightly dry-roasted to enhance their nutty, aromatic depth.

MEDICINAL & TRADITIONAL USES:

- Nigella sativa has one of the richest histories in herbal and traditional medicine of any plant on earth.
- The seeds contain thymoquinone — the principal bioactive compound, widely studied for its therapeutic properties.
- Mentioned in the Hadith (sayings of the Prophet Muhammad) as "a remedy for every disease except death" — making it one of the most revered plants in Islamic medicine (Tibb al-Nabawi).
- Used in Ayurveda for thousands of years to treat digestive, respiratory, and inflammatory conditions.
- Referenced in ancient Egyptian medical texts — seeds were found in the tomb of Tutankhamun.
- Also noted by the ancient Greek physician Dioscorides in De Materia Medica.
- Modern research has identified the following potential therapeutic properties of thymoquinone and the seed oil:
    - Anti-inflammatory
    - Antimicrobial and antifungal
    - Antioxidant
    - Immunomodulatory (supports immune function)
    - Antidiabetics (may help regulate blood sugar)
    - Bronchodilator (used for asthma and respiratory conditions)
    - Anti-cancer (under active research)
- Commonly consumed as black seed oil — taken directly or mixed into honey.
- Used topically for skin conditions, hair growth, and scalp health.

NUTRITIONAL & PHYTOCHEMICAL PROFILE

- Nigella sativa seeds are rich in:
    - Thymoquinone: Primary bioactive compound; powerful antioxidant and anti-inflammatory
    - Fixed oils: Linoleic acid (omega-6), oleic acid, palmitic acid
    - Volatile oils: Thymol, carvacrol, p-cymene
    - Proteins and amino acids
    - Dietary fiber
    - Vitamins: B1, B2, B3, and folate
    - Minerals: Iron, calcium, potassium, magnesium, zinc, and phosphorus
    - Alkaloids:Nigellicine and nigellidine

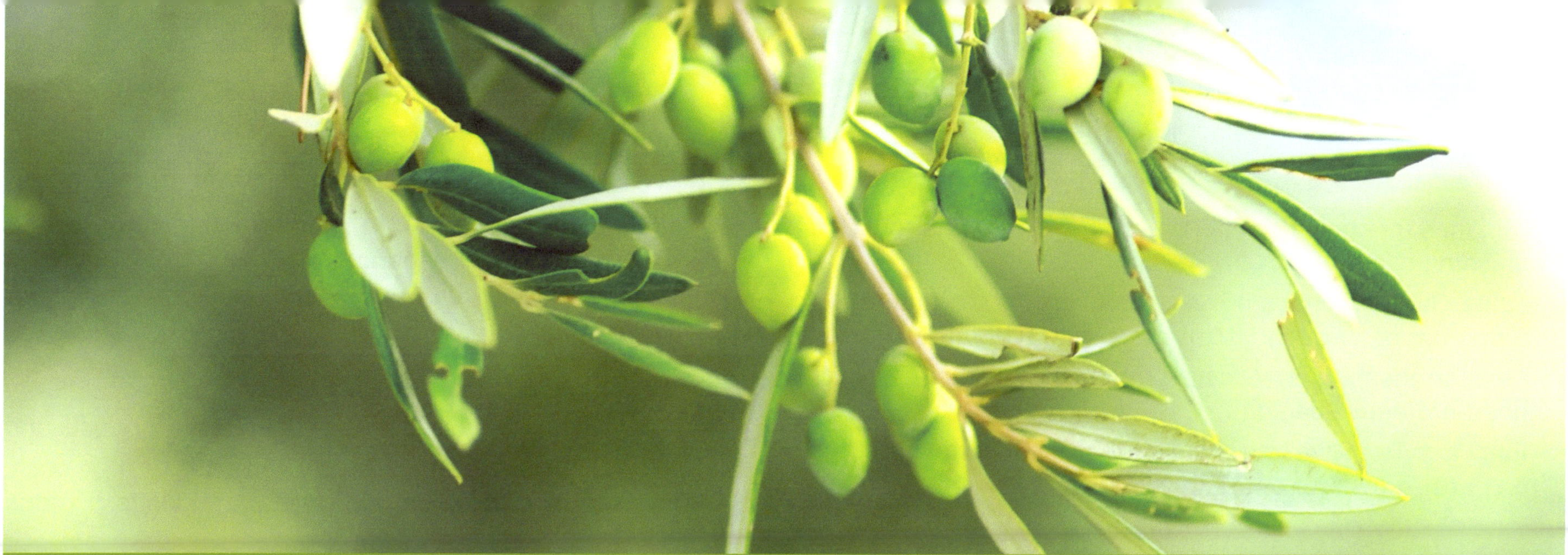

OLIVE (OLEA EUROPAEA)

GENERAL OVERVIEW

- Common Names: Olive (English), Zeytun (Arabic), Jaitun (Hindi), Oliva (Spanish, Italian)
- Native Range: Mediterranean Basin – Southern Europe, Northern Africa, and Western Asia
- Tree Type: Evergreen, long-lived (some trees live over 1,000 years)
- Fruit: Small oval drupe – green when unripe, turning purplish-black when mature

NUTRITIONAL & CHEMICAL COMPOSITION

- Main constituents of olive fruit and oil:
- Monounsaturated fatty acids (MUFA): Especially oleic acid (55–83%)
- Polyphenols: Oleuropein, hydroxytyrosol, tyrosol
- Vitamin E (tocopherols) – antioxidant
- Phytosterols: β-sitosterol
- Squalene: A natural antioxidant compound
- Small amounts of Omega-3 and Omega-6 fatty acids

MAJOR TYPES & FORMS

- Olive Fruit: Green (unripe) or black (ripe), eaten whole or pickled.
- Olive Oil: Extracted by cold-pressing the fruit; grades include:
    - Extra Virgin Olive Oil (EVOO): First cold press, highest quality
    - Virgin Olive Oil
    - Refined Olive Oil
    - Pomace Oil (from residual pulp)

CULINARY USES

- Oil: Used for cooking, salad dressings, marinades, and as a finishing oil.
- Table Olives: Consumed as appetizers or toppings after fermentation or curing (to remove natural bitterness).
- Mediterranean Diet: A central component known for its heart-protective benefits.
- Fun Fact: The olive tree is one of the oldest cultivated trees on Earth, grown for over 6,000 years.

B. MEDICINAL & HEALTH USES

1. **Cardiovascular Health**

- Olive oil's monounsaturated fats lower LDL ("bad") cholesterol and raise HDL ("good") cholesterol.
- Reduces blood pressure and improves arterial function.

2. **Anti-Inflammatory & Antioxidant Effects**

- Polyphenols like oleuropein and hydroxytyrosol combat oxidative stress, reducing inflammation and aging-related damage.

3. **Diabetes Support**

- Helps improve insulin sensitivity and control blood sugar levels.

4. **Digestive Health**

- Stimulates bile flow and supports liver function.
- Mildly laxative; helps regulate bowel movements.

5. **Skin & Hair**

- Olive oil nourishes and moisturizes the skin.
- Used in cosmetic products — soaps, creams, and hair treatments.
- Vitamin E helps repair and protect skin from UV damage.

6. **Immune Support**

- Regular consumption enhances body immunity and may lower risk of certain chronic diseases.

C. TRADITIONAL & RELIGIOUS SIGNIFICANCE

- Biblical & Religious Symbolism:
  - In the Bible, the olive branch symbolizes peace and reconciliation (Genesis 8:11 – Noah's dove).
  - Olive oil used for anointing priests and kings (Exodus 30:24).
  - In the New Testament, olive oil represents the Holy Spirit and healing.
- • Cultural Symbol: Peace, prosperity, and divine blessing.

OLIVE LEAF & ITS USES

- Olive leaf extract contains oleuropein, which has strong antibacterial, antiviral, and antioxidant properties.

USED AS:

- A natural immune booster
- Supportive treatment for hypertension
- A remedy for infections and inflammation

OTHER USES

- Cosmetic industry: Soaps, shampoos, creams, and lotions.
- Wood: Olive wood is hard, beautiful, and used for carvings, kitchenware, and religious artifacts.
- Aromatherapy: Olive oil serves as a carrier oil for essential oils.

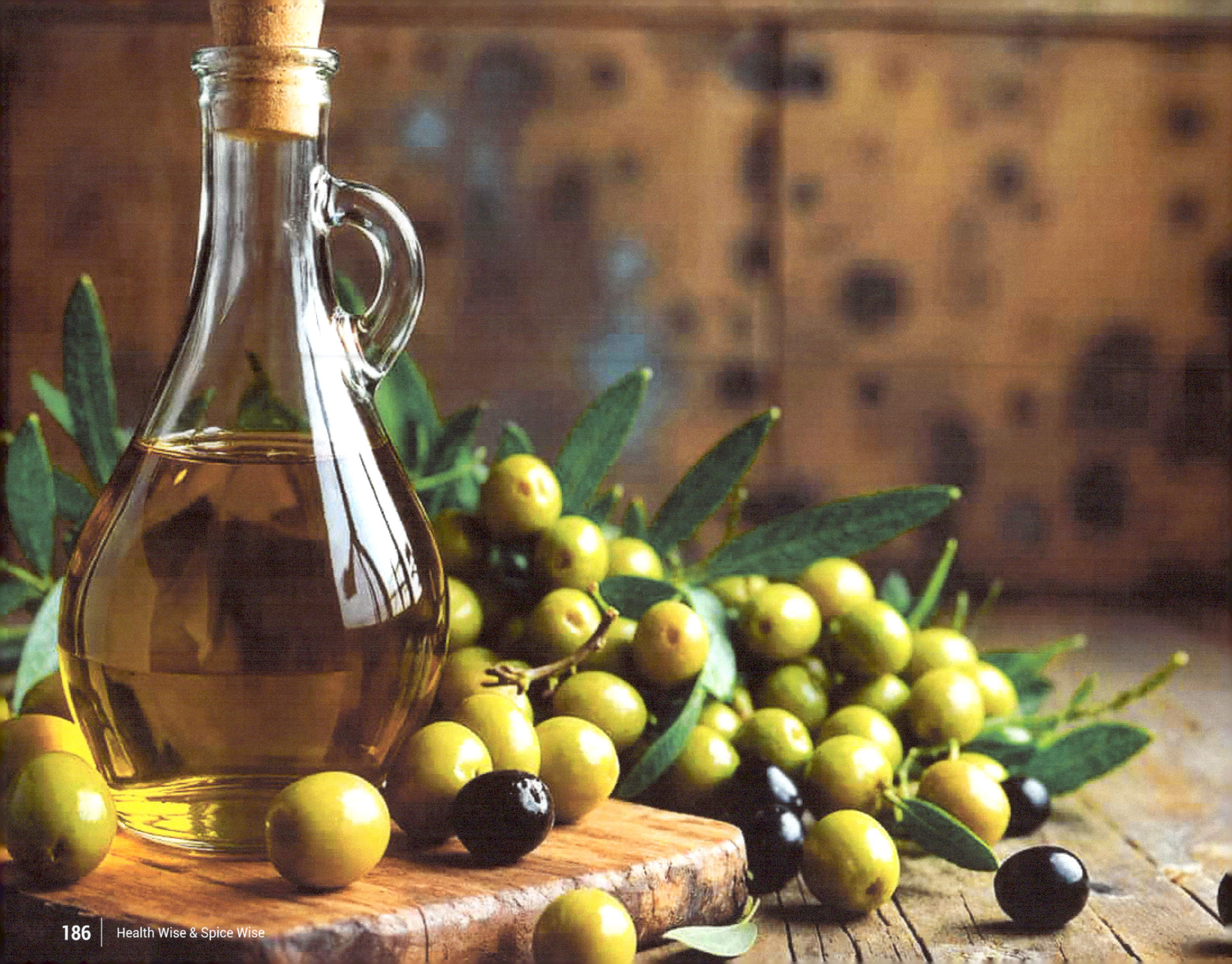

OLIVE OIL

TYPES OF OLIVE OIL

- Extra Virgin Olive Oil: Made from pure, cold-pressed olives, it has the highest quality, flavor, and nutrient content. Ideal for drizzling, salad dressings, and dipping.
- Virgin Olive Oil: Also made from cold-pressed olives but with slightly lower quality than extra virgin. Suitable for cooking and baking.
- Pure Olive Oil: A blend of virgin and refined olive oil, with a more neutral flavor. Good for frying and sautéing.
- Light Olive Oil: Refined olive oil with a light flavor and color. Suitable for high-heat cooking.

CULINARY USES

- Salad Dressings: Extra virgin olive oil is ideal for making flavorful salad dressings and vinaigrettes.
- Drizzling: Used as a finishing oil to drizzle over dishes like pasta, grilled vegetables, and bread.
- Cooking: Suitable for sautéing, roasting, grilling, and baking. The light and pure varieties are better for high-heat cooking.
- Marinades: Adds depth and richness to marinades for meats, poultry, and seafood.
- Dips: Mixed with herbs and spices to create delicious dipping oils for bread.
- Olive oil is a versatile and healthy ingredient that can enhance the flavor of many dishes.

HEALTH BENEFITS AND USES

Heart Health is the most well-studied benefit. Olive oil raises HDL ("good") cholesterol and lowers LDL ("bad") cholesterol, and is a cornerstone of the Mediterranean diet, which is strongly linked to reduced cardiovascular disease.

Anti-inflammatory effects come largely from oleocanthal, a compound that works similarly to ibuprofen by inhibiting the same enzymes involved in inflammation. This is thought to underline many of olive oil's broader health effects.

Brain health is an active research area. Studies suggest that regular consumption may lower the risk of cognitive decline and Alzheimer's disease, partly through reducing oxidative stress in brain tissue.

Blood sugar regulation — olive oil can slow glucose absorption and improve insulin sensitivity, making it beneficial for people managing or at risk of type 2 diabetes.

Cancer prevention is supported by several observational studies, particularly for breast and colorectal cancers. The antioxidants (polyphenols, vitamin E) help neutralize free radicals that can damage DNA.

Gut health is increasingly recognized — olive oil's polyphenols act as prebiotics, feeding beneficial gut bacteria and supporting a healthy microbiome.

Bone health — some research suggests that olive oil aids calcium absorption and may help preserve bone density, potentially reducing the risk of osteoporosis.

Skin and hair — used topically, it moisturizes deeply, reduces UV-related oxidative damage, and has antimicrobial properties useful for scalp health.

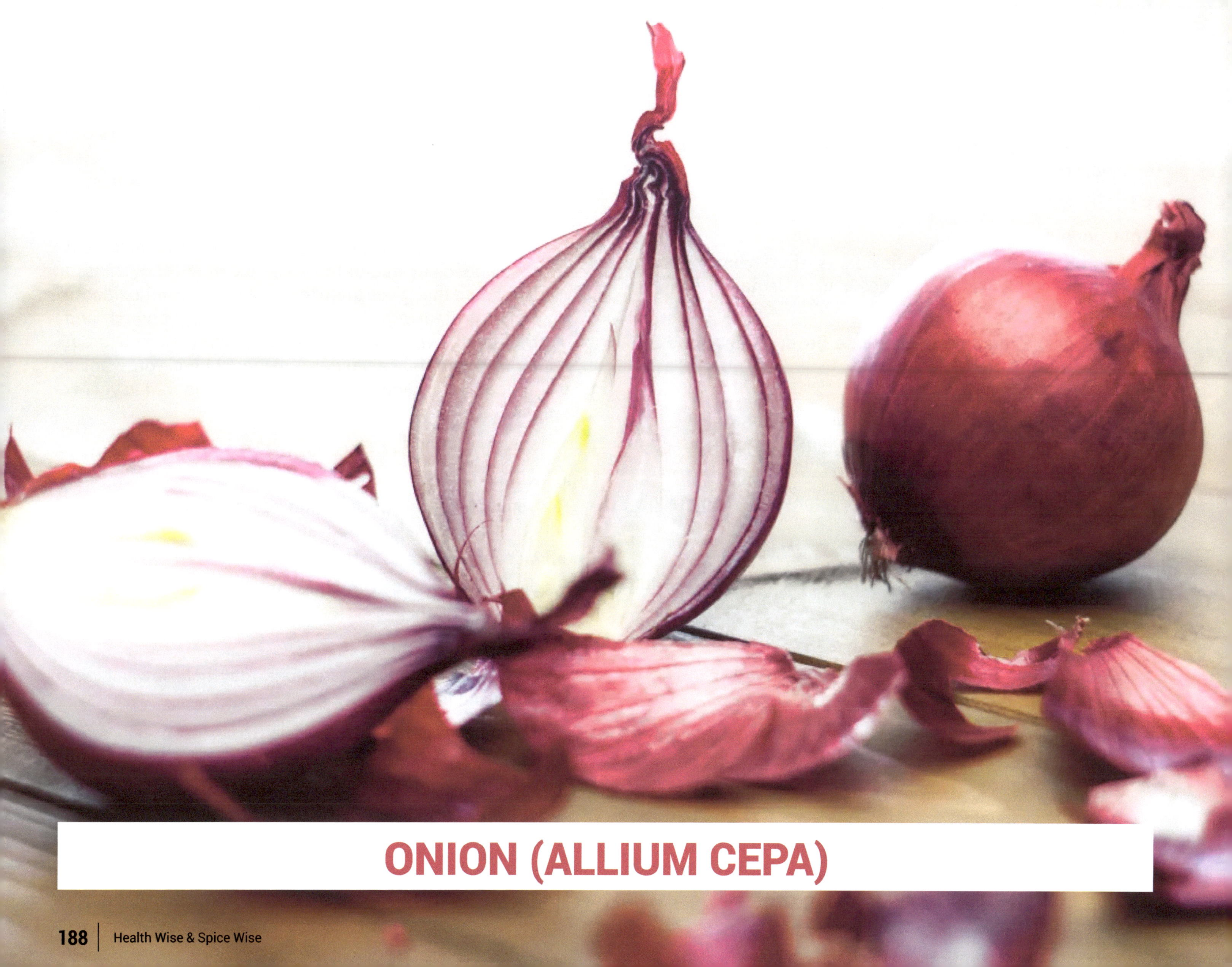

ONION (ALLIUM CEPA)

Red pearl onions are a variety of onions that have reddish-purple skin and are full of nutrients and antioxidants. They can be eaten raw or cooked, and are often used in grilling, roasting, and pickling.

PROPERTIES

Antioxidants

- Pearl onions contain antioxidants that help boost the immune system and protect cells from damage.

Anti-inflammatory

- Pearl onions contain quercetin, a flavonoid that has anti-inflammatory properties.

Vitamins and minerals

- Pearl onions are rich in vitamins C and B6, as well as essential minerals like potassium and manganese.

Anthocyanins

- Red onions contain anthocyanins, plant pigments that give red onions their deep color.

Flavor

- Red pearl onions are usually milder in flavor than white pearl onions.

USES

- Pearl onions can be used in stir fry mixes, salsas, sandwiches, and salads
- They can be grilled, roasted, or pickled
- The small bulbs are most commonly used whole

HEALTH BENEFITS

- Onions may help:
  - Regulate blood sugar levels
  - Improve digestive health
  - Reduce the risk of Alzheimer's disease
  - Lower the risk of colorectal cancer
  - Protect against diabetes and certain types of cancer

RED ONION

- Red onions are particularly good for their high antioxidant content, especially due to the presence of anthocyanins, a plant pigment that gives them their color; these antioxidants may help protect against certain cancers, diabetes, and contribute to overall heart health, making them a great addition to salads, salsas, and dishes where you want a vibrant color and slightly sharper flavor compared to yellow onions.

KEY POINTS ABOUT RED ONIONS:

High in antioxidants:

- Red onions contain more antioxidants than other onion varieties due to their anthocyanin content.

Potential cancer protection:

- Studies suggest that the antioxidants in red onions may help reduce the risk of certain cancers.

HEART HEALTH BENEFITS:

- The quercetin found in red onions may help lower blood pressure and improve heart health.

FLAVOR PROFILE:

- Red onions have a slightly sharper, spicier flavor compared to yellow onions, making them ideal for raw dishes like salads and salsas.

OREGANO (ORIGANUM VULGARE)

Oregano (Origanum vulgare) is a popular herb known for its pungent, aromatic flavor and numerous health benefits. Here are some key properties and health benefits of oregano:

NUTRITIONAL CONTENT

- Essential Oils: Contains essential oils such as carvacrol, thymol, and limonene.
- Vitamins and Minerals: Rich in vitamins A, C, E, and K, as well as B-complex vitamins. Also contains minerals like calcium, magnesium, iron, and manganese.
- Antioxidants: High in antioxidants like flavonoids and phenolic acids, which help protect against oxidative stress and damage.
- Fiber: Provides dietary fiber, aiding in digestion and promoting gut health.

HEALTH BENEFITS

- Antimicrobial Properties: Has strong antibacterial, antiviral, and antifungal properties, which help fight infections.
- Anti-inflammatory: Reduces inflammation and can help alleviate conditions like arthritis and muscle pain.
- Digestive Aid: Aids in digestion, relieves gas, and helps alleviate digestive issues like bloating and indigestion.
- Immune System Support: High vitamin C content helps boost the immune system and protect against infections.
- Respiratory Health: Helps relieve respiratory conditions such as coughs, colds, and bronchitis.
- Antioxidant Properties: Contains compounds that help neutralize free radicals, promoting overall health and reducing the risk of chronic diseases.
- Cardiovascular Health: Supports heart health by reducing blood pressure and cholesterol levels.
- Pain Relief: Has analgesic properties that help alleviate minor aches and pains.

USAGE

- Culinary Uses: Oregano is used to flavor a wide variety of dishes, including pizzas, pastas, soups, stews, and meat dishes. It's a staple in Mediterranean and Italian cuisine.
- Medicinal Uses: Consumed as a tea, tincture, or essential oil for its health benefits.
- Aromatherapy: Oregano essential oil is used in aromatherapy for its stimulating and clarifying effects.

Oregano is a versatile herb that not only enhances the flavor of your dishes but also offers numerous health benefits. Do you enjoy using oregano in your cooking, or do you have any favorite recipes that feature this herb?

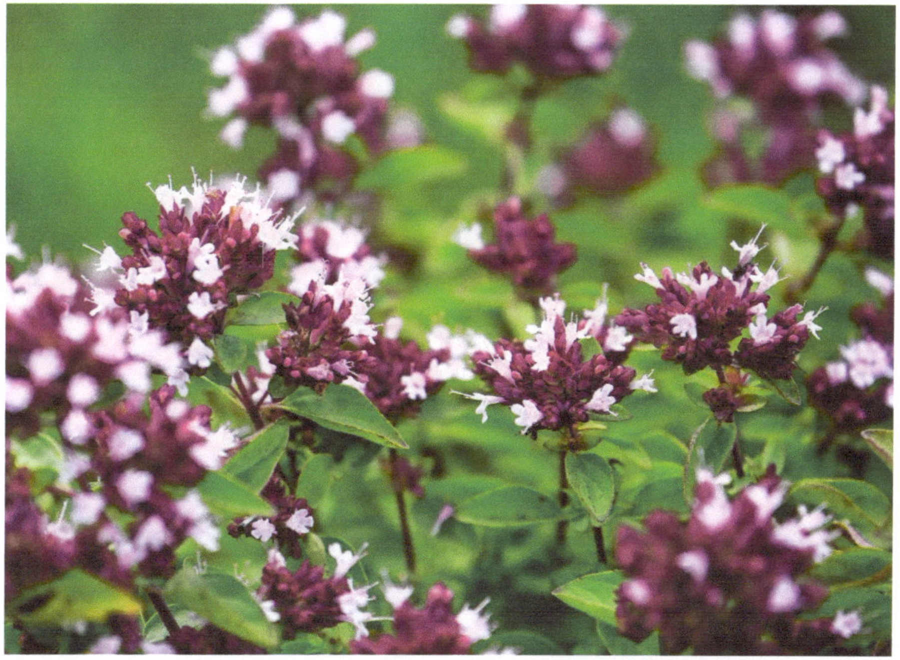

PARACRESS (SPILANTHES ACMELLA)

Paracress (Spilanthes acmella), also known as the toothache plant, is a medicinal herb prized for its tingling sensation and powerful therapeutic properties. It's used in traditional medicine, culinary applications, and skincare.

BOTANICAL OVERVIEW

- Scientific name: Spilanthes acmella (also known as Acmella oleracea)
- Family: Asteraceae
- Common names: Paracress, toothache plant, buzz buttons, electric daisy, jambu
- Appearance: Small, erect herb with broad leaves and distinctive gold-red flower heads
- Native origin: Likely Brazil, but cultivated widely in tropical and subtropical regions
- Key Bioactive Compound
- Spilanthol: Found in the roots, leaves, and flowers
- Responsible for the plant's tingling, numbing effect
- Offers analgesic, anti-inflammatory, antiseptic, and antimicrobial benefits

TRADITIONAL AND MEDICINAL USES

- Toothache relief: Chewing flower heads or leaves numbs pain
- Oral health: Treats mouth ulcers, gum infections, and stomatitis
- Digestive aid: Used for candida, thrush, and digestive discomfort
- Skin care: Treats fungal infections and supports anti-aging through collagen stimulation
- Anti-aging: Spilanthol helps reduce wrinkles and improve skin elasticity

CULINARY USES

- Leaves: Used raw or cooked in salads and stews
- Flower buds: Known for their grassy taste followed by a strong tingling sensation
- Flavoring agent: Used in chewing gum and tobacco in India

PHARMACOLOGICAL PROPERTIES

- Antimicrobial: Effective against bacteria like Streptococcus mutans, Staphylococcus aureus, and fungi like Candida albicans
- Anti-inflammatory: Reduces cytokine expression and supports wound healing
- Antiparasitic: Shows activity against Plasmodium species (malaria)

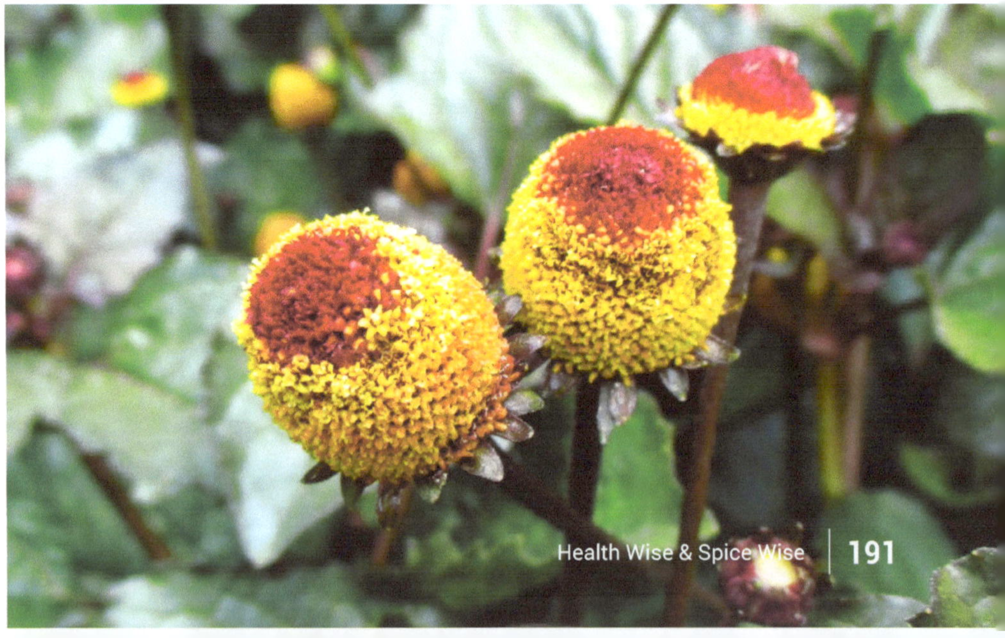

PERILLA (PERILLA FRUTESCENS)

- Perilla (Perilla frutescens) is a versatile herb from the mint family, widely used in Asian cuisine and traditional medicine for its aromatic leaves and health-promoting compounds.

Here's a detailed overview of this fascinating plant:

BOTANICAL OVERVIEW

- Scientific name: Perilla frutescens
- Family: Lamiaceae (mint family)
- Common names: Perilla, shiso (Japan), deulkkae (Korea), tía tô (Vietnam)
- Varieties:
  - P. frutescens var. crispa – crinkled leaves, often red or purple (shiso)
  - P. frutescens var. hirtella – lemon-scented variety
- Appearance: Oval, serrated leaves in green, red, or purple; aromatic with hints of mint, basil, and anise

KEY BIOACTIVE COMPOUNDS

- Perillaldehyde: Gives the plant its distinctive aroma
- Rosmarinic acid: Anti-inflammatory and antioxidant
- Omega-3 fatty acids: Found in perilla seeds, especially alpha-linolenic acid (ALA)

MEDICINAL AND HEALTH BENEFITS

- Anti-inflammatory: Helps reduce inflammation and allergic responses
- Antioxidant: Protects cells from oxidative stress
- Respiratory support: Used in traditional Chinese medicine for asthma and colds
- Digestive aid: Supports gut health and reduces bloating
- Skin health: Used in cosmetics for its soothing and anti-aging properties.

CULINARY USES

- Japan: Shiso leaves used in sushi, tempura, and pickles
- Korea: Deulkkae leaves wrap grilled meats; seeds used for oil and powder
- Vietnam: Tía tô leaves added to soups and salads
- Perilla oil: Nutty flavor, rich in omega-3s, used in cooking and dressings.

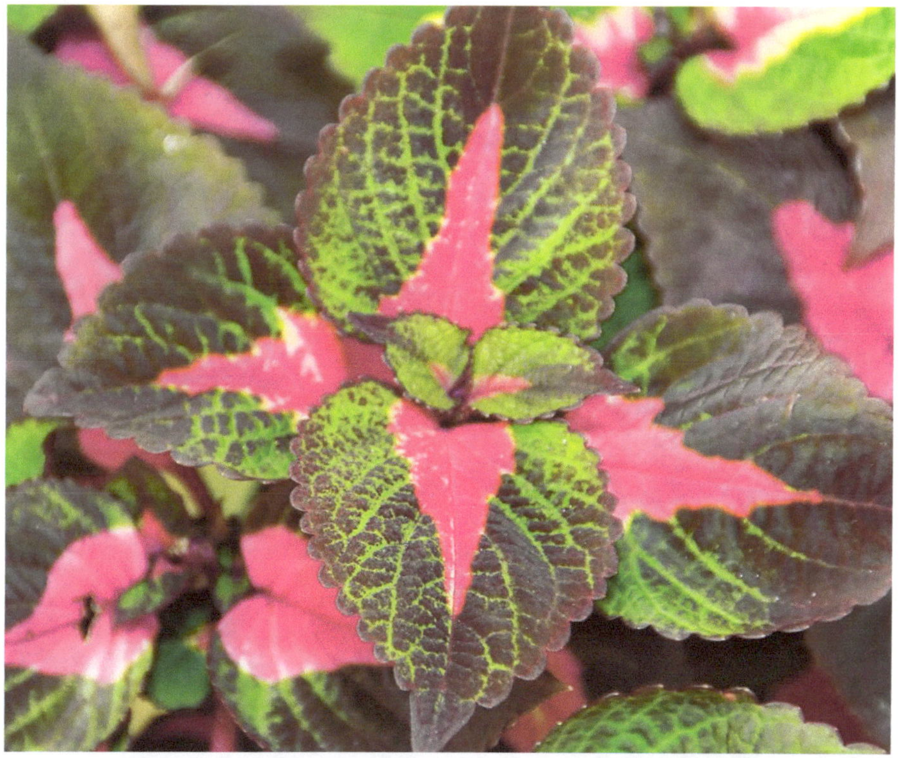

PINK PEPPER (SCHINUS TEREBINTHIFOLIUS)

Pink peppercorns come from the berries of the Schinus genus and are prized for their vibrant color, delicate heat, and aromatic complexity. Though not true pepper, they're widely used in culinary and traditional medicinal contexts.

Here's a detailed overview of pink pepper:

BOTANICAL OVERVIEW

- Scientific names: Schinus molle (Peruvian pepper tree), Schinus terebinthifolia (Brazilian pepper tree)
- Family: Anacardiaceae (same family as cashews and poison ivy)
- Common names: Pink peppercorn, false pepper, baie rose
- Appearance: Small, round berries with a rosy-pink hue; trees are evergreen and often ornamental

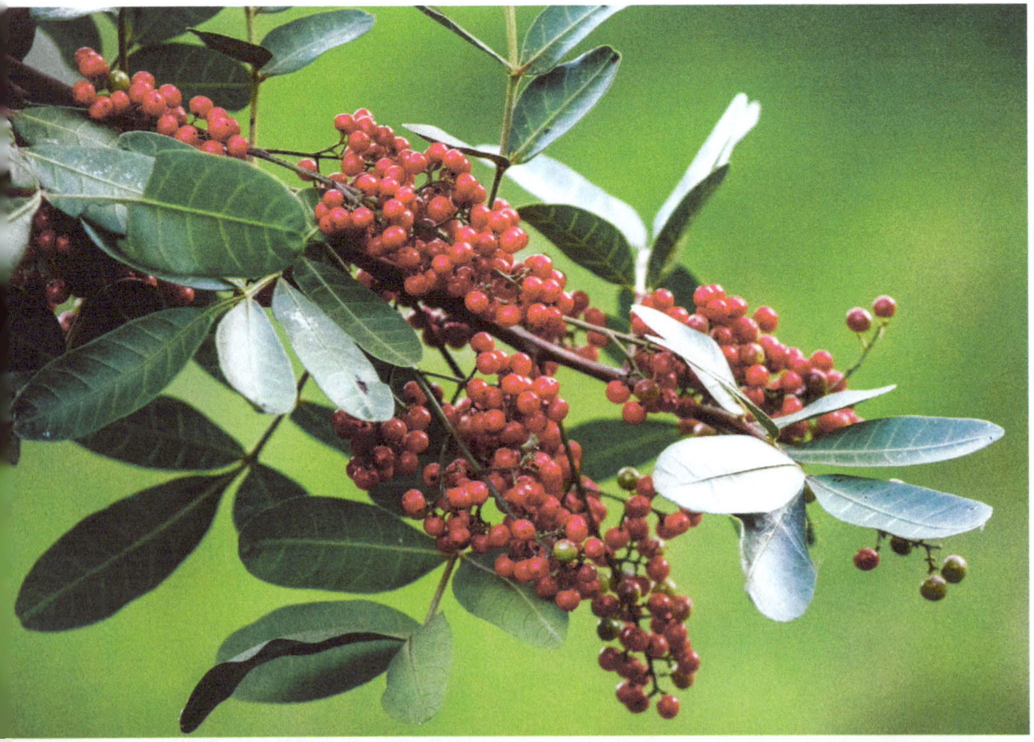

Essential oils: Includes pinene and limonene

- Tannins and resins: Offer mild antimicrobial and anti-inflammatory properties
- Fatty acids: Contains omega-6 (linoleic acid) and omega-9 (oleic acid) in small amounts

MEDICINAL AND TRADITIONAL USES

- Antiseptic and wound healing: Used in traditional medicine to treat infections and skin conditions
- Digestive aid: Helps relieve bloating and mild gastrointestinal discomfort
- Diuretic and antidepressant: Historically used in Andean cultures for urinary and mood-related issues
- Toothache relief: Bark and berries used in folk remedies

CULINARY USES

- Flavor profile: Mild fruity heat, subtle sweetness, with citrus and floral notes
- Applications:
  - Sprinkled on salads, meats, and desserts for color and aroma
  - Blended with black, white, and green peppercorns in gourmet mixes
  - Used in vinaigrettes, sauces, and even chocolates

POPPY (PAPAVER SOMNIFERUM)

BOTANICAL OVERVIEW

- Scientific name:Papaver somniferum (opium poppy)
- Family: Papaveraceae
- Common types: Opium poppy, corn poppy (Papaver rhoeas), oriental poppy (Papaver orientale), California poppy (Eschscholzia californica)
- Appearance: Delicate flowers in red, white, pink, or purple; seed pods contain tiny black or blue seeds

CULINARY USES

- Poppy seeds are used in baking (bagels, muffins, cakes) for their nutty flavor and crunchy texture.
- Poppy seed oil is valued for its light taste and high smoke point, used in dressings and marinades.
- Seeds are also added to salads, curries, and traditional dishes across Europe, India, and the Middle East.

MEDICINAL USES

- Opium alkaloids (morphine, codeine, thebaine) are extracted from Papaver somniferum for:
  - Pain relief: Morphine is a potent analgesic used post-surgery and for chronic pain.
  - Cough suppression: Codeine is used in cough syrups and mild pain medications.
  - Sedation and sleep aid: Opium has historically been used to treat insomnia.
- California poppy is used in herbal medicine for its mild sedative and anti-anxiety effects.

ORNAMENTAL USES

- Poppies are popular in gardens for their vibrant blooms and delicate petals.
- Varieties like oriental and corn poppies are grown for aesthetic appeal and pollinator attraction.

RECREATIONAL AND REGULATORY NOTES

- Opium has a long history of recreational use due to its euphoric effects, but it is highly addictive and regulated in most countries.
- Cultivation of opium poppy is controlled due to its potential for misuse.

OTHER APPLICATIONS

- Traditional remedies: Used in folk medicine for calming nerves and treating respiratory issues.

RECREATIONAL AND REGULATORY NOTES

- Opium has a long history of recreational use due to its euphoric effects, but it is highly addictive and regulated in most countries.
- Cultivation of opium poppy is controlled due to its potential for misuse.

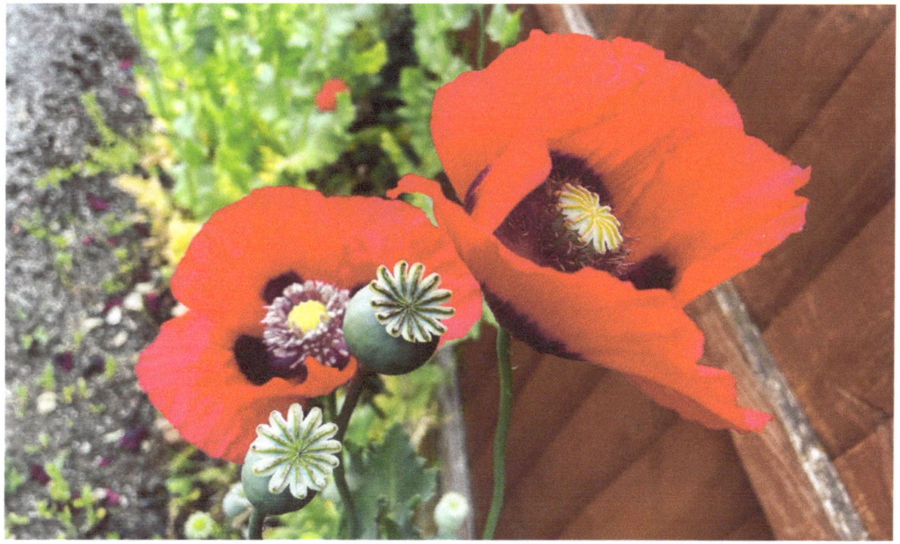

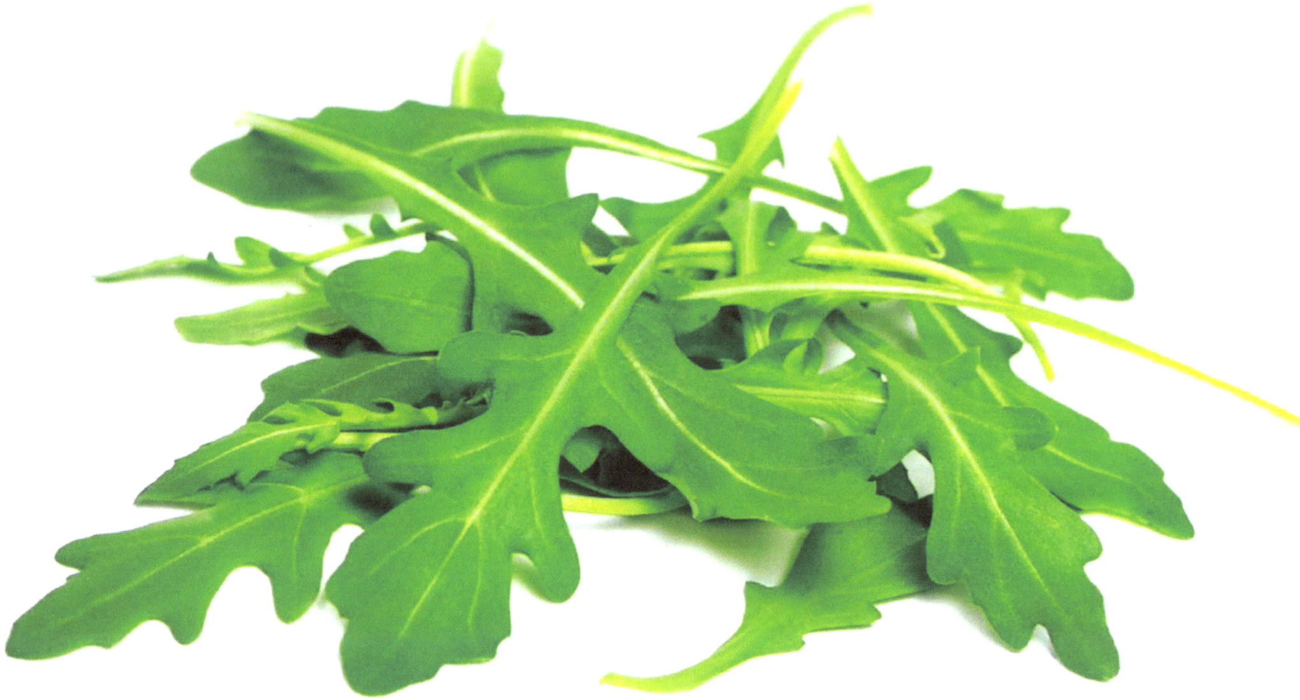

ROCKET (ERUCA SATIVA)

BOTANICAL BACKGROUND

- Also called arugula or rucola.
- Belongs to the Brassicaceae (mustard) family.
- Annual leafy green native to the Mediterranean.
- Distinct peppery, slightly bitter flavor.

COMMON CULINARY APPLICATIONS

- Used fresh in salads, sandwiches, and wraps.
- Added to pasta, pizzas, and risottos.
- Blended into pestos and dressings.

TYPES / VARIETIES

- Eruca sativa (salad rocket): common, mild flavor.
- Wild rocket (Diplotaxis tenuifolia): stronger, spicier taste.
- Baby rocket: tender, less pungent leaves.

CULINARY USES

- Eaten raw as salad greens.
- Lightly wilted in pasta or sautéed dishes.
- Used as a garnish for meats and seafood.

HEALTH BENEFITS

- • Rich in vitamins A, C, and K.

ROSE (ROSA DAMASCENA)

BOTANICAL BACKGROUND

- Deciduous shrub, family Rosaceae.
- Native to the Middle East; widely cultivated in Europe, India, and Iran.
- Produces fragrant pink to red flowers; petals and rose hips are used.
- Known for aromatic oils and culinary extracts.

COMMON CULINARY APPLICATIONS

- Rose water and rose petals used in desserts, sweets, and beverages.
- Added to syrups, jams, jellies, and baked goods.
- Used to flavor teas, drinks, and festive dishes.

TYPES / VARIETIES

- Damask Rose (Rosa damascena) – highly aromatic, used for oil and culinary purposes.
- Cabbage Rose (Rosa centifolia) – used in perfumes and desserts.
- Tea Rose (Rosa hybrida) – ornamental and sometimes culinary use.

CULINARY USES

- Flavoring for desserts, cakes, and pastries.
- Infused in beverages, teas, and milk-based drinks.
- Used in jams, jellies, and traditional sweets.

HEALTH BENEFITS

- Rich in antioxidants; supports skin and overall health.
- Possesses anti-inflammatory and antimicrobial properties.
- Traditionally used for digestion, relaxation, and stress relief.
- May support cardiovascular health and hormonal balance.

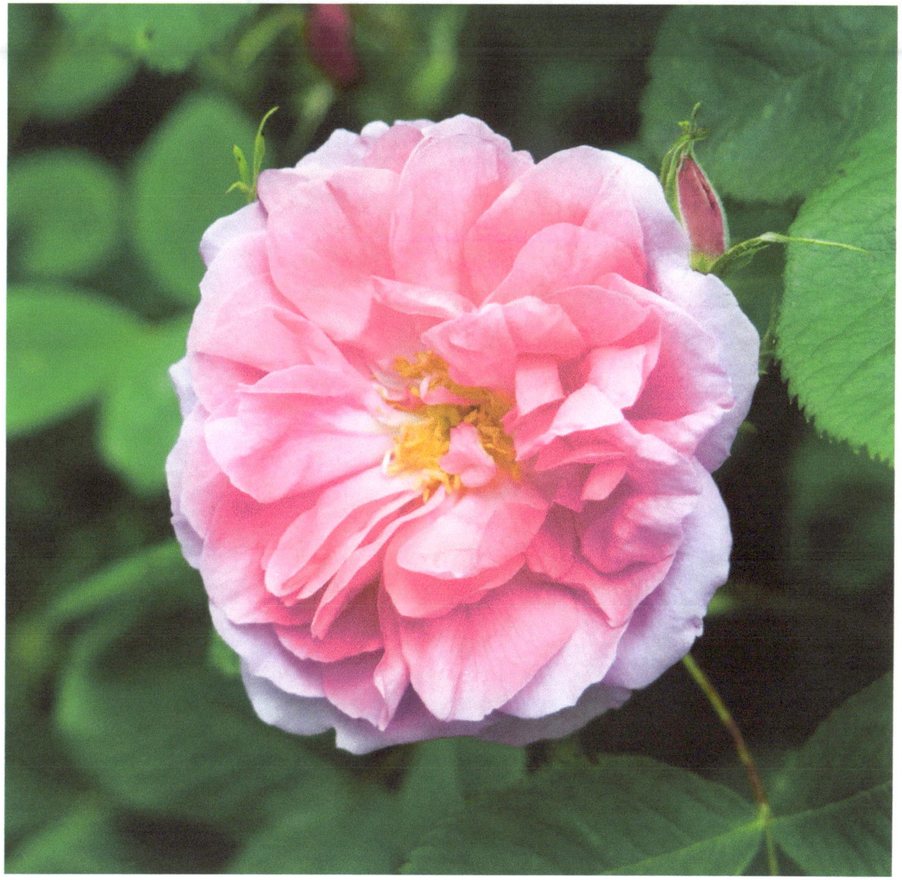

ROSEMARY (ROSMARINUS OFFICINALIS)

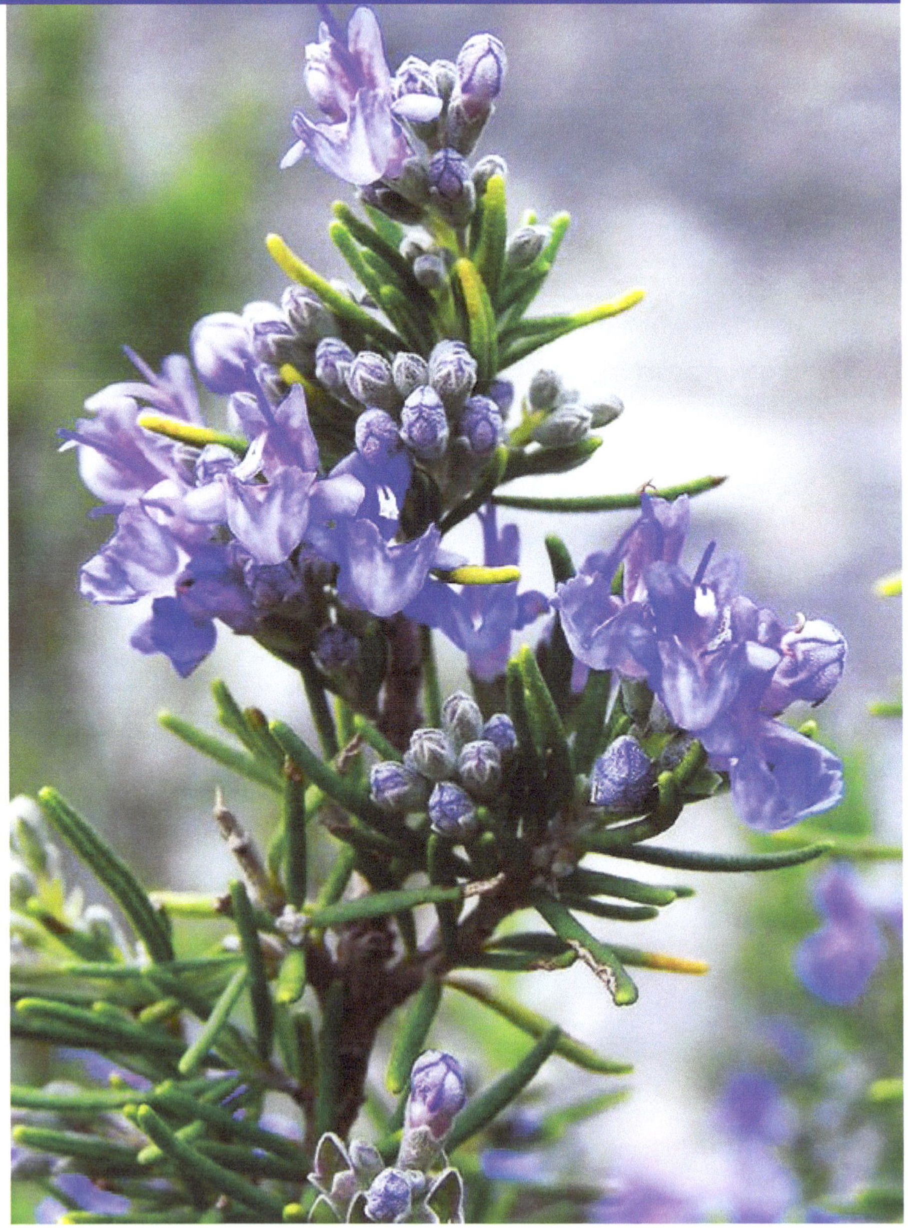

BOTANICAL BACKGROUND

- Woody, evergreen perennial shrub.
- Member of the mint family (Lamiaceae).
- Native to the Mediterranean region.
- Needle-like leaves, strong pine-like aroma.

COMMON CULINARY APPLICATIONS

- Seasoning for roasted meats (lamb, chicken, pork).
- Flavoring for potatoes, bread, soups, and stews.
- Infused into oils, vinegars, and marinades.

TYPES / VARIETIES

- R. officinalis (common rosemary).
- 'Tuscan Blue' – tall, aromatic.
- 'Prostratus' – creeping variety.
- 'Arp' – cold-hardy type.

CULINARY USES

- Fresh or dried leaves used in cooking.
- Add whole sprigs during roasting or grilling.
- Pairs with garlic, lemon, and olive oil.

HEALTH BENEFITS

- Rich in antioxidants and anti-inflammatory compounds.
- May improve memory and concentration.
- Supports digestion and circulation.

RUE (RUTA GRAVEOLENS)

BOTANICAL BACKGROUND

- Perennial evergreen shrub, member of the Rutaceae family.
- Native to Southern Europe and the Mediterranean.
- Strong, bitter aroma with bluish-green leaves.
- Historically used in folk medicine and rituals.

COMMON CULINARY APPLICATIONS

- Used sparingly due to bitterness and toxicity in high doses.
- Traditional flavoring in Ethiopian cuisine (coffee & beverages).
- Occasionally added to grappa or liqueurs in Italy.

TYPES / VARIETIES

- Common Rue (Ruta graveolens) – culinary and medicinal.
- Ornamental Rue varieties used mainly for gardens.

CULINARY USES

- Fresh leaves used in very small amounts to flavor food or drink.
- Infused in oils, wines, or spirits for bitterness.
- Pairs with strong flavors (garlic, chili, coffee).

HEALTH BENEFITS

- Traditionally used for digestion and as an anti-inflammatory.
- Contains antioxidants and alkaloids.
- Historically valued for reducing anxiety and muscle spasms.
- Must be used with caution – high doses can be toxic.

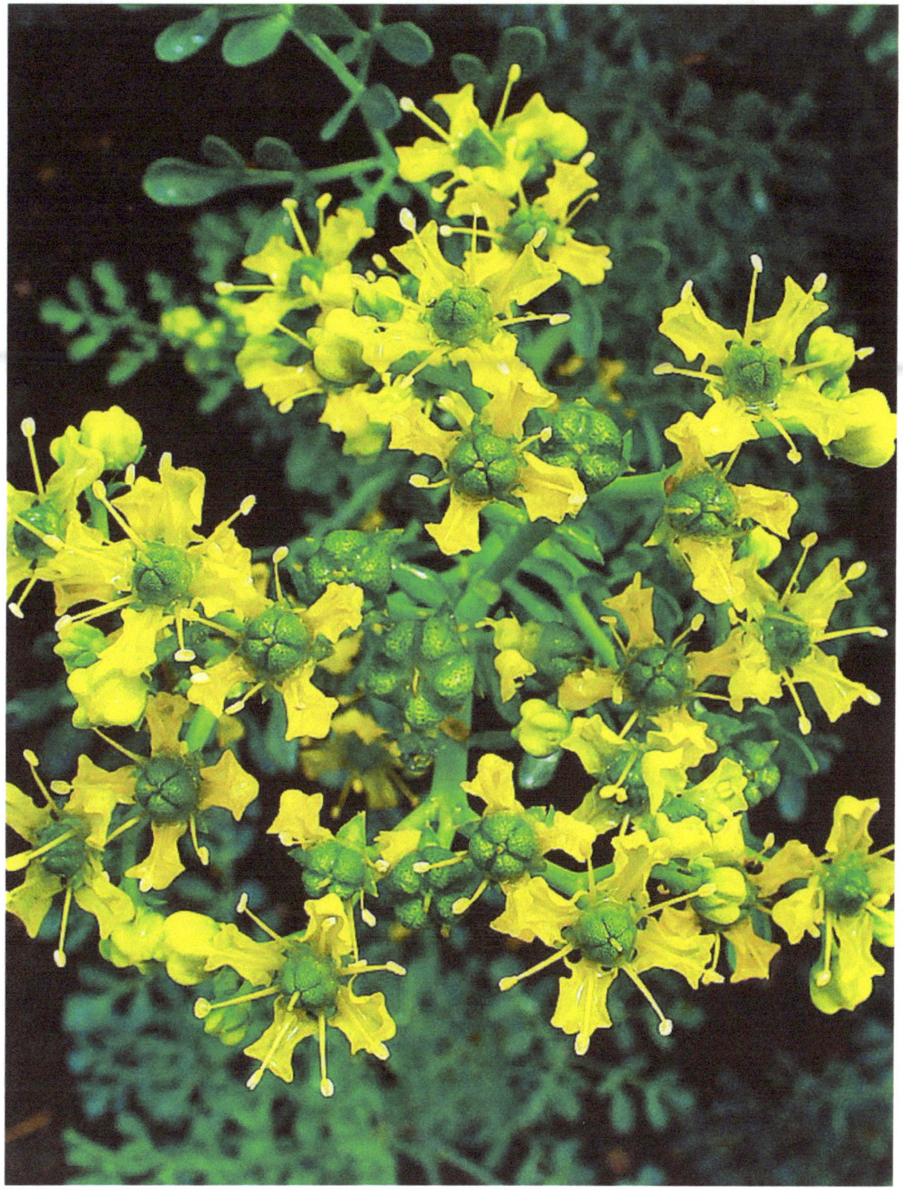

SAFFRON (CROCUS SATIVUS)

BOTANICAL BACKGROUND

- Perennial in Iridaceae.
- Native to SW Asia; grown in Iran, Kashmir, Spain, Greece.
- Spice from dried red stigmas; very labor-intensive harvest.

CULINARY APPLICATIONS

- Flavoring & coloring agent.
- Key in Mediterranean, Middle Eastern, Indian dishes.
- Used in paella, risotto, biryani, bouillabaisse.

TYPES / VARIETIES

- Kashmiri – deep red, aromatic, prized.
- Spanish (La Mancha) – mild, sweet.
- Iranian – largest production, intense.
- Greek (Kozani) – strong aroma, high quality.

CULINARY USES

- Soaked in warm liquid before use.
- Enhances rice, stews, desserts, teas.
- Used in syrups, sweets, liqueurs.

HEALTH BENEFITS

- Rich in antioxidants.
- May lift mood, ease anxiety.
- Supports digestion & appetite.
- Traditionally used for memory, PMS relief.

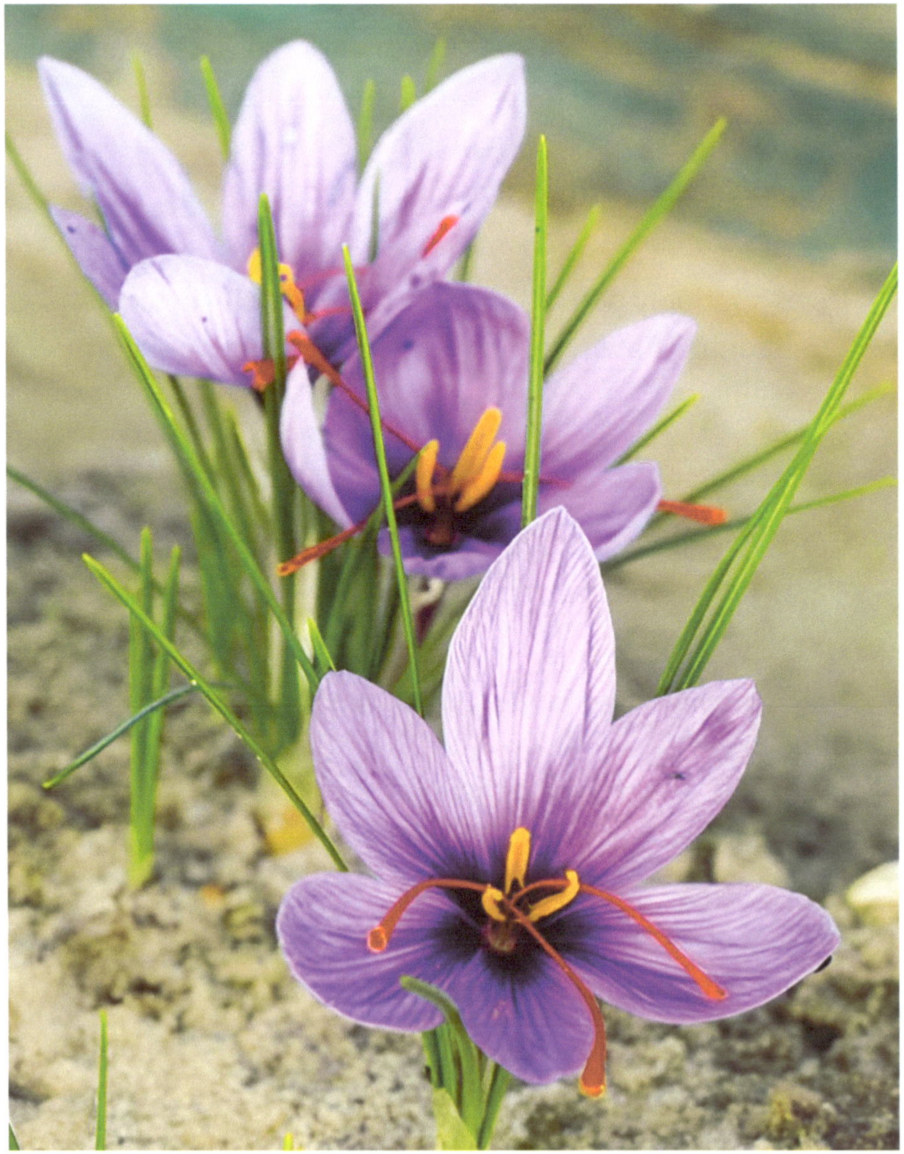

SAGE (SALVIA OFFICINALIS)

Sage (Salvia officinalis) is a popular herb known for its culinary, medicinal, and ornamental uses. Here are some of its key properties and health benefits:

NUTRITIONAL CONTENT

- Essential Oils: Sage contains essential oils such as thujone, camphor, cineole, and borneol.
- Vitamins and Minerals: It's rich in vitamins A, C, K, and B-complex vitamins, as well as minerals like calcium, iron, magnesium, and manganese.
- Antioxidants: Contains potent antioxidants like rosmarinic acid, which help protect cells from damage.

HEALTH BENEFITS

- Cognitive Health: Sage is known to improve memory and brain function, which can be beneficial for conditions like Alzheimer's disease.
- Anti-inflammatory: Helps reduce inflammation and alleviate conditions like arthritis.
- Antimicrobial Properties: Has antiseptic and antimicrobial properties that help fight infections.
- Digestive Aid: Aids in digestion, relieves stomach cramps, and reduces bloating.
- Menopausal Symptoms: Helps alleviate symptoms of menopause, such as hot flashes and night sweats.
- Oral Health: Used in mouth rinses to promote oral health and treat conditions like gingivitis and sore throat.
- Blood Sugar Regulation: Can help regulate blood sugar levels, which is beneficial for people with diabetes.
- Skin Health: Applied topically, sage can help with conditions like acne and eczema.

USAGE

- Culinary Uses: Sage leaves are used to flavor meats, sausages, stuffing, and sauces. It's a staple in many culinary traditions.
- Medicinal Uses: Consumed as a tea, tincture, or essential oil for its health benefits.
- Aromatherapy: Sage essential oil is used in aromatherapy for its calming and clarifying scent.

Sage is a versatile herb with a rich history of use in various cultural practices. Do you enjoy using sage in your cooking or for its health benefits?

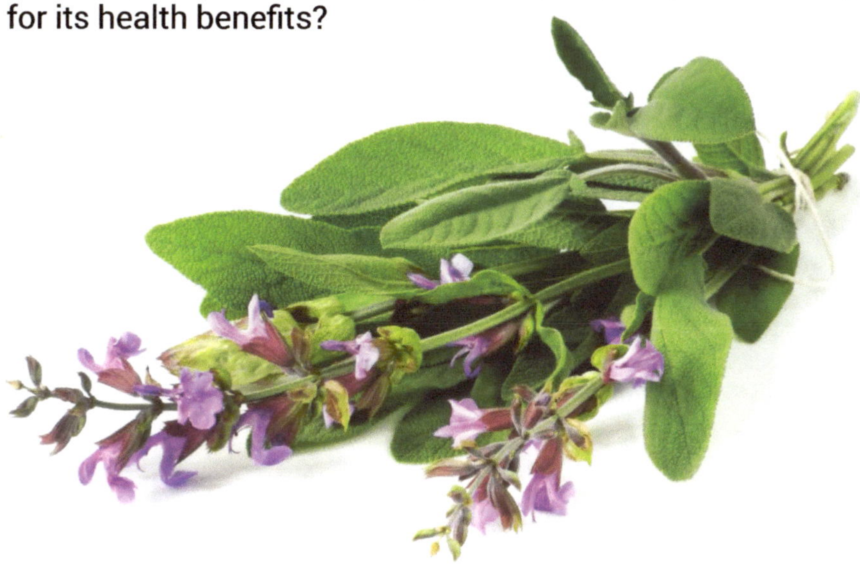

SAVORY (SATUREJA HORTENSIS)

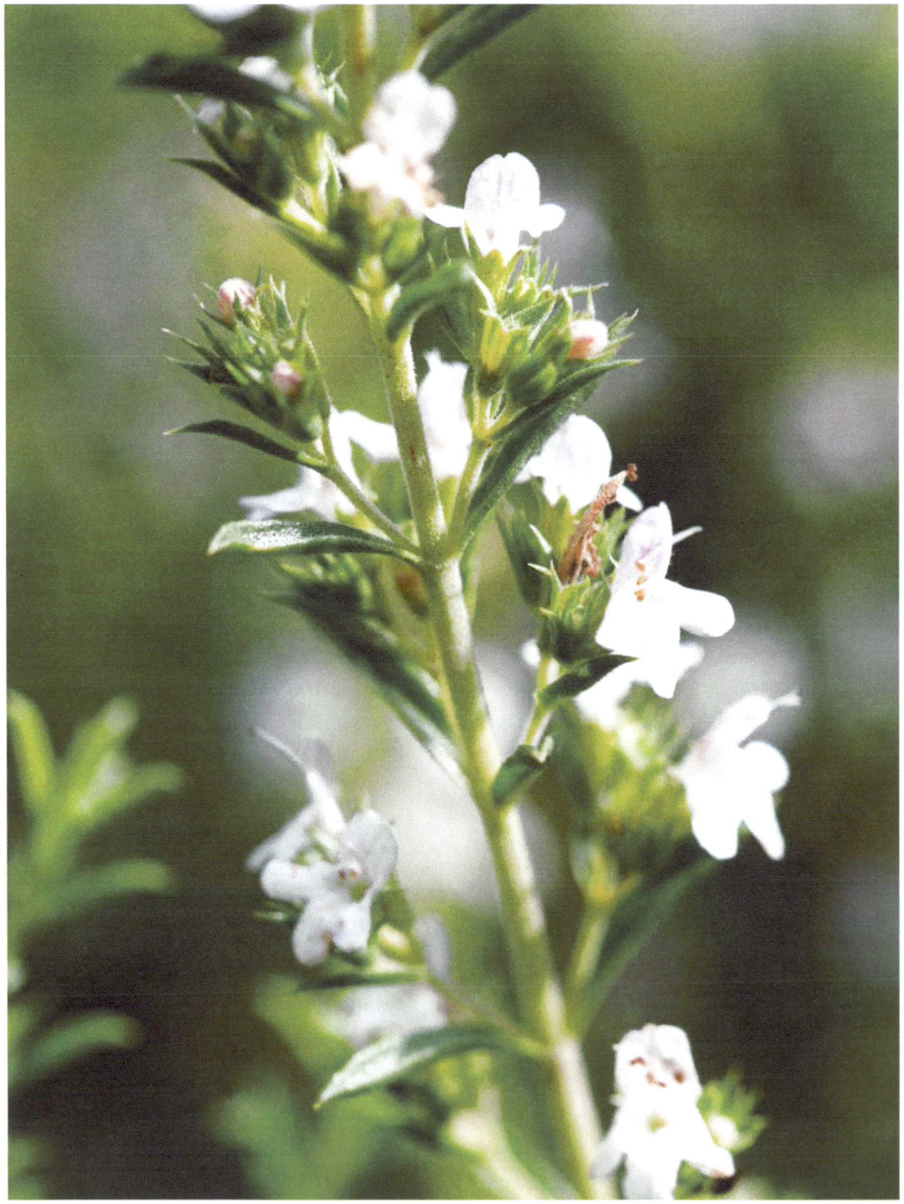

- Annual herb in the mint family (Lamiaceae).
- Native to the Eastern Mediterranean and Western Asia.
- Known as summer savory; aromatic with peppery taste.
- Related to winter savory (Satureja montana), a perennial.

COMMON CULINARY APPLICATIONS

- Used fresh or dried as seasoning.
- Popular in Mediterranean and Balkan cuisines.
- Classic herb for bean dishes, soups, and sausages.
- Often included in spice blends (e.g., Herbes de Provence).

TYPES / VARIETIES

- Summer Savory (S. hortensis) – mild, delicate, widely used.
- Winter Savory (S. montana) – stronger, slightly bitter, evergreen.

CULINARY USES

- Enhances meats, stews, and roasted vegetables.
- Combines well with thyme, rosemary, and parsley.
- Used in marinades, stuffings, and bread.
- Traditional seasoning for beans to reduce gas.

HEALTH BENEFITS

- Contains antioxidants and essential oils.
- Traditionally used for digestive issues and sore throats.
- Mild antibacterial and anti-inflammatory properties.

SCREW PINE (PANDANUS) FLOWER (PANDANUS ODORATISSIMUS)

BOTANICAL BACKGROUND

- Tropical perennial plant, family Pandanaceae.
- Native to Southeast Asia and the Indian subcontinent.
- Produces long, narrow, fragrant leaves and distinctive flowers.
- Flowers are large, cream to yellow, and highly aromatic.
- Grown for ornamental, culinary, and traditional medicinal uses.

COMMON CULINARY APPLICATIONS

- Leaves and flowers used for flavoring rice, desserts, and beverages.
- Infused in coconut milk, sweets, and traditional cakes.
- Used to wrap foods for steaming, imparting aroma.
- Extracts and syrups made for flavoring drinks and desserts.

TYPES / VARIETIES

- Pandanus odoratissimus var. odoratissimus – most common culinary type.
- Regional cultivars with variations in aroma intensity and flower size.
- Some ornamental varieties grown for fragrance rather than consumption.

CULINARY

- flowers used to flavor rice, desserts, drinks; leaves wrapped around meats or cakes for aroma; extracts used in syrups, custards, and traditional sweets.

HEALTH

- contains antioxidants; traditionally used to reduce fever and headaches; may support digestion; used in aromatherapy for stress relief; anti-inflammatory and antimicrobial properties.

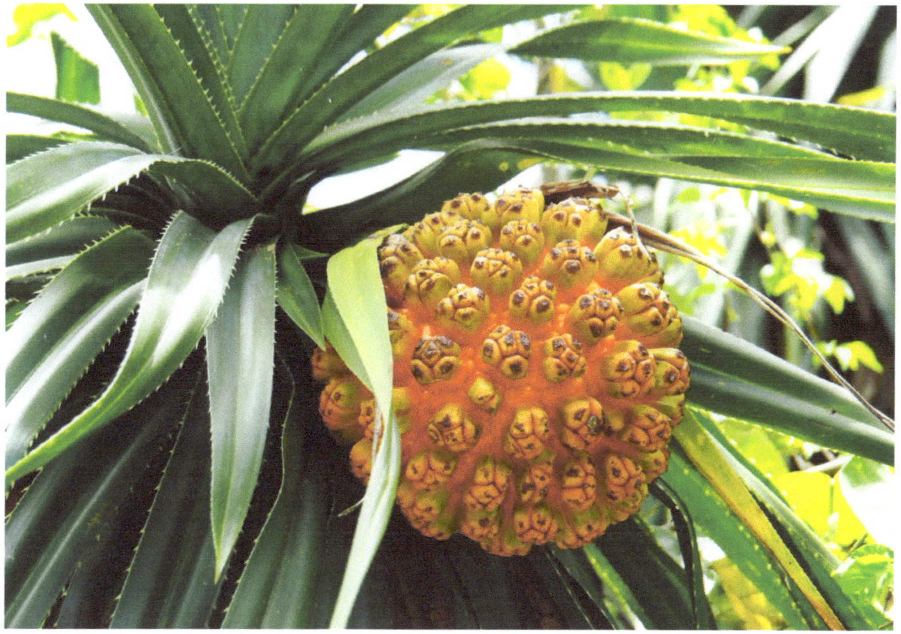

SESAME (SESAMUM INDICUM)

Sesame (Sesamum indicum) is one of the oldest oilseed crops known to humanity, valued for its nutrient-rich seeds, versatile oil, and cultural significance across Asia, Africa, and the Middle East.

Here's a detailed overview of its uses and characteristics:

BOTANICAL OVERVIEW

- Scientific name : Sesamum indicum
- Family : Pedaliaceae
- Origin : Believed to be native to Africa or India
- Growth habit : Erect annual plant, 60 cm to 2.5 meters tall, with tubular flowers and seed pods

CULINARY USES

- Sesame seeds (white, black, or brown) are used in:
- Baked goods (buns, crackers, cookies)
- Traditional sweets (e.g., til laddoos in India)
- Asian dishes (e.g., sushi, stir-fries, tahini)
- Sesame oil:
- Used for cooking, especially in Korean, Chinese, and Indian cuisines
- Adds nutty flavor and aroma
- Cold-pressed oil used in dressings and marinades

MEDICINAL AND HEALTH BENEFITS

- Rich in nutrients: High in calcium, magnesium, iron, zinc, and vitamin B1
- Heart health: Contains lignans and phytosterols that help lower cholesterol
- Antioxidant properties: Due to sesamol and sesamin compounds
- Anti-inflammatory: Used in Ayurvedic and traditional medicine for joint pain and skin conditions
- Digestive aid: Helps relieve constipation and supports gut health

COSMETIC AND TOPICAL USES

- Sesame oil is used in:
- Massage therapy (Ayurveda: abhyanga)
- Skin moisturizers and hair oils
- Natural sunscreens and anti-aging products

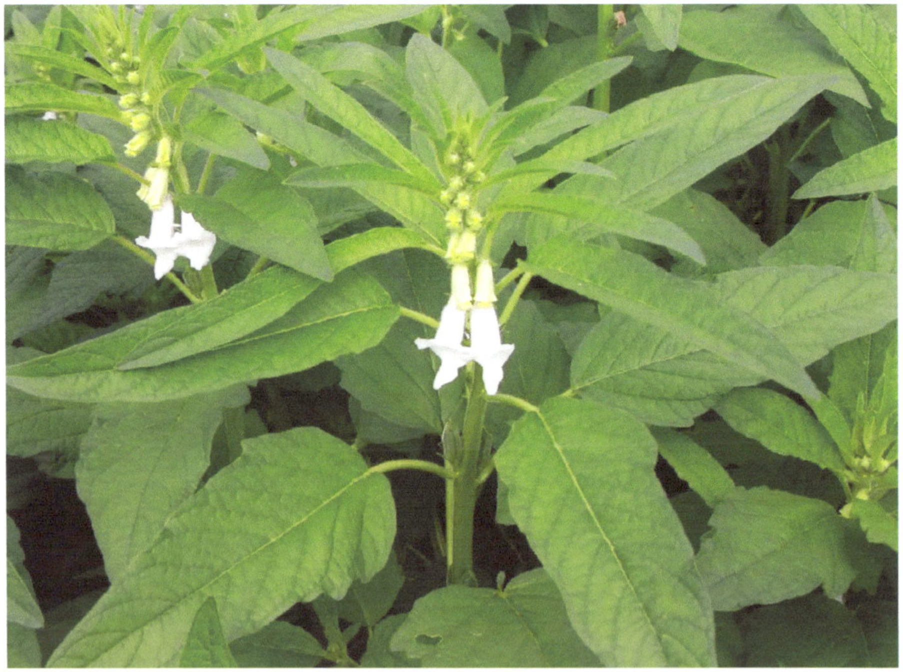

SICHUAN PEPPER (ZANTHOXYLUM PIPERITUM)

Sichuan pepper (Zanthoxylum piperitum) is a unique spice known for its tingling, numbing sensation and citrusy aroma, widely used in Asian cuisine and traditional medicine. It's not related to black pepper or chili but belongs to the citrus family.

BOTANICAL OVERVIEW

- Scientific name:Zanthoxylum piperitum (Japanese prickly ash)
- Family : Rutaceae (same as citrus)
- Common names: Sichuan pepper, Japanese pepper, prickly ash, huājiāo (in Chinese)
- Appearance: Shrub or small tree (2–5 meters tall) with pinnate leaves and reddish-brown fruit capsules that split open to reveal black seeds.

CULINARY USES

- Flavor profile: Citrusy, slightly woody, with a tingling and numbing effect due to hydroxy-α-sanshool.
- Key ingredient in Chinese cuisine, especially Sichuan dishes like:
    - Mapo tofu
    - Chongqing hot pot
    - Five-spice powder (includes Sichuan pepper, star anise, cloves, cinnamon, fennel).
- Used in Japanese (shichimi togarashi) and Indian spice blends.
- Young leaves and flower buds are used in soups, miso, soy sauce, and rice vinegar.

MEDICINAL AND HEALTH BENEFITS

- Analgesic and anti-inflammatory: Helps relieve joint pain and digestive discomfort.
- Antioxidant-rich: High ORAC value (118,400 per 100g), supports cellular health.
- Traditional uses: Employed in Chinese, Ayurvedic, and Native American medicine for cardiovascular support and wound healing.

CULTIVATION AND GROWTH

- Native regions: East Asia and parts of North America
- Safety and Usage Tips
- Texture caution: Hard shells can be irritating or pose a choking risk—recommended to roast and grind before use.
- Add at end of cooking: Preserves aroma and flavor
- Not related to true pepper (Piper nigrum)—no capsaicin or piperine

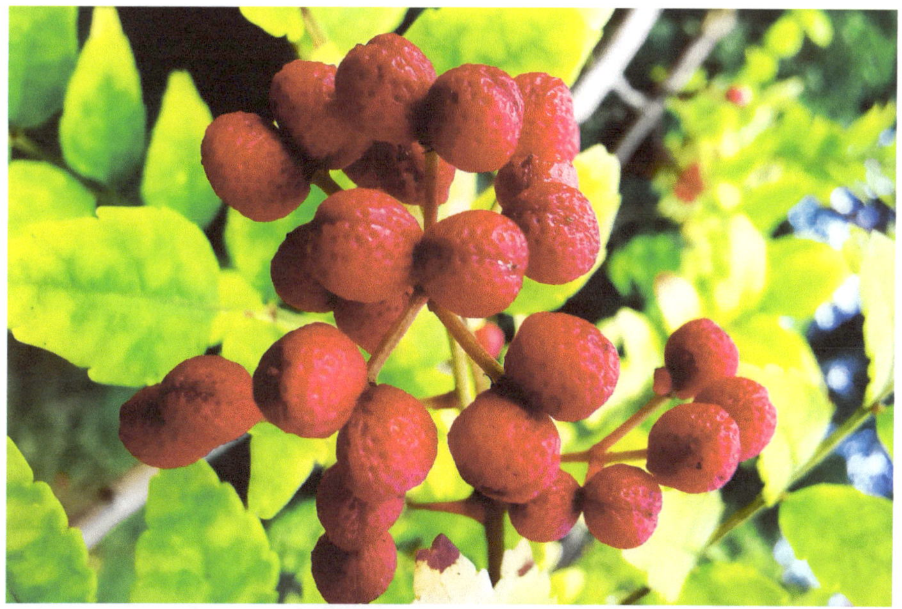

SILPHION (SILPHIUM)

Silphion (Silphium) was a legendary plant of classical antiquity, famed for its medicinal, culinary, and symbolic value—so prized that it was once worth its weight in silver and gold.

BOTANICAL IDENTITY AND MYSTERY

- Scientific uncertainty: The exact species of Silphion is unknown; it's believed to be related to the genus Ferula, possibly Ferula drudeana.

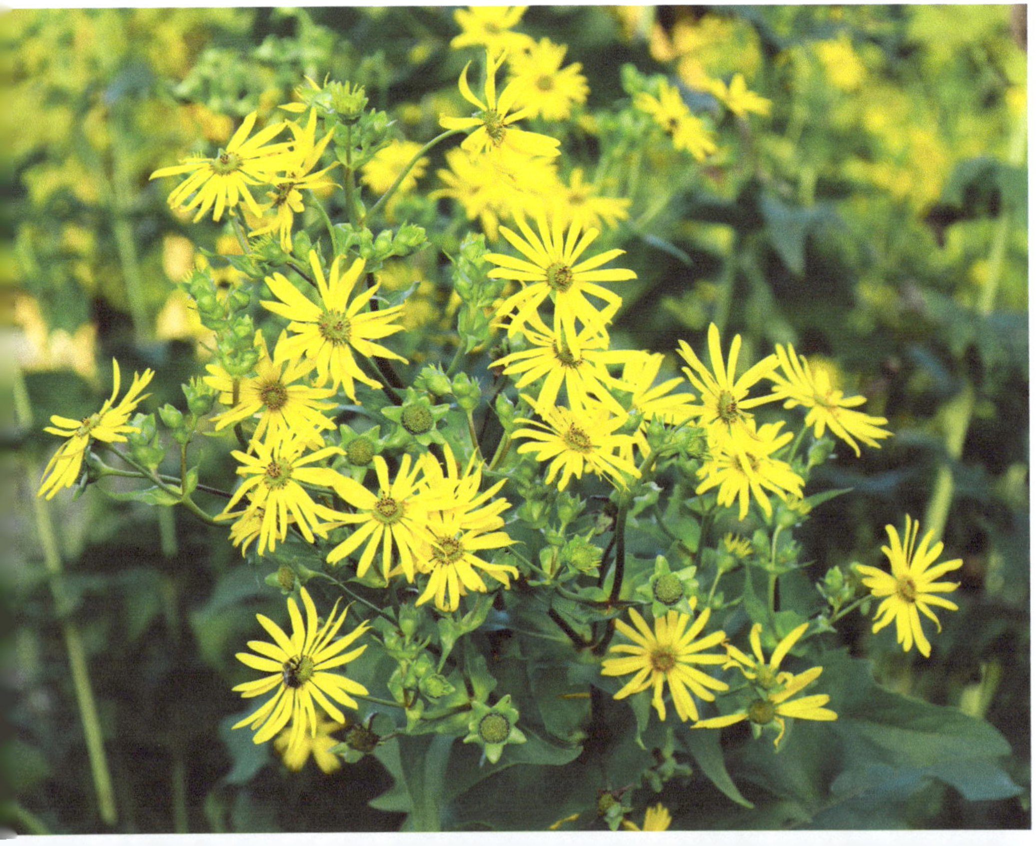

- Extinct or rediscovered?: Thought to be extinct since Roman times, but recent discoveries in Turkey suggest Ferula drudeana may be a surviving relative.
- Appearance: Described as having thick branching roots, yellow flowers, and a tall stalk—similar to fennel or asafoetida.

HISTORICAL SIGNIFICANCE

- Origin: Native to the region around Cyrene (modern-day Libya), where it was central to the economy.
- Trade and currency: So valuable that Cyrenian coins bore its image; Julius Caesar reportedly stored 1,500 pounds of its resin in Rome's treasury.
- Cultural symbolism: Celebrated in poetry and song; considered a symbol of love and luxury.

MEDICINAL AND CULINARY USES

- **Medicinal properties**
  - Used as an aphrodisiac, contraceptive, and digestive aid
  - Treatcoughs, sore throats, and various infections
  - Resin (called laserpicium) was the most valued part
- **Culinary uses:**
  - Crushed, roasted, sautéed, and boiled for flavoring food
  - Used as a spice and condiment in Greek and Roman cuisine

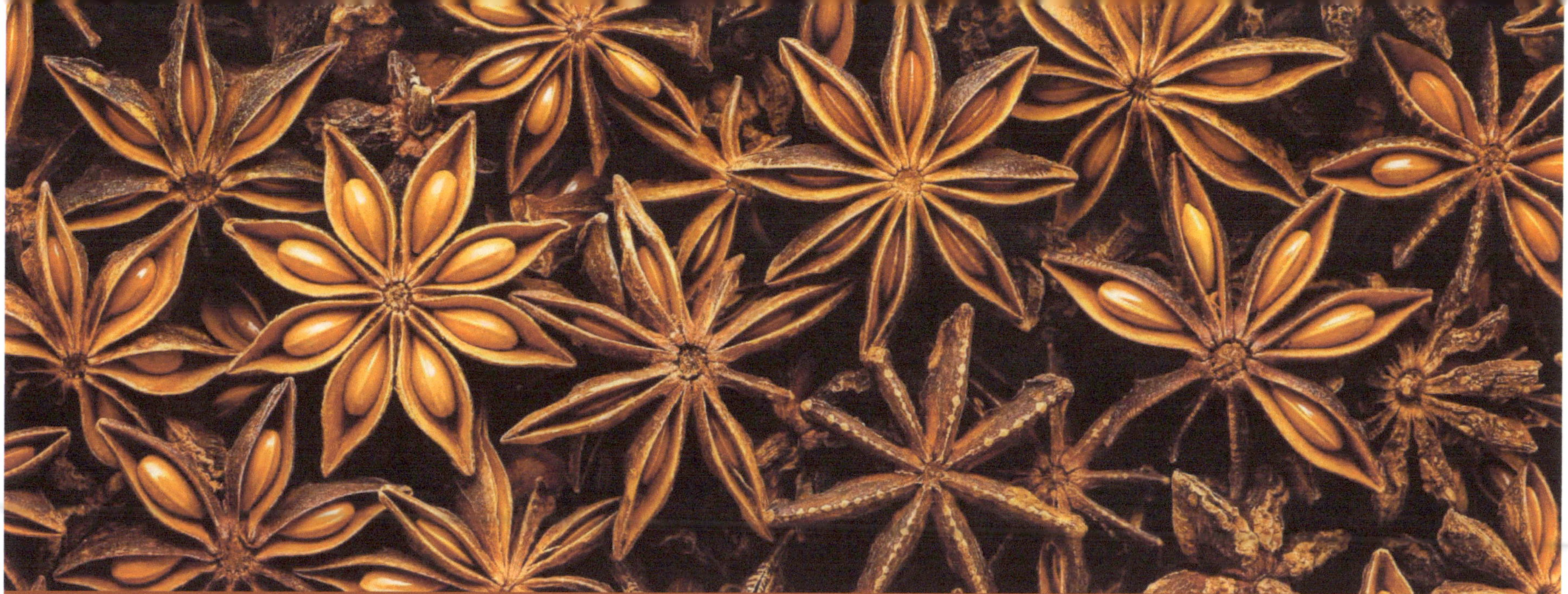

STAR ANISE (ILLICIUM VERUM)

- Common Name and Botanical Name Star Anise (Illicium verum)
- Part of the Plant Used Dried pods and seeds
- Country or Region of Origin Asia
- Common Use Asian cooking, especially with meats

ANTIMICROBIAL PROPERTIES

- Star anise contains anethole, which is effective against bacteria, yeast, and fungal strains
- Star anise essential oil (SAO) contains trans-anethole, which may help protect against damage caused by E. coli
- Antioxidant properties
- Star anise has high antioxidant content, which may protect cells from damage that can lead to cancer

ANTIFUNGAL PROPERTIES

- Star anise has broad-spectrum antifungal activity, which can inhibit food spoilage caused by Aspergillus and Fusarium

OTHER PROPERTIES

- Star anise contains shikimic acid, which is used to make oseltamivir (Tamiflu), an antiviral medication for influenza A and B
- Star anise has been used in traditional Chinese medicine
- Star anise has been used as a spice in food .

Star anise has been used to treat respiratory infections, stomach disorders, and colic in babies

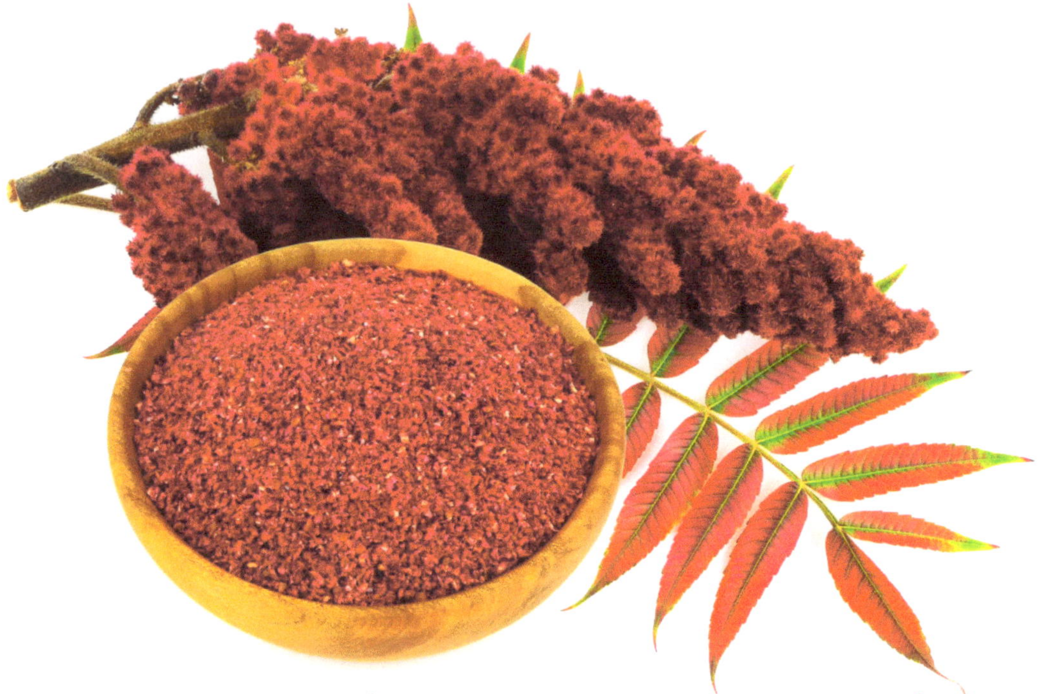

SUMAC (RHUS CORIARIA)

- **Antioxidant** : Sumac has powerful antioxidant properties that may help with cardiovascular disease, diabetes, and cancer
- **Anti-inflammatory** : Sumac has anti-inflammatory properties
- **Antibacterial** : Sumac has antibacterial properties
- **Anti-diabetic** : Sumac has anti-diabetic properties
- **Hepatoprotective** : Sumac has hepatoprotective properties
- **Cardioprotective** : Sumac has cardioprotective properties
- **Neuroprotective** : Sumac has neuroprotective properties
- **Digestive aid** : Sumac has been used traditionally to aid digestion
- Vitamins and minerals Vitamin C, Vitamin A, Potassium, Calcium, and Magnesium.

FIBER

- Sumac contains fiber, which supports healthy digestion, heart health, and blood sugar regulation

FLAVOR

- Sumac has a sour and light flavor

USES

- Sumac is a commonly used spice, condiment, and flavoring agent
- Sumac has been used in traditional medicine to treat hemorrhoids, wound healing, diarrhea, ulcer, and eye inflammation.

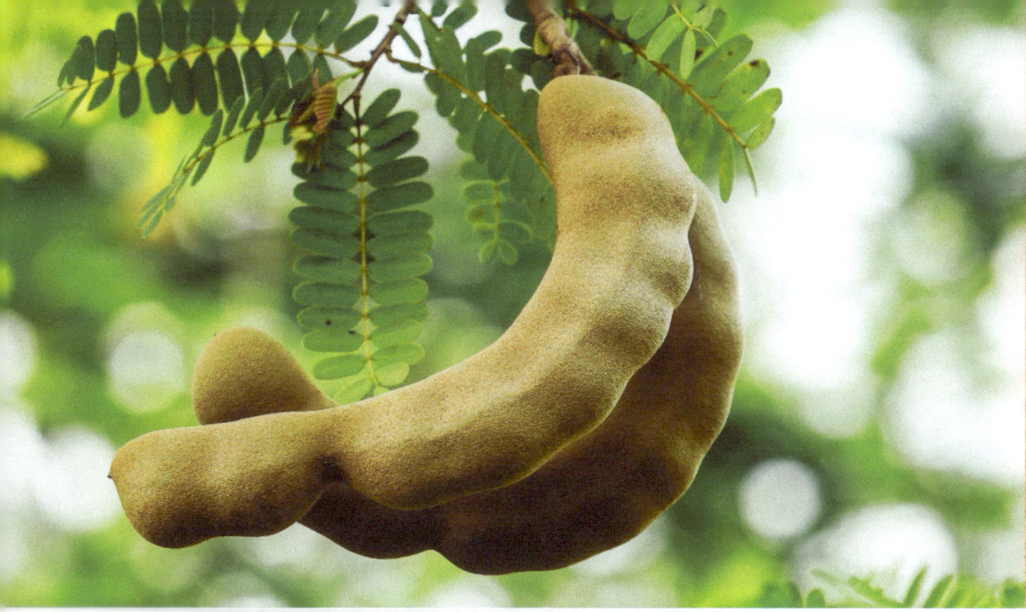
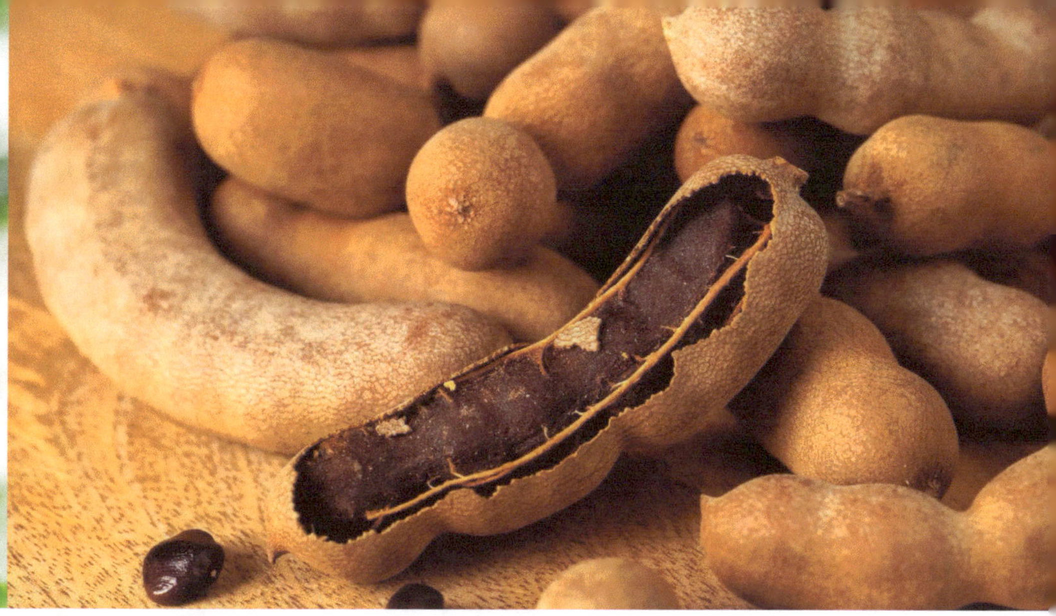

TAMARIND (TAMARINDUS INDICA)

- This fruit has many uses, including cooking, health, and household purposes.

CULINARY USES

- Tamarind pulp is widely used for cooking in South and Southeast Asia, Mexico, the Middle East, and the Caribbean. The seeds and leaves are also edible.
- It is used in sauces, marinades, chutneys, drinks, and desserts. It's also one of the ingredients of Worcestershire sauce.

MEDICINAL PROPERTIES

- Tamarind has played an important role in traditional medicine.
- In beverage form, it was commonly used to treat diarrhea, constipation, fever, and malaria. The bark and leaves were also used to promote wound healing.
- Modern researchers are now studying this plant for potential medicinal uses, such as helping prevent peptic ulcer.
- The polyphenols in tamarind have antioxidant and anti-inflammatory properties. These can protect against diseases such as heart disease, cancer, and diabetes.

OTHER USES

- Tamarind pulp can also be used as a metal polish. It contains tartaric acid, which helps remove tarnish from copper and bronze.
- Tamarind is used as a flavoring in many dishes. It may also have medicinal properties and can be used as a tarnish remover.
- It is an effective way to deal with allergic asthma and cough because of its antihistaminic properties. It's also a rich source of vitamin C and can boost the immune system to prevent cold and cough.

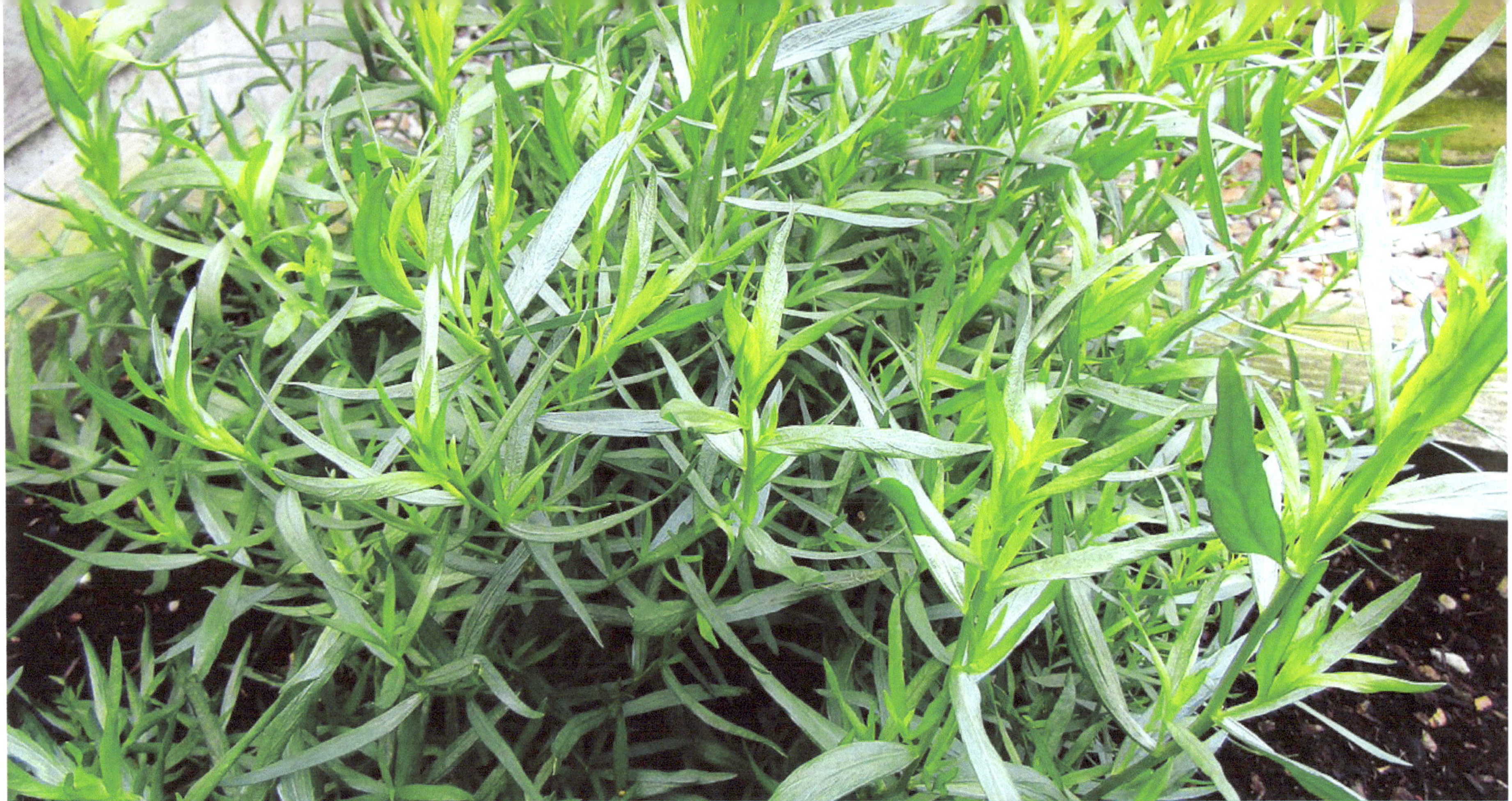

TARRAGON (ARTEMISIA DARACUNCULUS)

- Tarragon (Artemisia dracunculus) is one of the most refined and aromatic culinary herbs, prized especially in French cuisine for its delicate, anise-like flavor. It's also valued in traditional herbal medicine for its digestive and restorative properties.
- Here's a complete, structured summary in the same style as before

BOTANICAL OVERVIEW

- Common Name : Tarragon
- Scientific Name : Artemisia dracunculus
- Family : Asteraceae (Daisy family)
- Plant Type : Perennial aromatic herb
- Native to : Central Asia and Siberia; now widely grown in Europe and North America
- Related species : Artemisia absinthium (wormwood), Artemisia vulgaris (mugwort).

TYPE	DESCRIPTION	USE
French Tarragon (A. dracunculus var. sativa)	True culinary type; rich, refined flavor; sterile (grown from cuttings)	Cooking and herbal use
Russian Tarragon (A. dracunculoides)	Hardier, coarser leaves, less aromatic	Grown in colder regions; less used in fine cooking

CULINARY USES

- Tarragon is a signature herb in French cuisine, especially in the famous "fines herbes" blend (with parsley, chervil, and chives).

COMMON USES :

- Sauces: Béarnaise, tartar, hollandaise, and creamy dressings
- Vinegars: Tarragon vinegar for salads and marinades
- Poultry & Fish: Adds delicate flavor to chicken, fish, and eggs
- Egg Dishes: Omelets, quiches, and scrambled eggs
- Soups & Vegetables: Especially with carrots, mushrooms, and potatoes

FLAVOR NOTE:

- Because it's potent, it's best added near the end of cooking to preserve its aroma.

MEDICINAL AND HEALTH BENEFITS

- Traditionally used in European and Russian folk medicine for digestive and metabolic support.

KEY BENEFITS:

- Digestive stimulant: Increases appetite and aids digestion
- Mild analgesic: Chewing leaves can relieve toothache (due to eugenol)
- Sedative: Mildly calming, helps relieve insomnia and anxiety
- Circulatory booster: Improves blood flow and reduces water retention
- Antibacterial: Helps prevent microbial infections
- Metabolic aid: May help regulate blood sugar and improve appetite
- Rich in antioxidants: Supports overall cellular health

ACTIVE COMPOUNDS

- Estragole (methyl chavicol) — gives the characteristic anise flavor
- Eugenol — mild analgesic and antiseptic
- Cineole & ocimene — aromatic terpenes aiding respiration
- Flavonoids & coumarins — antioxidants and circulation enhancers
- Vitamins & minerals: A, C, B-complex, calcium, iron, magnesium

Note: Estragole in very high doses may be toxic — culinary amounts are perfectly safe.

TARRAGON ESSENTIAL OIL

- Uses:
  - Aromatherapy for stress relief and sleep
  - Massage oils for muscle relaxation
  - Flavoring in foods and liqueurs (like Chartreuse and vermouth)

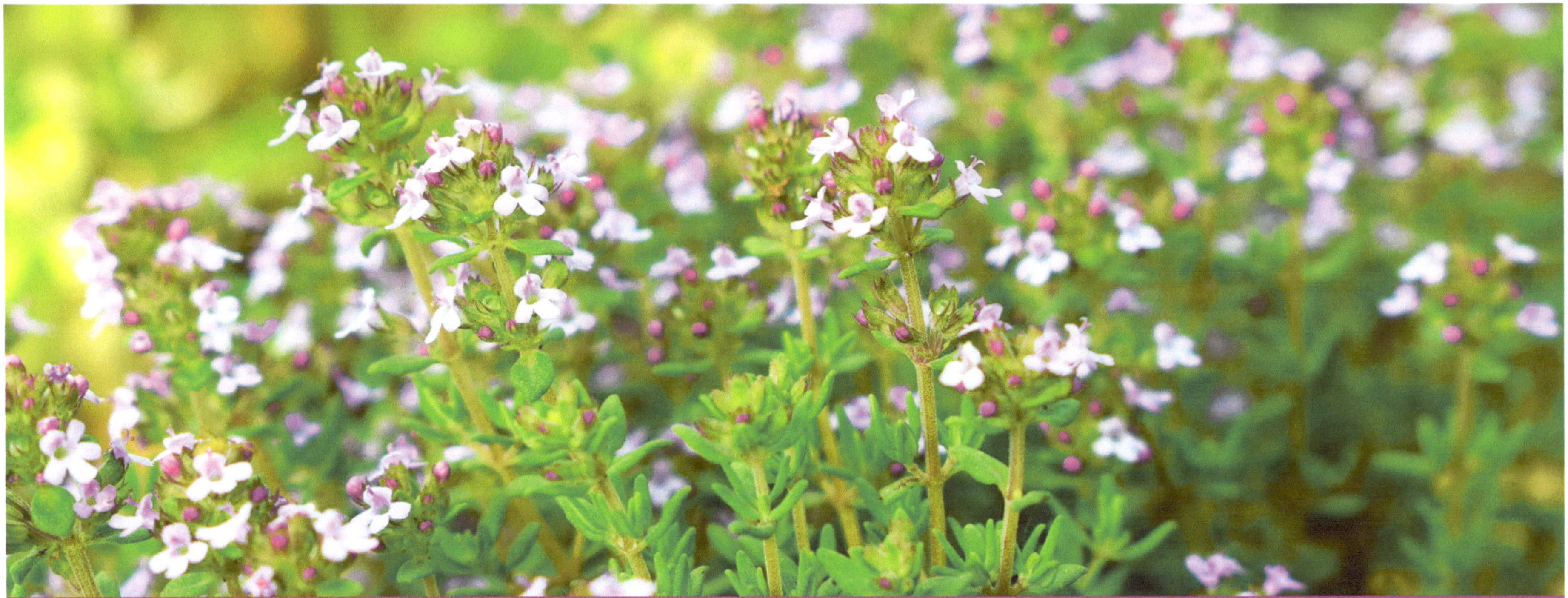

THYME (THYUMUS VULGARIS)

- Thyme – a common flavoring agent in western cooking
- Thyme has many properties, including antioxidants, anti-inflammatory, and antimicrobial properties. It's also rich in vitamins, minerals, and phytonutrients.

PROPERTIES

- Antimicrobial: Thyme has antibacterial, antifungal, and antiviral properties.
- Anti-inflammatory: Thyme can help with inflammation.
- Antioxidant: Thyme contains antioxidants that can help prevent food from oxidizing.
- Relaxing: Thyme can have a relaxing effect on the nervous system.
- Expectorant: Thyme can help with coughs and respiratory conditions.
- Bactericidal: Thyme can help with bacterial infections.
- Anti-Alzheimer's disease: Thyme may help delay the onset of Alzheimer's disease.

USES

- Food: Thyme can be used to flavor meat, fish, and vegetables.
- Tea: Thyme can be used to make tea.
- Aromatherapy: Thyme can be used in aromatherapy.
- Medicine: Thyme can be used as a medicine to treat conditions like acne, infections, and high blood pressure.

PRECAUTIONS

- You should speak with a healthcare professional before taking thyme supplements or using thyme oil for health.

TONKA BEANS (DIPTERYX ODORATA)

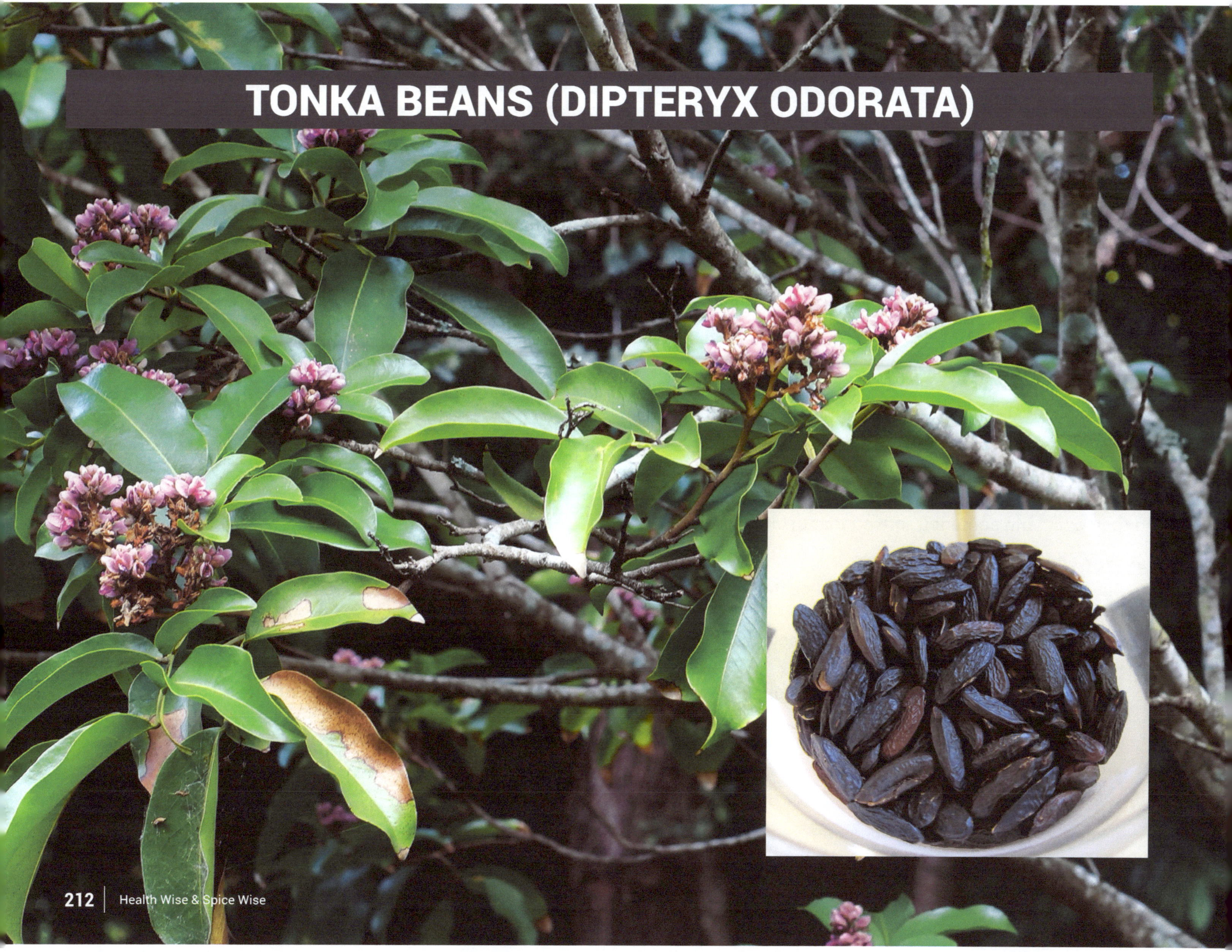

Tonka Beans - one of the most exotic and fragrant spices in the world — mysterious, luxurious, and deeply aromatic. They are used in fine perfumery, gourmet desserts, and traditional medicine, often as a vanilla or almond substitute.

- Here's a complete, structured overviewsimilar to the earlier herbal profiles.

BOTANICAL OVERVIEW

- Common Name: Tonka Bean
- Scientific Name:Dipteryx odorata
- Family: Fabaceae (Legume family)
- Native to: Northern South America — especially Venezuela, Brazil, Guyana, and French Guiana
- Other Names: Cumaru, Tonquin Bean, Tonka Seed

CULINARY USES

Tonka beans are highly aromatic and used in fine desserts and luxury flavorings, though regulated in some countries due to their coumarin content (more on that below).

COMMON USES:

- Flavoring: Vanilla-like substitute in custards, ice creams, chocolates, pastries, and macarons.
- Beverages: Adds depth to coffee, cocktails, rum, and liqueurs.
- Spice blends: Used sparingly in fusion and molecular gastronomy.
- French cuisine: Featured in haute pâtisserie (e.g., crème brûlée, ganache, or mousse).

FLAVOR PROFILE:

Sweet, warm, complex — blending vanilla, almond, hay, caramel, and tobacco notes. A single bean can flavor dozens of desserts — it's shaved or infused, never eaten whole.

MEDICINAL AND TRADITIONAL USES

- Tonka beans have long been used in folk medicine and perfumery for their calming, antispasmodic, and aphrodisiac qualities.

TRADITIONAL BENEFITS:

- Sedative and calming: Used for relaxation and to reduce anxiety or insomnia.
- Circulatory aid: Stimulates blood flow and eases cramps.
- Anti-inflammatory: Soothes muscle pain and joint inflammation.
- Respiratory relief: Used in aromatic balms for cough and chest congestion.
- Aphrodisiac: Long believed to promote love and attraction (used in perfumes).

In traditional South American medicine, tonka beans were carried as good luck charms or talismans for prosperity.

TONKA BEAN ESSENTIAL OIL & EXTRACT

- Extraction: Solvent or alcohol extraction from cured beans.
- Main constituents: Coumarin, vanillin, benzaldehyde, cinnamic acid derivatives.
- Aroma: Sweet, warm, and sensual.

USES:

- Fine perfumery (base notes in oriental and amber scents).
- Aromatherapy (calming, grounding).
- Flavoring (trace amounts in liqueurs, desserts, tobacco).

TURMERIC (CURCUMA LONGA)

BOTANICAL BACKGROUND

- Perennial herb, family Zingiberaceae.
- Native to South Asia; widely cultivated in tropical regions.
- Grows 1 m tall with broad green leaves and underground rhizomes.
- Produces small yellow-green flowers; rhizomes harvested for spice.
- Known for bright yellow-orange color and earthy aroma.

COMMON CULINARY APPLICATIONS

- Used as ground powder or fresh rhizome in curries, stews, and rice dishes.
- Key ingredient in spice blends (curry powder, garam masala).
- Adds color and flavor to soups, sauces, pickles, and marinades.
- Used in beverages like golden milk and teas.
- Provides warm, earthy, slightly bitter, peppery flavor.

TYPES / VARIETIES

- Alleppey Turmeric – highly aromatic, deep color, from Kerala, India.
- Madras Turmeric – milder flavor, commonly exported.
- Erode Turmeric – bright color, medium pungency, India.
- Regional cultivars differ in curcumin content, flavor, and color intensity.

CULINARY

- resh or powdered rhizome in curries, rice, sauces, soups, pickles, teas, and spice blends; adds color and flavor.

HEALTH

- rich in curcumin, a potent antioxidant and anti-inflammatory; supports joint and digestive health; may improve liver function and immunity; traditionally used for skin care and wound healing; may support cardiovascular and cognitive health.

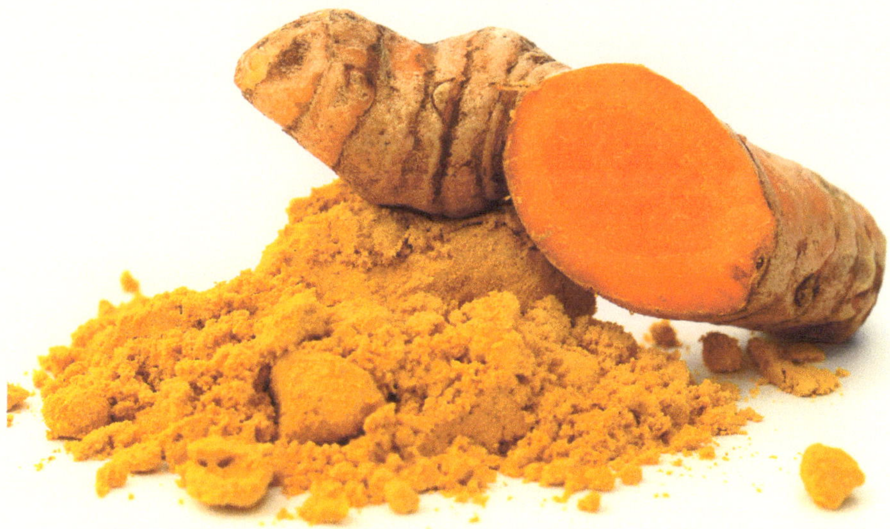

VANILLA (VANILLA PLANIFOLIA)

Vanilla (Vanilla planifolia) is a beloved spice derived from the pods of vanilla orchids. Known for its sweet, aromatic flavor and scent, vanilla is widely used in culinary and perfumery applications. Here are some key properties and health benefits of vanilla:

NUTRITIONAL CONTENT

- Vanillin: The primary compound responsible for vanilla's characteristic flavor and aroma.
- Antioxidants: Contains antioxidants like vanillic acid and vanillin, which help protect against oxidative stress and damage.
- Vitamins and Minerals: Contains trace amounts of vitamins B2 and B3, as well as small amounts of minerals like magnesium, calcium, and potassium.

HEALTH BENEFITS

- Antioxidant Properties: Helps neutralize free radicals, reducing oxidative stress and promoting overall health.
- Anti-inflammatory: Reduces inflammation and can help alleviate conditions like arthritis.
- Mood Enhancement: Known for its calming and mood-enhancing properties, which can help reduce stress and anxiety.
- Digestive Aid: Aids in digestion and can help alleviate nausea and stomach discomfort.
- Pain Relief: Has mild analgesic properties that can help alleviate minor aches and pains.
- Skin Health: Used in skincare products for its soothing and anti-aging properties.

USAGE

- Culinary Uses: Vanilla is used to flavor a wide variety of dishes, including desserts, beverages, and savory dishes. It is a key ingredient in baking and confectionery.
- Perfumery: Widely used in perfumes and fragrances for its sweet and warm scent.
- Medicinal Uses: Consumed as an extract or infused in teas for its health benefits.
- Aromatherapy: Vanilla essential oil is used in aromatherapy for its calming and soothing effects.

Vanilla is not only a delightful addition to your culinary creations but also offers a range of health benefits. Have you ever used vanilla in your cooking, or do you have any favorite recipes that feature this aromatic spice?

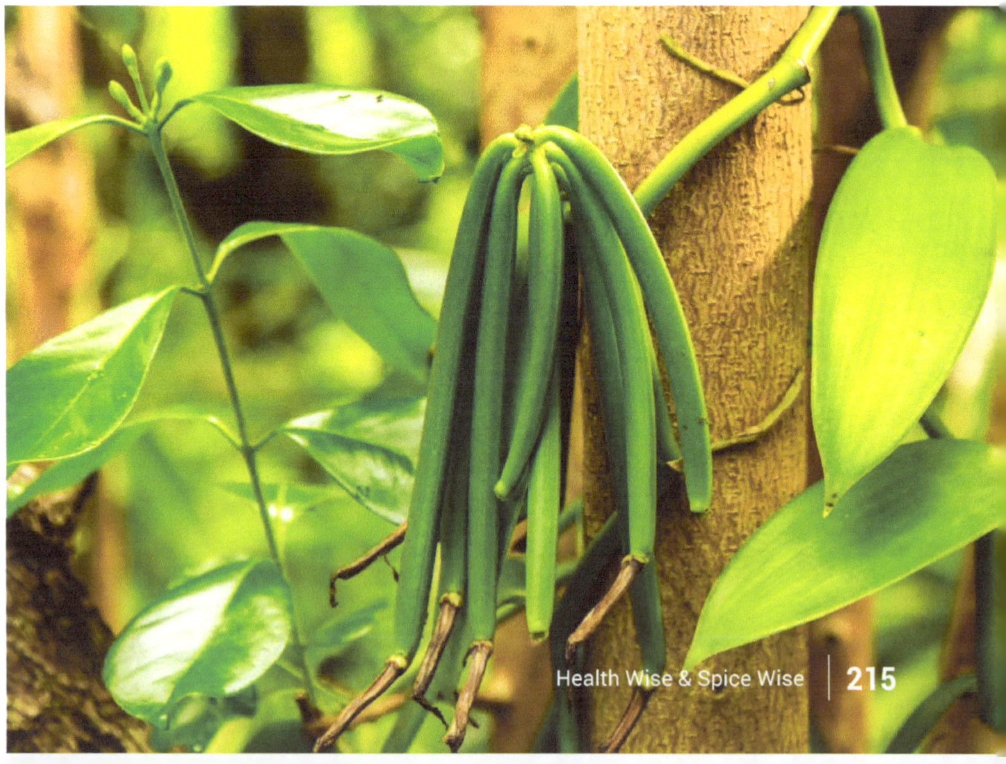

WASABI (WASABIA JAPONICA)

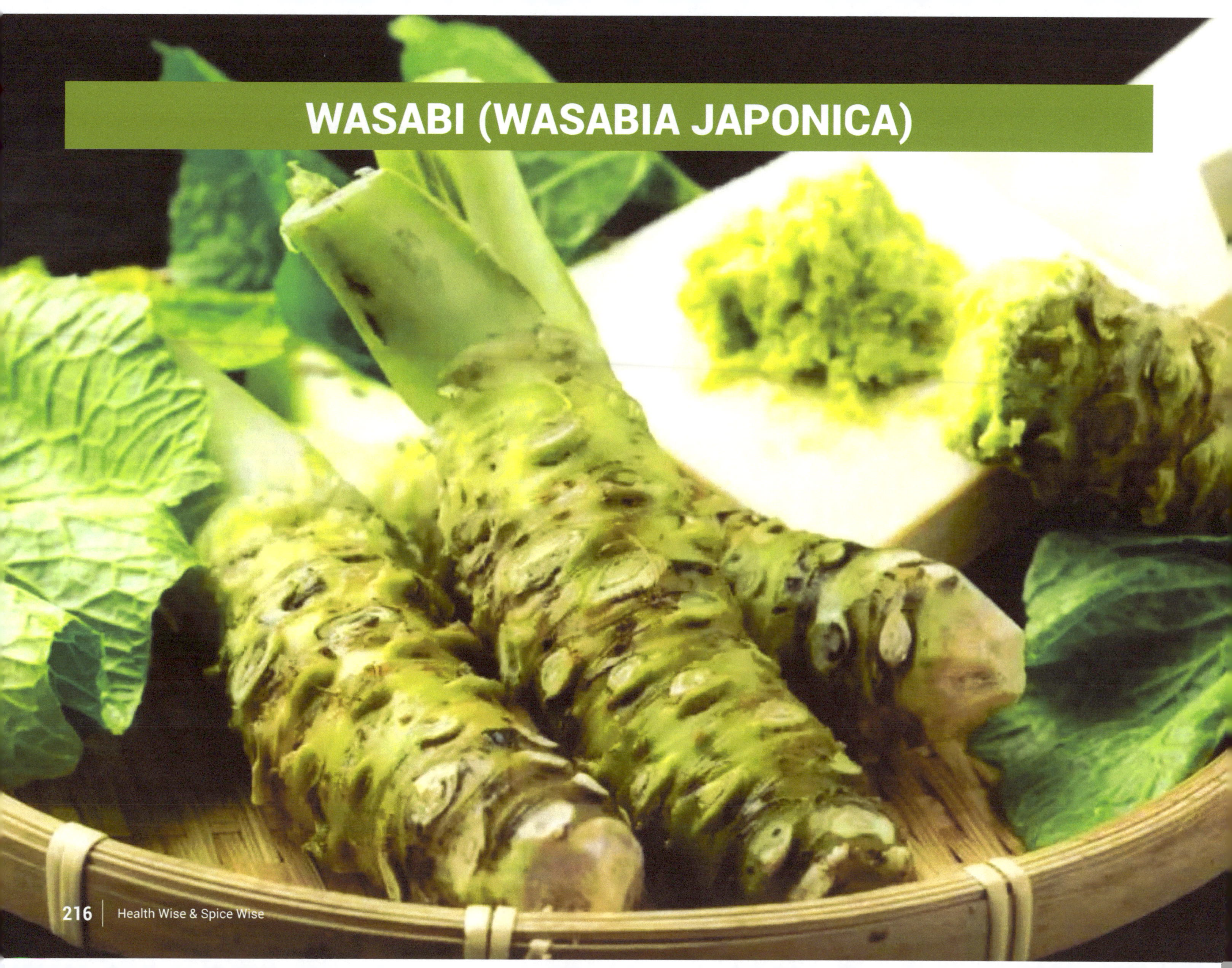

Wasabi is one of the most distinctive and pungent plants used in global cuisine — famed for its fiery, aromatic "heat" that quickly rises to the nose rather than burning the tongue like chili. It's not just a condiment for sushi — it's a rare medicinal herb with fascinating chemistry and powerful antimicrobial properties.

BOTANICAL OVERVIEW

- Common Name: Wasabi
- Scientific Name:Wasabia japonica (syn. Eutrema japonicum)
- Family: Brassicaceae (Mustard family — same as horseradish, mustard, cabbage)
- Plant Type: Perennial herb
- Native to: Japan (mountainous river valleys)
- Common Names: Japanese Horseradish, Mountain Wasabi
- Aroma: Sharp, fresh, nasal-clearing, like a mix of horseradish and mustard — but more refined.
- True wasabi only grows in cool, running mountain streams — hence the name "Sawa Wasabi" ("stream wasabi").

CULINARY USES

Forms Used:

- Fresh Rhizome: Grated finely into a paste (most authentic form).
- Powder or Paste: Commercial forms often made from horseradish, mustard, and green coloring (since true wasabi is expensive and perishable).

FLAVOR PROFILE:

- Hot, sharp, but quickly fading — unlike chili heat.
- The pungency is due to isothiocyanates, which evaporate quickly — giving a flash of heat to the sinuses.

COMMON USES:

- Japanese cuisine: Served with sushi, sashimi, soba noodles, and grilled meats.
- Fusion cooking: Mixed into mayonnaise, dressings, mashed potatoes, or marinades.
- Snacks: Flavoring for peas, nuts, and chips.
- Fresh wasabi must be grated just before use — its aroma and heat fade within 15 minutes.

MEDICINAL AND HEALTH BENEFITS

Wasabi is not just a flavor — it's a functional food with strong antimicrobial, anti-inflammatory, and detoxifying properties.

KEY BENEFITS:

- Antibacterial & Antiviral: Natural protection against microbes — reason it's paired with raw fish.
- Respiratory cleanser: Clears sinuses and nasal congestion.
- Circulation enhancer: Stimulates blood flow and prevents platelet clumping.
- Anti-inflammatory: May help with arthritis and joint pain.
- Anticancer potential: Isothiocyanates shown to inhibit cancer cell growth in studies.
- Cardiovascular support: Helps lower cholesterol and reduce clot risk.
- Digestive aid: Stimulates enzyme secretion and bile flow.

Wasabi's power comes from isothiocyanates (ITCs) sulfur-containing compounds released when the rhizome is grated.

MOST COMMON PEPPERS USED IN COOKING

Peppers are one of the most diverse and widely used ingredients in cooking worldwide. They range from completely mild and sweet to intensely hot and fiery, with the heat measured on the Scoville scale. Here's a comprehensive guide to the various types of peppers used in cooking:

SWEET PEPPERS (0 SCOVILLE HEAT UNITS)

BELL PEPPERS

Bell peppers are the most common sweet pepper variety, available in green, red, yellow, orange, and purple colors. They have a crisp texture and mild, sweet flavor. Red peppers are fully ripened green peppers and tend to be sweeter. They're excellent raw in salads, stuffed, roasted, grilled, or sautéed in stir-fries and fajitas.

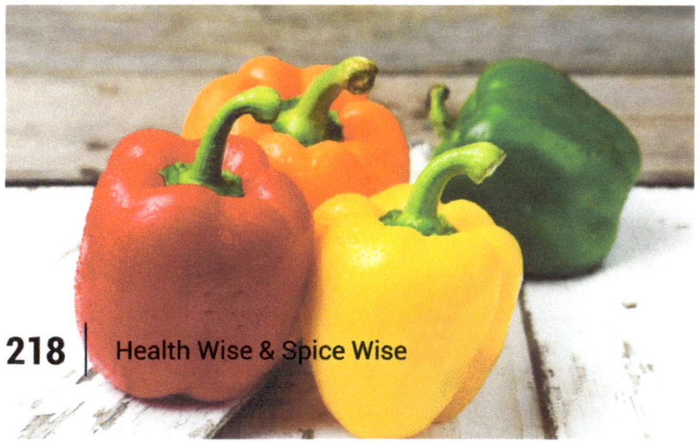

SWEET ITALIAN PEPPERS

Also called cubanelle peppers, these are thin-walled, mild peppers that are perfect for frying. They have a sweet, mild flavor and are commonly used in Italian cooking.

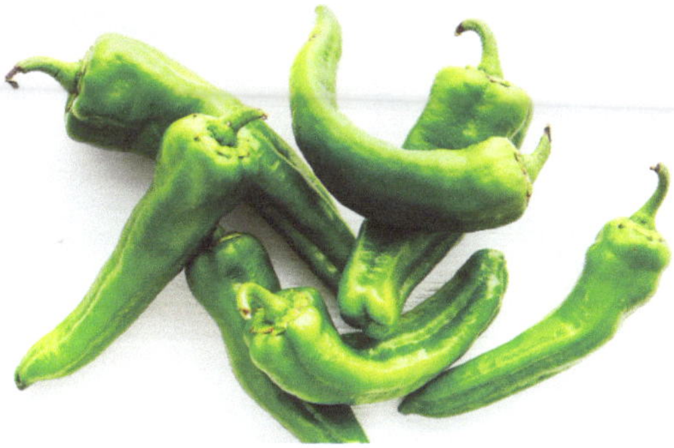

PIMENTO PEPPERS

These small, heart-shaped red peppers are very sweet and are often used stuffed in olives or processed into pimento cheese.

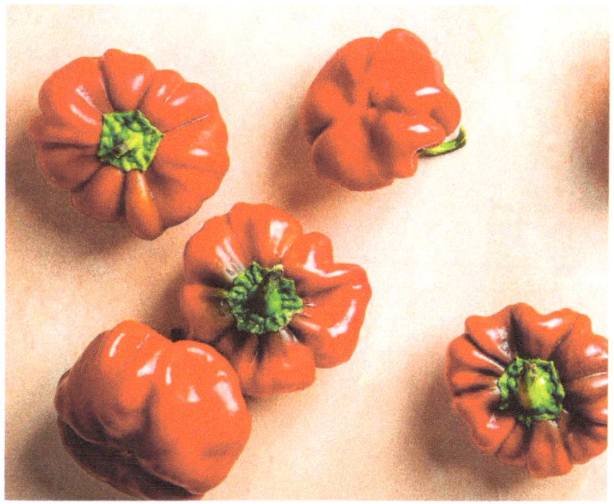

MILD HOT PEPPERS (1,000-8,000 SHU)

POBLANO PEPPERS

Large, dark green peppers with thick walls and mild heat. When dried, they become ancho chiles. Poblanos are perfect for stuffing (chiles rellenos) or roasting. They have a rich, earthy flavor with subtle heat.

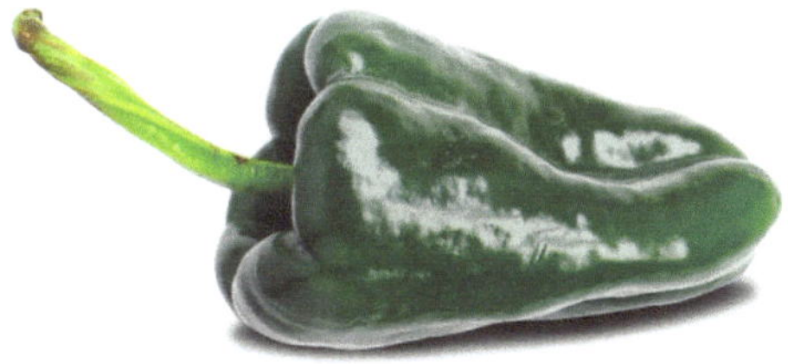

ANAHEIM PEPPERS

Also called New Mexico chiles, these are mild, long green peppers commonly used in Southwestern cuisine. They're excellent for roasting and have a slightly sweet flavor with minimal heat.

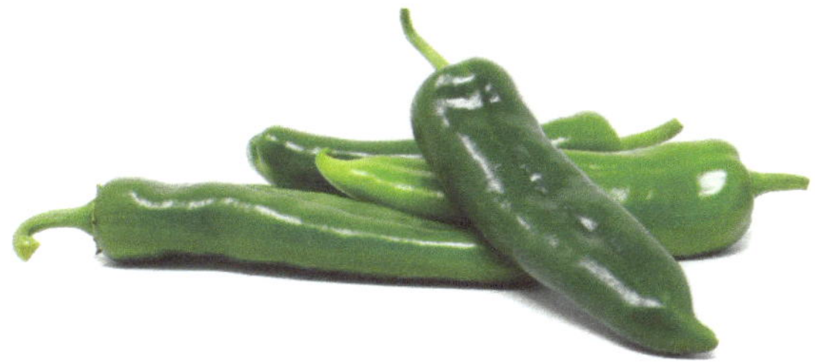

BANANA PEPPERS

Yellow, waxy peppers that are mild and slightly sweet. They're popular, pickled, and used on pizzas, sandwiches, and in salads.

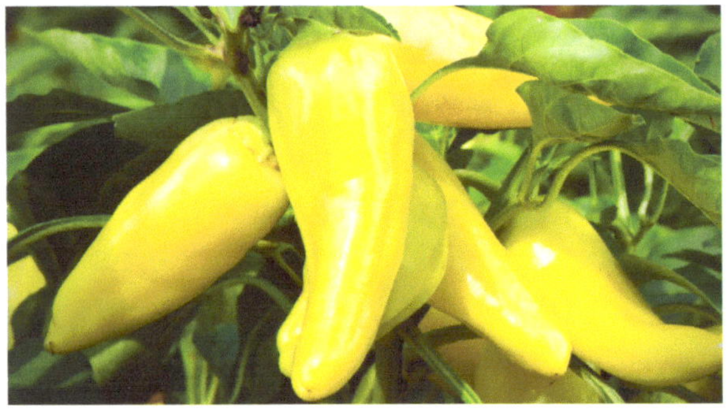

PEPPERONCINI

Small, yellow-green Italian peppers that are typically pickled. They have a tangy, mildly spicy flavor and are common in Mediterranean dishes and antipasto platters.

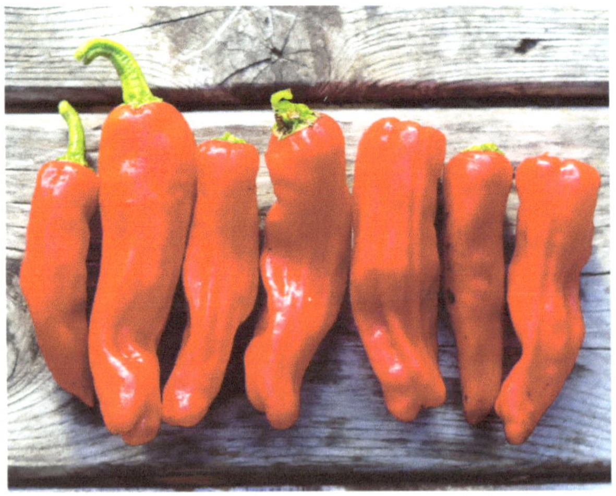

MEDIUM HOT PEPPERS (2,500-30,000 SHU)

JALAPEÑO PEPPERS

Perhaps the most well-known hot pepper, jalapeños are medium-sized green peppers (red when fully ripe) with moderate heat and a fresh, bright flavor. They're used in salsas, nachos, poppers, and countless Mexican and Tex-Mex dishes.

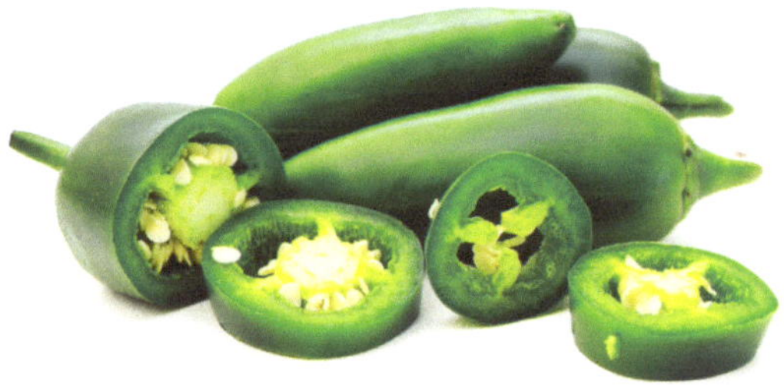

FRESNO PEPPERS

Similar in heat to jalapeños but with a fruitier flavor. They're often red and used in hot sauces and salsas.

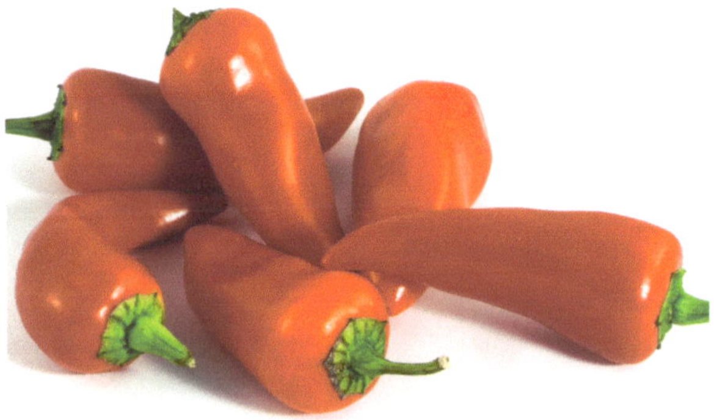

SERRANO PEPPERS

Smaller and hotter than jalapeños, Serranos have a crisp texture and bright, intense heat. They're commonly used in Mexican cuisine, particularly in salsas and guacamole.

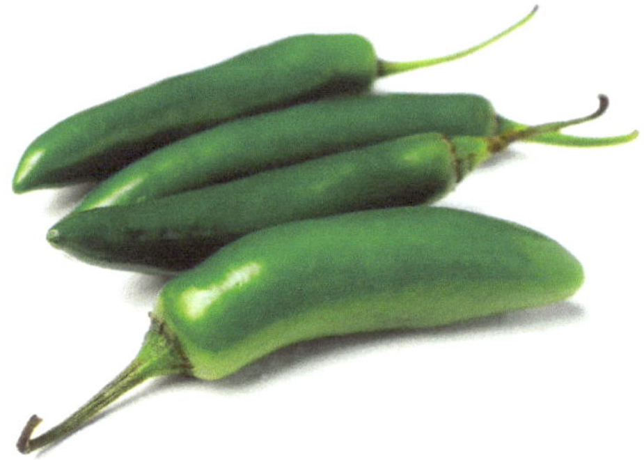

CHIPOTLE PEPPERS

These are jalapeños that have been smoked and dried, giving them a distinctive smoky, earthy flavor along with moderate heat. They're often sold in adobo sauce.

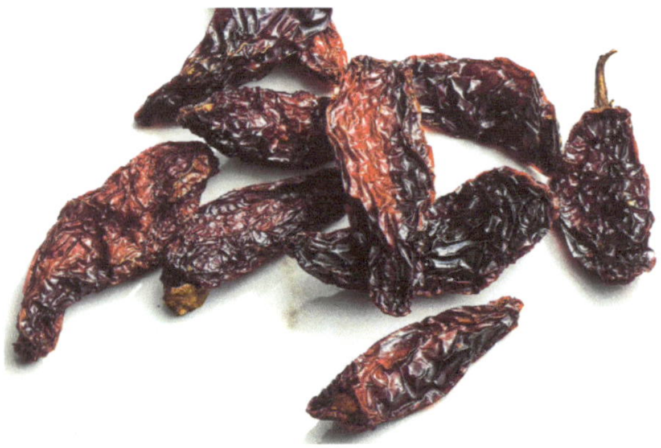

HOT PEPPERS (30,000-100,000 SHU)

CAYENNE PEPPERS

Thin, red peppers that are very hot and often ground into powder. They're used worldwide to add heat to dishes without changing the flavor profile significantly.

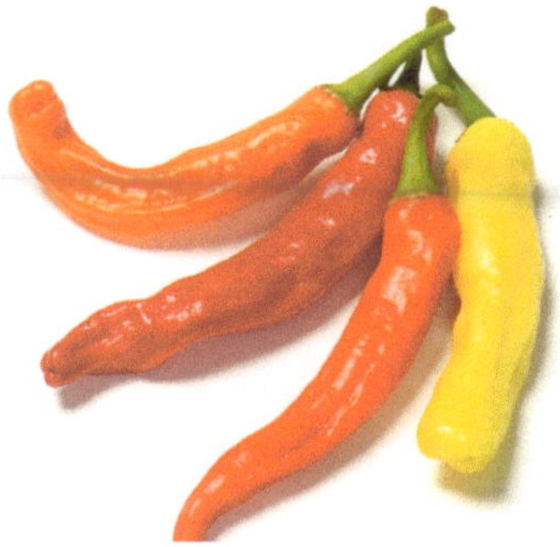

Thai Chili Peppers (Bird's Eye)

Very small but extremely hot peppers used extensively in Southeast Asian cuisine. They have clean, intense heat and are often used whole in curries and stir-fries.

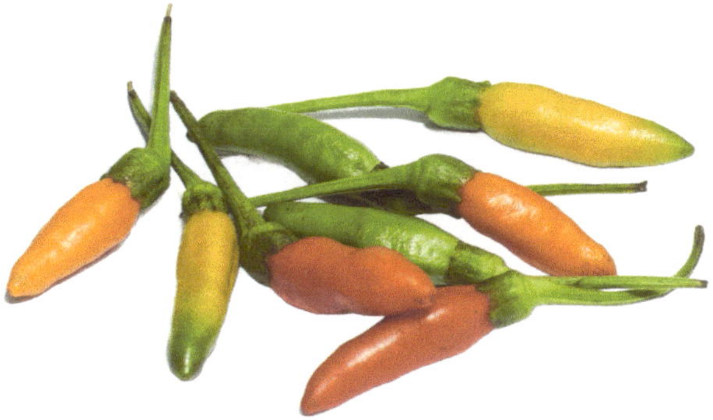

TABASCO PEPPERS

Small, tapered peppers are used to make the famous Tabasco sauce. They have sharp, vinegary heat.

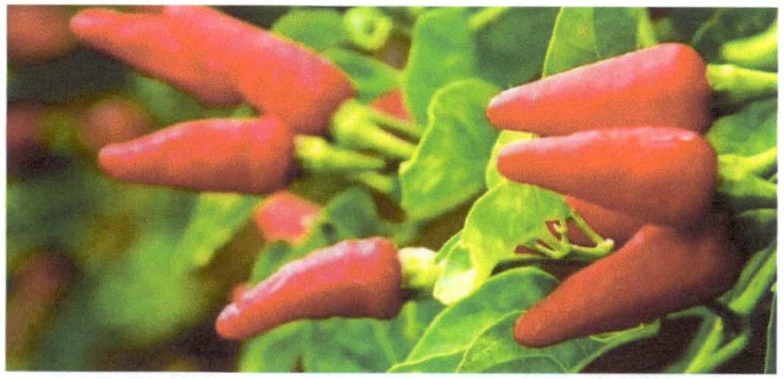

VERY HOT PEPPERS (100,000-350,000 SHU)

HABANERO PEPPERS

Small, lantern-shaped peppers that are extremely hot but also have a distinctive fruity, citrusy flavor. They come in various colors, including orange, red, and chocolate brown. Popular in Caribbean and Mexican cuisine.

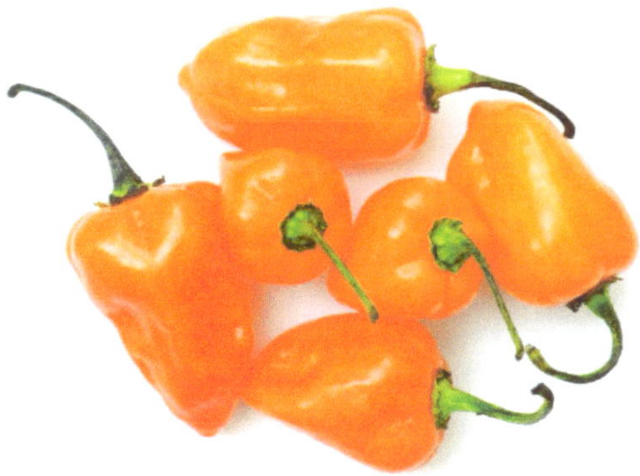

SCOTCH BONNET PEPPERS

Similar in heat to habaneros but with a slightly different flavor profile. They're essential in Caribbean cooking, particularly Jamaican jerk seasoning.

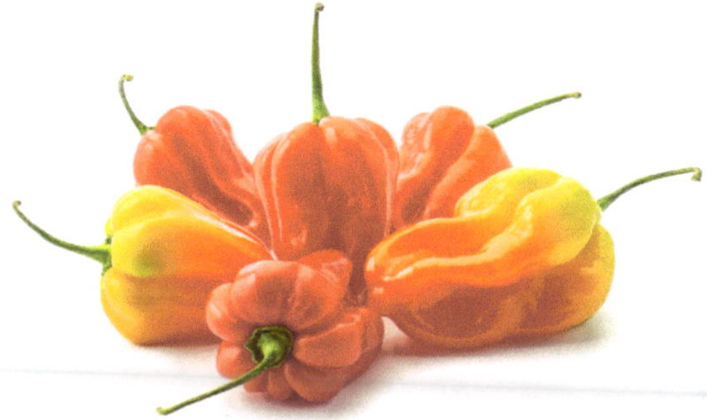

Extremely Hot Peppers (350,000+ SHU)

Ghost Peppers (Bhut Jolokia)

Once considered the world's hottest pepper, ghost peppers are used sparingly in Indian cuisine and hot sauces. They have intense heat with a slightly sweet, smoky flavor.

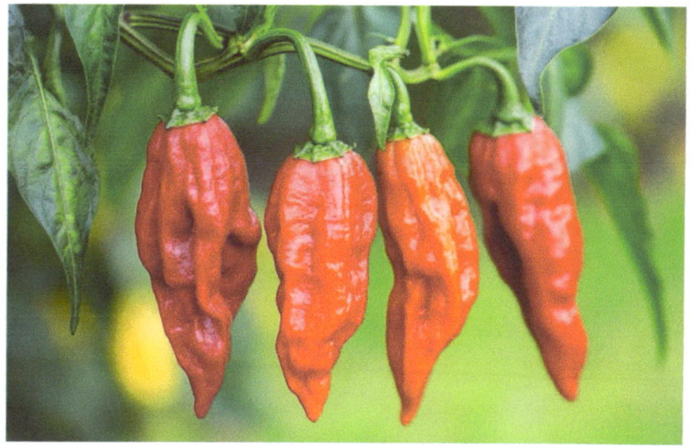

CAROLINA REAPER

Currently, the world's hottest pepper measures over 2 million SHU. These are used primarily in extreme hot sauces and should be handled with extreme caution.

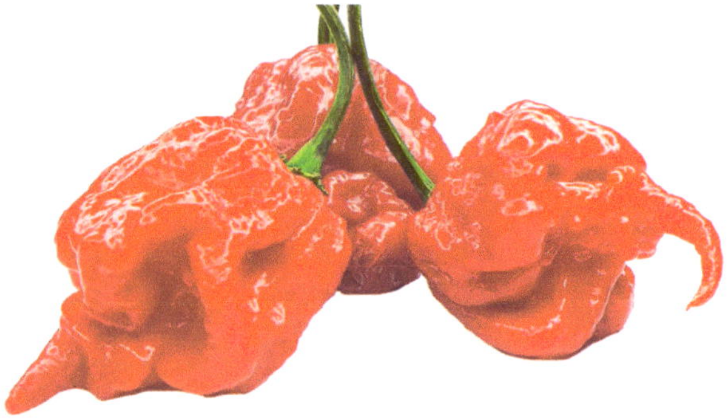

DRIED AND SPECIALTY PEPPERS

ANCHO CHILES

Dried poblano peppers have a sweet, fruity flavor and mild heat. Essential in Mexican mole sauces.

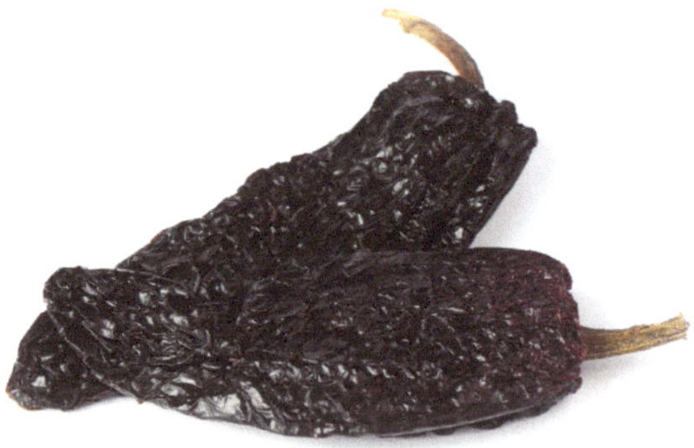

CHIPOTLE

Smoked jalapeños with earthy, complex flavor.

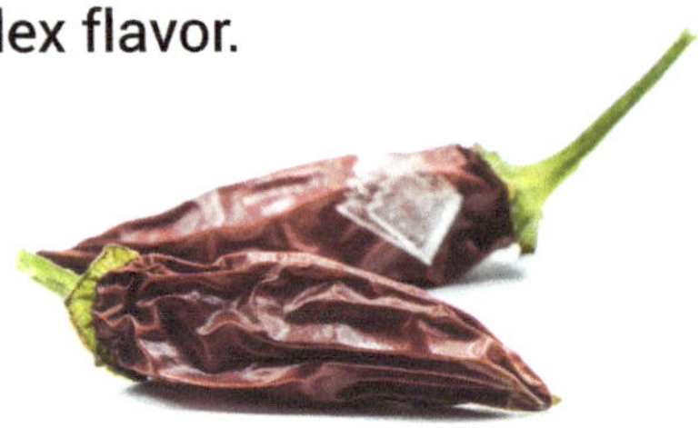

GUAJILLO

Dried mirasol peppers with mild heat and fruity flavor, commonly used in Mexican sauces.

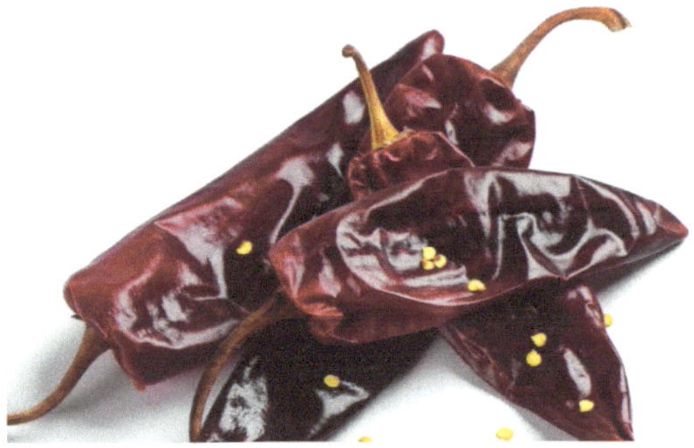

PASILLA

Dried chilaca peppers have mild heat and a rich, complex flavor.

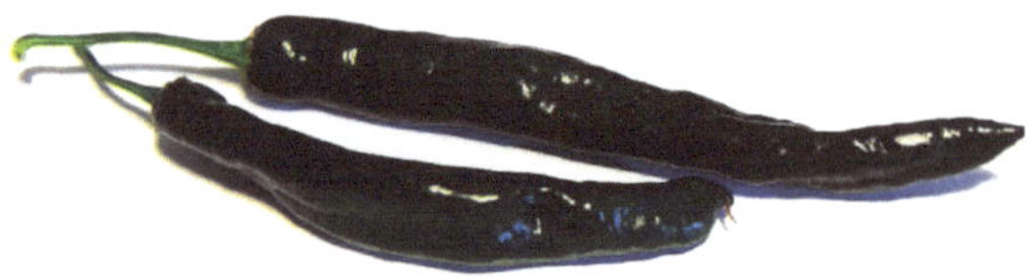

COOKING APPLICATIONS

Peppers can be prepared in numerous ways: roasted, grilled, stuffed, pickled, sautéed, or used raw. The cooking method often affects both flavor and heat level. Roasting tends to sweeten peppers and can reduce heat slightly, while cooking with seeds and membranes intact increases the heat level.

When working with hot peppers, wear gloves and avoid touching your eyes. The capsaicin that creates heat is concentrated in the seeds and white membranes, so removing these reduces the heat while maintaining flavor.

Paprika is a spice made from ground sweet pepper pods, primarily from the Capsicum annuum plant. It's widely used in various cuisines for its flavor, color, and health benefits. Here are some key properties and health benefits of paprika:

NUTRITIONAL CONTENT

- Capsaicin: Contains capsaicin, which gives it mild heat and has numerous health benefits.
- Vitamins and Minerals: Rich in vitamins A, C, E, and B-complex vitamins, as well as minerals like iron, magnesium, and potassium.
- Antioxidants: High in antioxidants such as beta-carotene and lutein, which help protect against oxidative stress and damage.

HEALTH BENEFITS

- Antioxidant Properties: Helps neutralize free radicals, reducing oxidative stress and promoting overall health.
- Anti-inflammatory: Reduces inflammation and can help alleviate conditions like arthritis.
- Immune System Support: High vitamin C content helps strengthen the immune system and fight off infections.
- Eye Health: Beta-carotene and lutein contribute to maintaining good vision and overall eye health.
- Digestive Aid: Stimulates digestion and promotes healthy gut function.
- Cardiovascular Health: Supports heart health by improving blood circulation and reducing cholesterol levels.
- Skin Health: Antioxidants help maintain healthy skin and protect against damage from free radicals.

USAGE

- Culinary Uses: Paprika is used to add color, flavor, and mild heat to a wide variety of dishes, including soups, stews, sauces, and meat rubs. It's a staple in Hungarian, Spanish, and other Mediterranean cuisines.
- Medicinal Uses: Can be consumed as a supplement or used in traditional remedies for its health benefits.
- Aromatherapy: Paprika is not typically used in aromatherapy, but its essential oil can be found in some topical applications for its anti-inflammatory properties.

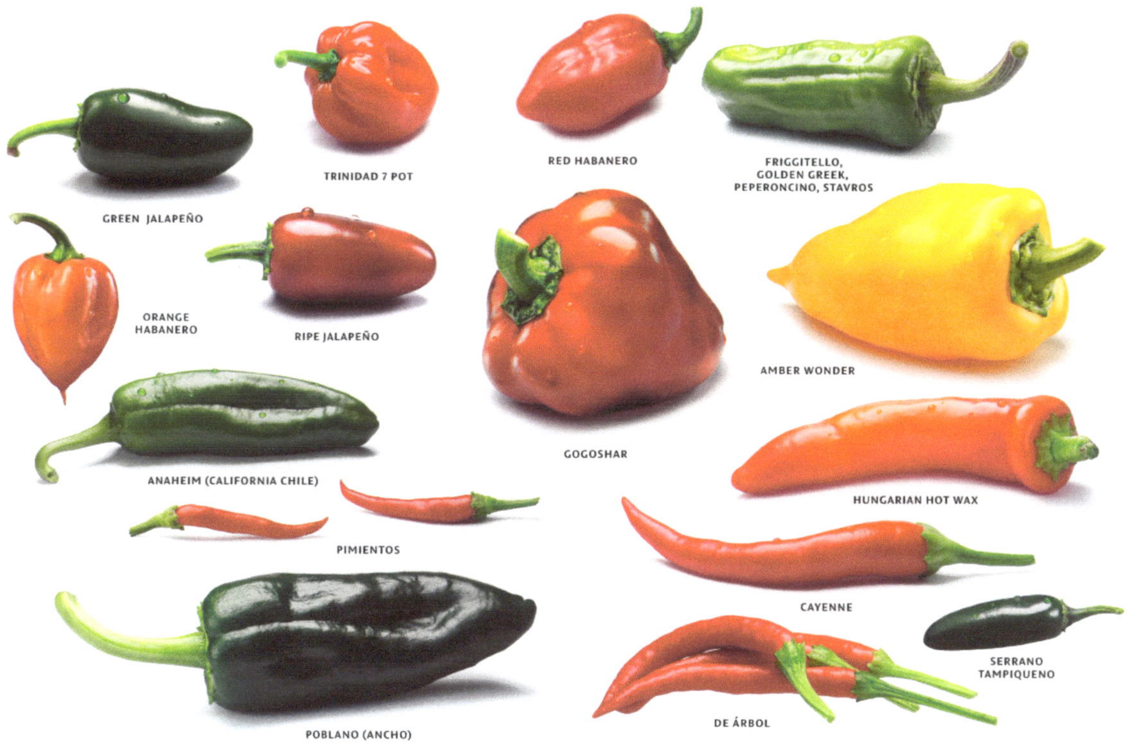

WINES

Cooking wine is a type of wine specifically formulated for use in cooking. It typically has a higher salt content and other additives to enhance flavor and preserve its shelf life. Here are some key properties and uses of cooking wine:

PROPERTIES

- Alcohol Content: Contains alcohol, which helps to enhance flavors in the food. However, the alcohol usually evaporates during cooking, leaving behind the rich flavors.
- Salt Content: Higher salt content compared to regular drinking wine, which acts as a preservative and flavor enhancer.
- Flavor: Available in various flavors, including red, white, sherry, and marsala. Each type adds a distinct flavor profile to dishes.
- Additives: May contain additional preservatives and flavor enhancers to maintain quality over time.

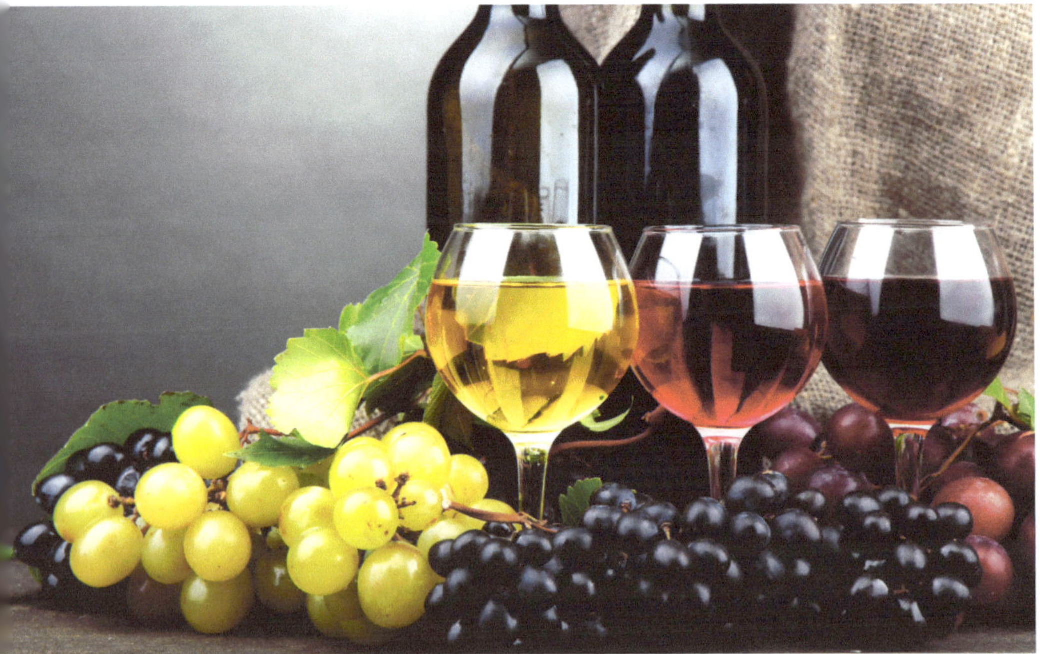

CULINARY USES

- Deglazing: Used to deglaze pans, helping to dissolve the browned bits stuck to the bottom of the pan and create a flavorful base for sauces.
- Marinades: Adds depth of flavor to marinades for meats, poultry, and seafood, helping to tenderize the protein.
- Sauces: Integral in making a variety of sauces, such as red wine reduction or white wine cream sauce, adding complexity and richness.
- Stews and Soups: Enhances the flavor of stews, soups, and braises by contributing acidity and depth.
- Baking: Used in certain baking recipes to add moisture and flavor, particularly in savory baked goods.

TYPES OF COOKING WINE

- Red Cooking Wine: Best for hearty dishes like beef stews, tomato-based sauces, and reductions.
- White Cooking Wine: Suitable for lighter dishes, such as chicken, seafood, and cream-based sauces.
- Sherry Cooking Wine: Adds a nutty, slightly sweet flavor to sauces, soups, and desserts.
- Marsala Cooking Wine: Commonly used in Italian dishes, such as chicken marsala, and adds a rich, sweet flavor.

Cooking wine is a versatile ingredient that can elevate the flavor of your dishes. However, it's important to note that due to its high salt content, it should be used judiciously to avoid overly salty dishes.

CITRUS JUICE AND RIND

Citrus juice and zest (commonly called the "rind") are fantastic additions to many culinary creations, offering both flavor and functional benefits. Here are some ways to incorporate them into your cooking:

CULINARY USES OF CITRUS JUICE

- Marinades: Citrus juice, such as lemon, lime, or orange, helps tenderize meat, poultry, and seafood while adding a fresh, tangy flavor.
- Salad Dressings: Fresh citrus juice can be combined with olive oil, herbs, and spices to create vibrant and tangy salad dressings.
- Sauces and Glazes: Adds brightness and acidity to sauces, glazes, and reductions, enhancing the overall flavor profile.
- Beverages: Used in cocktails, mocktails, and refreshing drinks like lemonade and limeade.
- Desserts: Adds a zesty flavor to desserts like sorbets, cakes, pies, and fruit salads.
- Cooking Vegetables: Adds a fresh tang to steamed or roasted vegetables.
- Fish and Seafood: Perfect for drizzling over grilled or baked fish and seafood dishes to brighten flavors.

CULINARY USES OF CITRUS ZEST (RIND)

- Baking: Adds intense citrus flavor to baked goods like cakes, muffins, cookies, and breads.
- Seasoning: Can be mixed with herbs, spices, and salt to create flavorful seasoning blends for meats, poultry, and vegetables.
- Garnishing: Provides a colorful and aromatic garnish for dishes, cocktails, and desserts.
- Infusing: Infuses flavor into oils, vinegars, syrups, and spirits, creating unique and aromatic ingredients.
- Cooking Rice and Grains: Adds a subtle citrus aroma and flavor when added to the cooking water for rice, quinoa, or couscous.
- Dairy: Enhances the flavor of dairy-based dishes like yogurt, cream cheese spreads, and panna cotta.

COMBINING CITRUS JUICE AND ZEST

- Citrus Marmalade: Combines both juice and zest to create a sweet and tangy spread.
- Citrus Butter: Mixes zest and a touch of juice into butter for a flavorful spread or cooking ingredient.
- Citrus Syrups: Combines juice and zest to make aromatic syrups for pancakes, waffles, and cocktails.
- Citrus Salsas: Uses both juice and zest to create fresh and vibrant salsas for topping fish, chicken, or tacos.

Incorporating citrus juice and zest can elevate your dishes with their bright, fresh, and aromatic qualities.

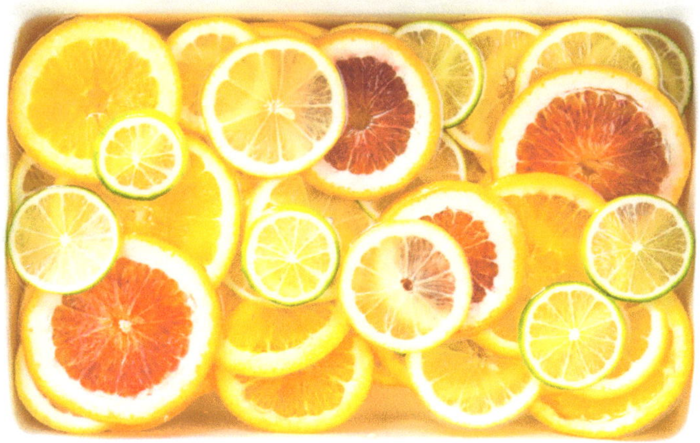

VINEGARS

Vinegars are a versatile ingredient that can enhance the flavor of many dishes. Here's a rundown of different types of vinegars and their culinary uses:

TYPES OF VINEGARS

- Apple Cider Vinegar: Made from fermented apple juice, it has a tangy, fruity flavor. Great for salad dressings, marinades, and sauces. It also adds a subtle sweetness to dishes.
- Balsamic Vinegar: Originating from Italy, it has a rich, complex flavor with a balance of sweet and sour. Ideal for salad dressings, glazes, marinades, and drizzling over fresh fruit or cheese.
- Red Wine Vinegar: Made from fermented red wine, it has a bold and tangy flavor. Perfect for vinaigrettes, marinades, and pickling.
- White Wine Vinegar: Made from fermented white wine, it has a mild, slightly fruity flavor. Great for salad dressings, sauces, and deglazing pans.
- Rice Vinegar: Common in Asian cuisine, it has a mild and slightly sweet flavor. Used in sushi rice, salads, and stir-fries.
- Malt Vinegar: Made from malted barley, it has a strong, tangy flavor. Commonly used with fish and chips and in pickling.
- Distilled White Vinegar: Made from distilled grain alcohol, it has a sharp, clean flavor. Used in pickling, cleaning, and preserving.
- Sherry Vinegar: Made from sherry wine, it has a nutty, complex flavor. Great for sauces, dressings, and marinades.
- Champagne Vinegar: Made from champagne, it has a light, delicate flavor. Ideal for light dressings and seafood dishes.

CULINARY USES

- Marinades: Vinegars help tenderize meat and add depth of flavor.
- Salad Dressings: Vinegars are a key component in vinaigrettes and other dressings, balancing oil and seasonings.
- Pickling: Used to preserve vegetables, adding a tangy flavor and extending shelf life.
- Sauces and Glazes: Adds acidity and complexity to sauces and glazes, enhancing the overall flavor.
- Deglazing: Vinegars help deglaze pans, dissolving browned bits to create flavorful bases for sauces.
- Baking: Can be used to add acidity to baked goods, helping with leavening and flavor balance.
- Condiments: Vinegars are often a key ingredient in condiments like ketchup, mustard, and hot sauces.

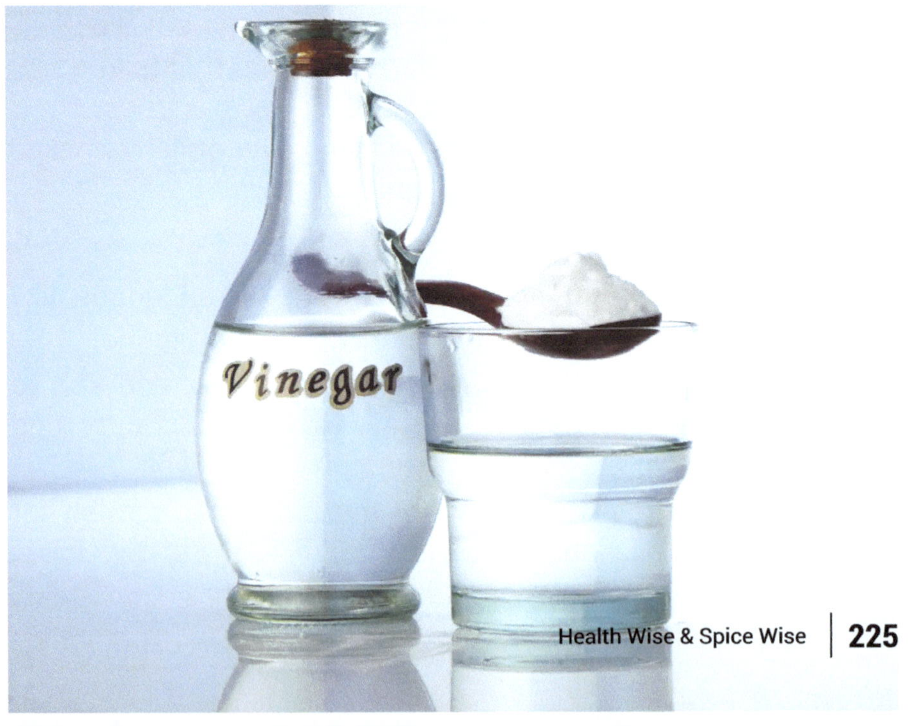

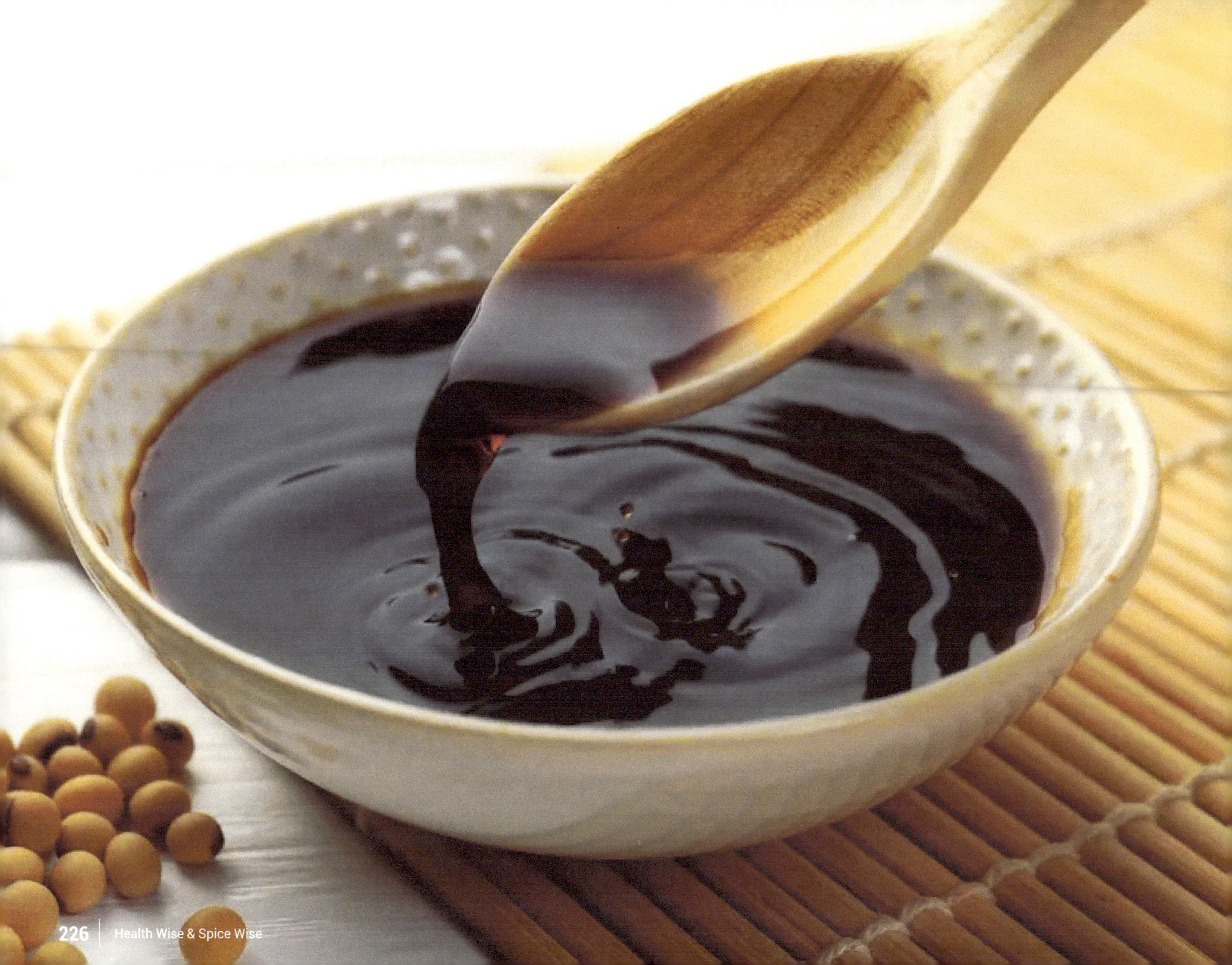

SOY SAUCE

Soy sauce is a fermented condiment traditionally made from soybeans, wheat, salt, and water. It is a staple in many Asian cuisines and is known for its rich, umami flavor. Here are some key properties and uses of soy sauce:

PROPERTIES

- Umami Flavor. Soy sauce is rich in glutamates, which give it a strong umami taste that enhances the overall flavor of dishes.
- Amino Acids: Contains various amino acids resulting from fermentation, which contribute to its complex flavor profile.
- Sodium Content: High in sodium, which acts as a natural preservative and flavor enhancer.
- Fermentation: Made through a fermentation process involving specific molds, yeasts, and bacteria that break down proteins and carbohydrates.

HEALTH BENEFITS

- Digestive Health: Fermented foods like soy sauce can promote healthy gut bacteria, aiding in digestion.
- Antioxidants: Contains antioxidants that help protect against oxidative stress and damage.
- Rich in Nutrients: Provides small amounts of proteins, vitamins, and minerals, including vitamin B12 and iron.
- Blood Pressure Regulation: Contains peptides that may help with blood pressure regulation (though its high sodium content should be consumed in moderation).

TYPES OF SOY SAUCE

- Light Soy Sauce: Lighter in color and saltier, commonly used in Chinese cuisine for seasoning and marinades.
- Dark Soy Sauce: Darker and thicker, often used for adding color and richness to dishes, such as in Chinese braised dishes.
- Tamari: A gluten-free version of soy sauce made primarily from soybeans, commonly used in Japanese cuisine.
- Shoyu: A Japanese soy sauce that is typically brewed with both soybeans and wheat, providing a balanced and slightly sweet flavor.
- Low-Sodium Soy Sauce: Contains less sodium than regular soy sauce, offering a healthier option without compromising too much on flavor.

CULINARY USES

- Marinades: Used to marinate meats, poultry, and seafood, adding depth and umami flavor.
- Stir-Fries: Essential for flavoring stir-fry dishes, providing a savory and rich taste.
- Dipping Sauce: Commonly used as a dipping sauce for sushi, dumplings, and spring rolls.
- Soups and Broths: Adds depth and richness to soups, broths, and stews.
- Salad Dressings: Combined with ingredients like vinegar, oil, and garlic to create flavorful dressings.
- Seasoning: Used to season various dishes, enhancing the overall flavor profile.

Soy sauce is a versatile condiment that can elevate the taste of many dishes.

HONEY

PROPERTIES

- Flavor: Sweet, floral, and varies based on the type of flowers visited by the bees.
- Texture: Thick, viscous, and sticky.
- Color: Ranges from light amber to dark brown, depending on the source of nectar.
- Nutrition: Contains vitamins (B6, thiamine, niacin, riboflavin) and minerals (calcium, copper, iron, magnesium, manganese, phosphorus, potassium, zinc).

HEALTH BENEFITS

- Antioxidant: Rich in antioxidants that help combat oxidative stress.
- Antibacterial and Antimicrobial: Contains natural antibacterial and antimicrobial properties, useful for wound healing and soothing sore throats.
- Digestive Health: Promotes healthy digestion and can relieve gastrointestinal issues.
- Energy Boost: Provides a natural source of energy due to its carbohydrate content.
- Allergy Relief: Local honey is believed to help alleviate seasonal allergies through gradual exposure to pollen.

CULINARY USES

- Sweetener: Used in beverages, baking, and cooking as a natural sweetener.
- Glazes and Marinades: Adds flavor and helps caramelize glazes for meats and vegetables.
- Dressings and Sauces: Enhances salad dressings, sauces, and dips.
- Topping: Drizzled over yogurt, oatmeal, pancakes, and toast.

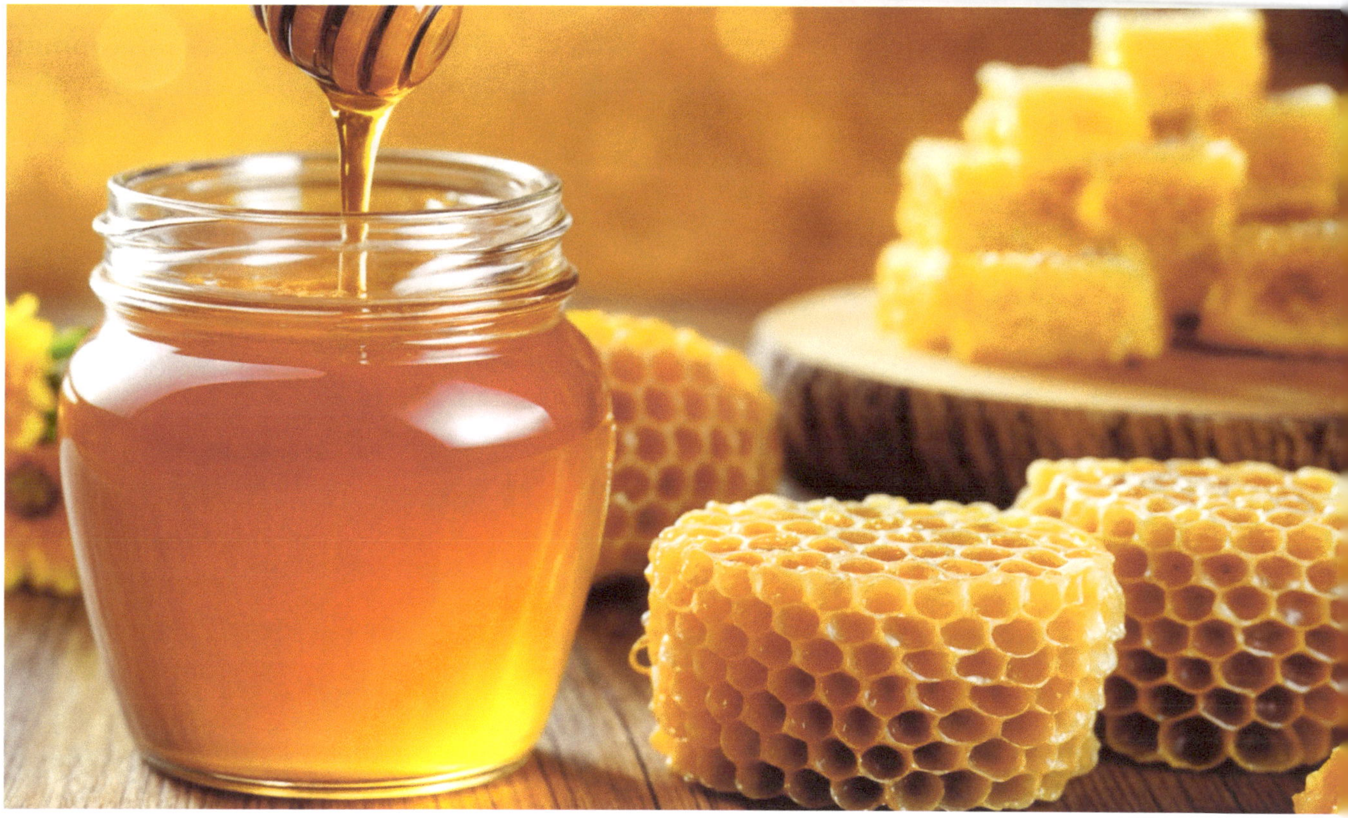

MAPLE SYRUP

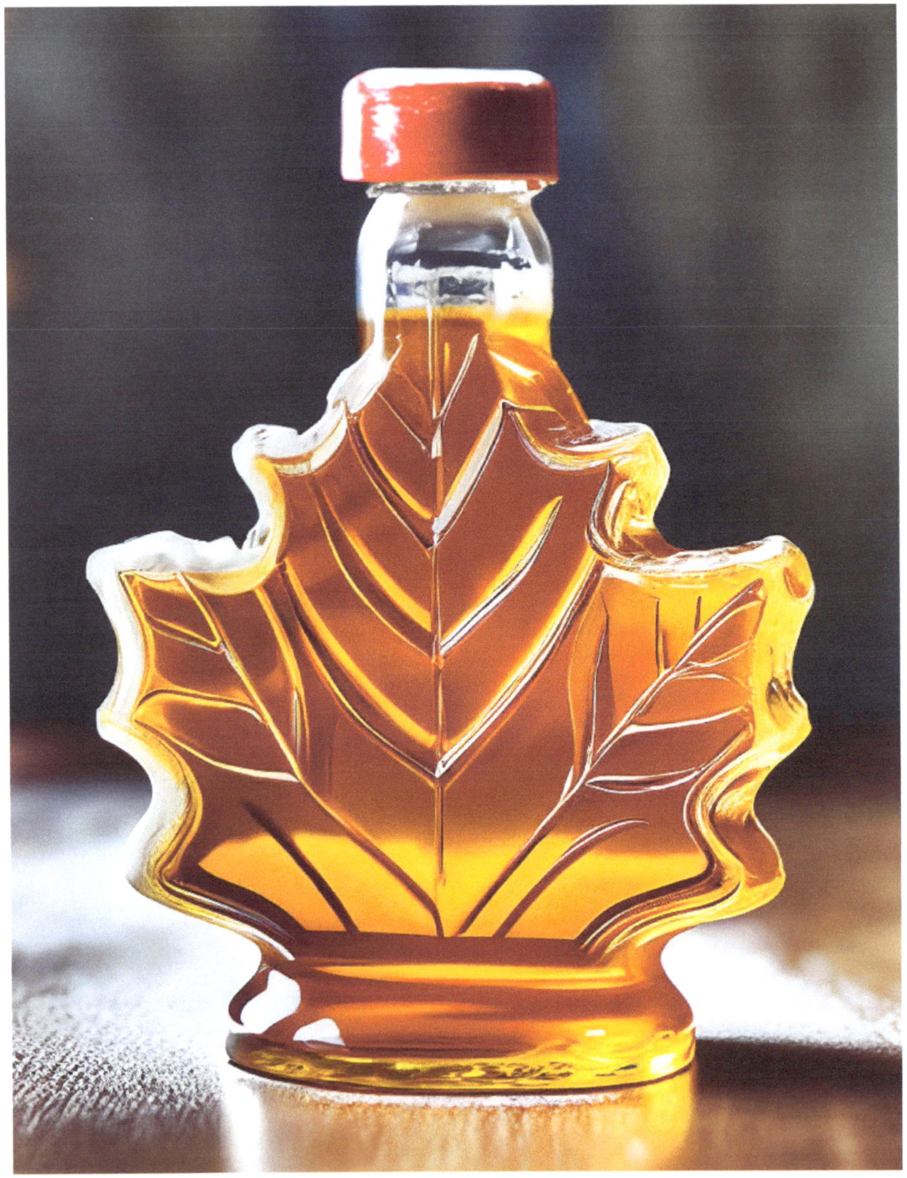

PROPERTIES

- Flavor: Rich, caramel-like, with a distinct maple flavor.
- Texture: Smooth, syrupy, and pourable.
- Color: Classified into grades ranging from golden (light) to very dark, depending on the time of the season it was harvested.
- Nutrition: Contains vitamins (riboflavin, thiamine) and minerals (calcium, potassium, iron, zinc, manganese).

HEALTH BENEFITS

- Antioxidant: Contains antioxidants that protect against oxidative stress.
- Anti-inflammatory: Provides anti-inflammatory benefits due to polyphenols.
- Bone Health: High manganese content supports bone health.
- Energy Boost: Offers a natural source of energy from its carbohydrate content.

CULINARY USES

- Sweetener: Commonly used as a sweetener in baking and cooking.
- Topping: Traditional topping for pancakes, waffles, and French toast.
- Flavoring: Adds flavor to desserts, granola, oatmeal, and yogurt.
- Glazes and Sauces: Used in marinades, glazes, and sauces for meats and vegetables.

Both honey and maple syrup are versatile, natural sweeteners that can enhance the flavor of a wide variety of dishes.

WORCESTERSHIRE SAUCE

Worcestershire sauce is a fermented condiment known for its complex, tangy, and savory flavor. It originates from England and is commonly used to enhance the taste of various dishes. Here are some key properties and uses of Worcestershire sauce:

PROPERTIES

- Ingredients: Typically made from a blend of vinegar, molasses, sugar, salt, anchovies, tamarind extract, onions, garlic, and various spices.
- Flavor Profile: A combination of sweet, salty, tangy, and umami flavors, resulting in a rich and complex taste.
- Fermentation: The fermentation process contributes to its depth of flavor and unique taste.

HEALTH BENEFITS

- Antioxidants: Contains antioxidants from ingredients like garlic, onions, and tamarind, which help protect against oxidative stress.
- Digestive Health: The vinegar content aids in digestion and can stimulate appetite.
- Vitamins and Minerals: Provides small amounts of vitamins and minerals such as vitamin B6, iron, and potassium.

CULINARY USES

- Marinades: Used to marinate meats, poultry, and seafood, adding depth and a savory flavor.
- Sauces and Stews: Enhances the flavor of sauces, stews, and casseroles by adding complexity.
- Dressings: Combined with other ingredients to create flavorful salad dressings and vinaigrettes.
- Bloody Mary: An essential ingredient in the classic Bloody Mary cocktail, adding a savory and spicy kick.
- Grilled and Roasted Dishes: Brushed onto meats and vegetables before grilling or roasting to enhance flavor.
- Seasoning: Used as a seasoning for various dishes, including burgers, meatloaf, and stir-fries.

Worcestershire sauce is a versatile condiment that can elevate the taste of many dishes with its unique and complex flavor.

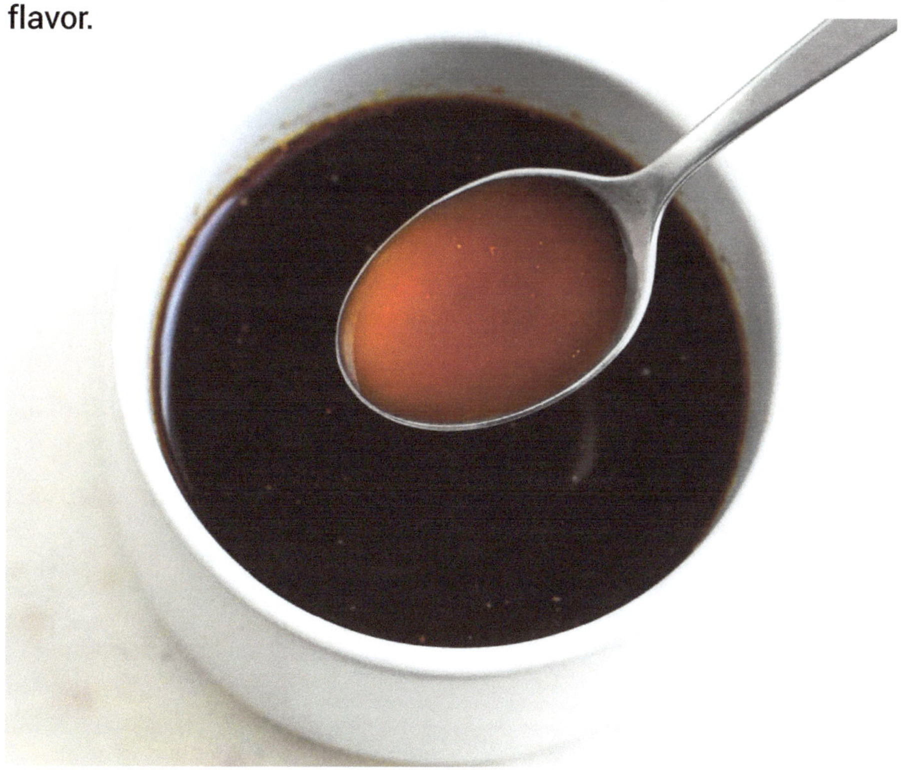

MISO PASTE

Miso paste is a traditional Japanese seasoning made from fermented soybeans. It is known for its rich umami flavor and numerous health benefits. Here are some key properties and uses of miso paste:

PROPERTIES

- Ingredients: Typically made from soybeans, salt, and a fermenting agent called koji (a type of mold), which can also include rice, barley, or other grains.
- Flavor: Has a salty, savory, and umami-rich flavor. The taste can vary from sweet and mild to rich and robust, depending on the fermentation process.
- Texture: Thick, smooth, and paste-like consistency.
- Types: Common types of miso include white miso (shiro miso), red miso (aka miso), and mixed miso (awase miso), each with varying flavors and fermentation times.

HEALTH BENEFITS

- Probiotics: Contains beneficial probiotics that support gut health and aid in digestion.
- Rich in Nutrients: Provides essential vitamins and minerals such as vitamin K, manganese, zinc, and protein.
- Antioxidants: Contains antioxidants that help protect against oxidative stress and inflammation.
- Low in Calories: Generally low in calories, making it a healthy addition to various dishes.

CULINARY USES

- Soups: The most well-known use is in miso soup, where it is dissolved in broth and combined with tofu, seaweed, and green onions.
- Marinades: Used as a marinade for meats, fish, and vegetables to add depth and umami flavor.
- Dressings and Sauces: Can be mixed into salad dressings, dips, and sauces to enhance flavor.
- Stews and Broths: Adds richness and umami to stews, broths, and hot pots.
- Glazes: Used as a glaze for roasting or grilling meats and vegetables, providing a savory and slightly sweet coating.
- Condiments: Can be used as a condiment or seasoning for various dishes, including rice, noodles, and stir-fries.

Miso paste is a versatile ingredient that can elevate the flavor of many dishes while offering numerous health benefits.

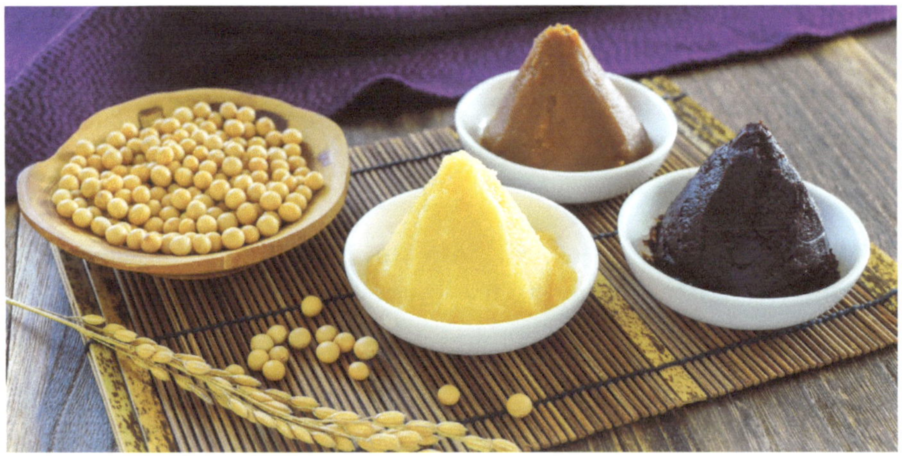

COMMON NUTS USED IN COOKING

Nuts are an excellent addition to many dishes, offering flavor, texture, and nutritional benefits. Here's a detailed look at various nuts commonly used in cooking:

ALMONDS

- Flavor: Mild and slightly sweet.
- Texture: Crunchy; available in whole, sliced, slivered, or ground forms.
- Uses: Baked goods, salads, granola, sauces, and as a snack.

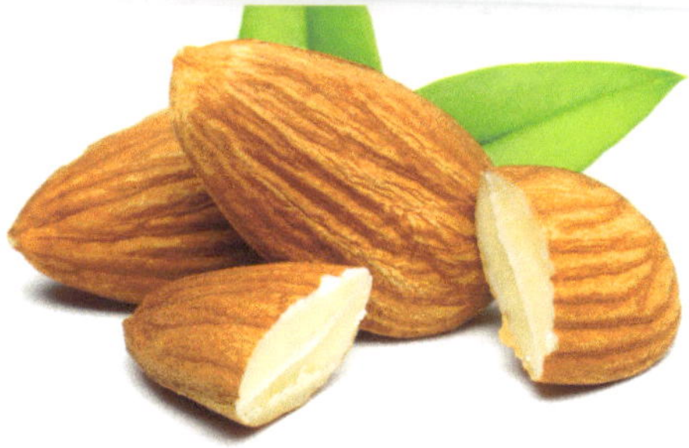

WALNUTS

- Flavor: Rich, slightly bitter, and earthy.
- Texture: Crunchy with a tender interior.
- Uses: Baked goods, salads, pestos, and as a snack.

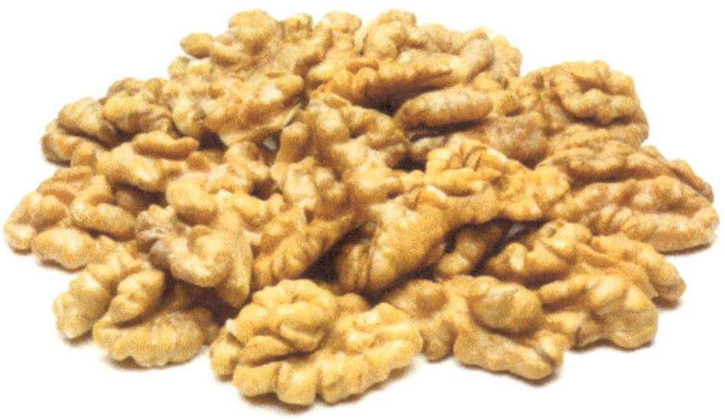

PECANS

- Flavor: Sweet, buttery, and rich.
- Texture: Crunchy with a creamy interior.
- Uses: Pies, baked goods, salads, and as a snack.

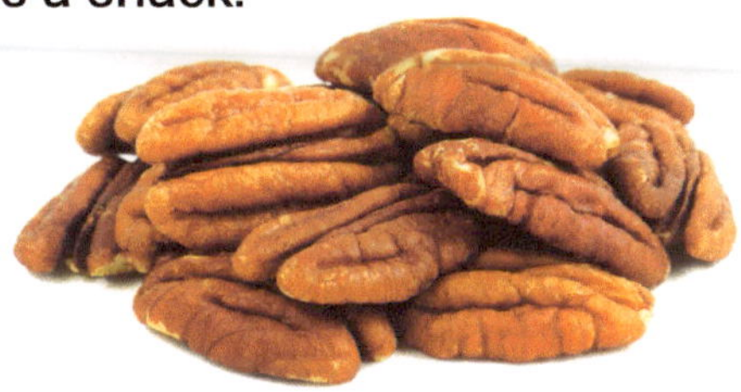

CASHEWS

- Flavor: Mild, buttery, and slightly sweet.
- Texture: Soft and creamy when cooked.
- Uses: Curries, stir-fries, sauces (especially vegan cheese sauces), and as a snack.

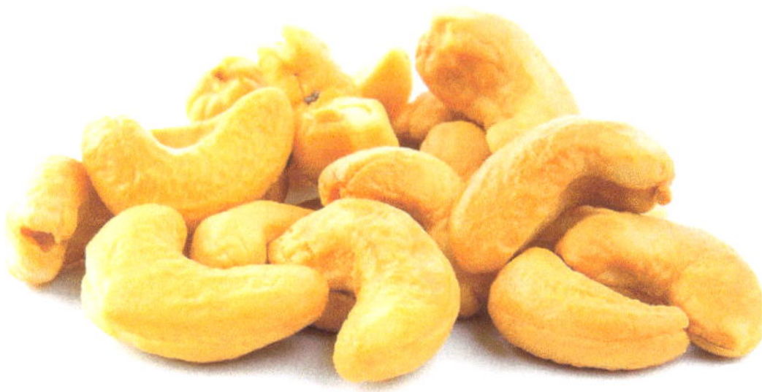

PISTACHIOS

- Flavor: Slightly sweet and nutty.
- Texture: Crunchy.
- Uses: Baked goods, salads, ice cream, and as a snack.

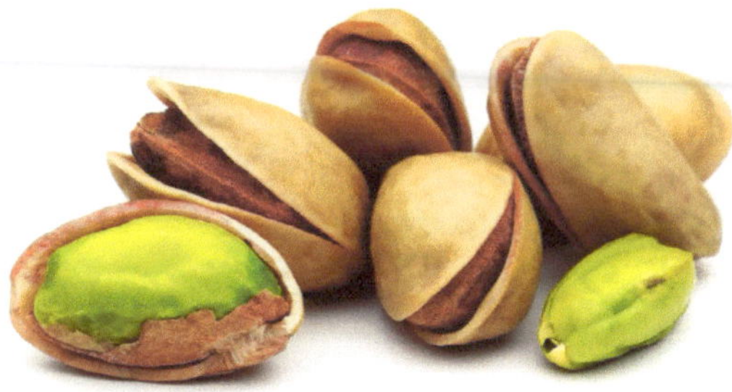

HAZELNUTS

- Flavor: Sweet, rich, and nutty.
- Texture: Crunchy.
- Uses: Chocolates, baked goods, spreads (like Nutella), and as a snack.

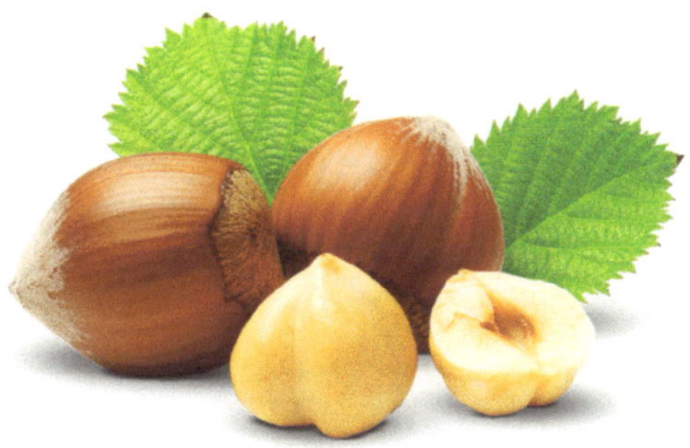

PINE NUTS

- Flavor: Mild and buttery.
- Texture: Soft and creamy.
- Uses: Pesto, salads, baked goods, and as a garnish.

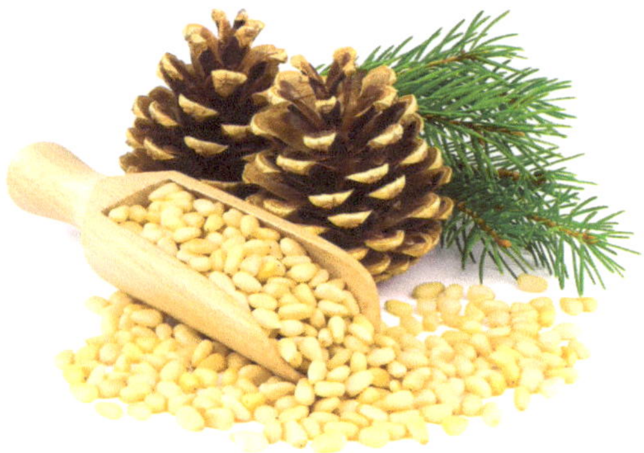

BRAZIL NUTS

- Flavor: Rich, earthy, and slightly creamy.
- Texture: Creamy and crunchy.
- Uses: Baked goods, granola, and as a snack.

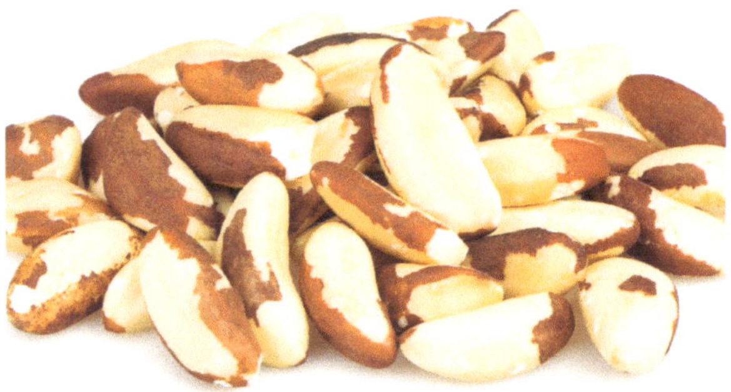

PEANUTS **(technically legumes, but often grouped with nuts)**

- Flavor: Rich, earthy, and slightly sweet.
- Texture: Crunchy.
- Uses: Peanut butter, baked goods, sauces, and as a snack.

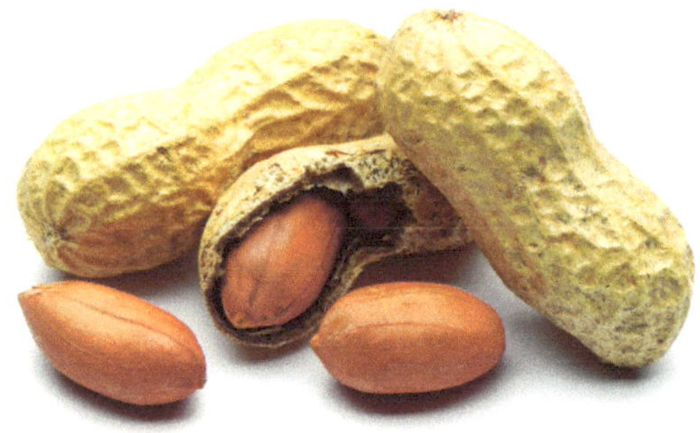

MACADAMIA NUTS

- Flavor: Rich, buttery, and slightly sweet.
- Texture: Creamy and crunchy.
- Uses: Baked goods, chocolates, and as a snack

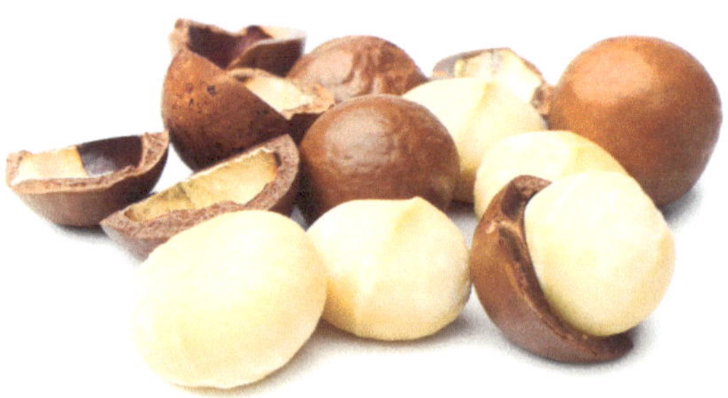

Nuts are incredibly versatile and can be used in both sweet and savory dishes.

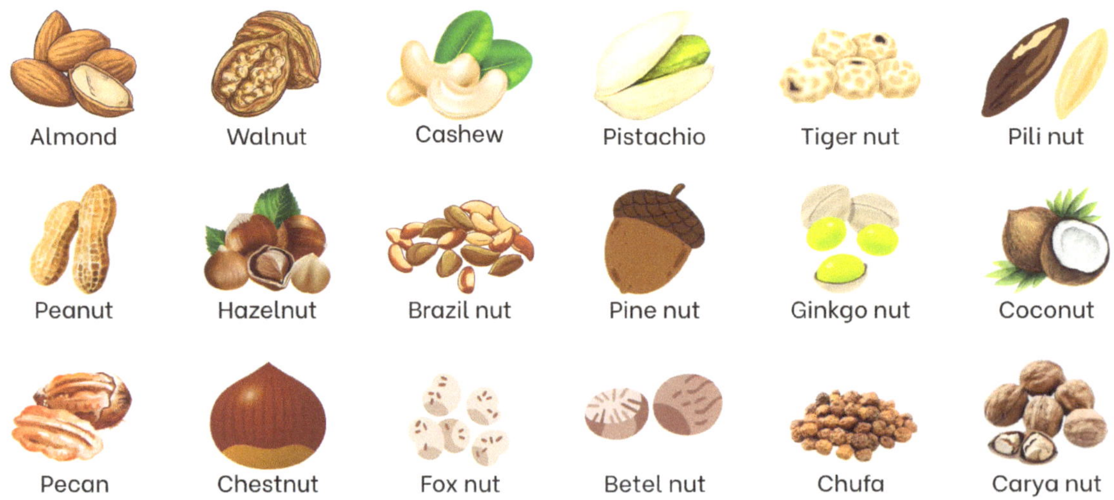

REFERENCES

1. Bower, J. E., & Crosswell, A. D. (2013). Mindfulness meditation and reward processing: Effects on negative affect and responses to self-relevant stimuli. Emotion, 13(3), 533–538. https://doi.org/10.1037/a0031892
2. Büssing, A., Michalsen, A., Khalsa, S. B. S., Telles, S., & Sherman, K. J. (2012). Effects of yoga on mental and physical health: A short summary of reviews. Evidence-Based Complementary and Alternative Medicine, 2012, 165410. https://doi.org/10.1155/2012/165410
3. Chiesa, A., &Serretti, A. (2010). A systematic review of neurobiological and clinical features of mindfulness meditations. Psychological Medicine, 40(8), 1239–1252. https://doi.org/10.1017/S0033291709991747
4. Cramer, H., Lauche, R., Langhorst, J., & Dobos, G. (2013). Yoga for depression: A systematic review and meta-analysis. Depression and Anxiety, 30(11), 1068–1083. https://doi.org/10.1002/da.22166
5. Davidson, R. J., Kabat-Zinn, J., Schumacher, J., Rosenkranz, M., Muller, D., Santorelli, S. F., Urbanowski, F., Harrington, A., Bonus, K., & Sheridan, J. F. (2003). Alterations in brain and immune function produced by mindfulness meditation. Psychosomatic Medicine, 65(4), 564–570. https://doi.org/10.1097/01.PSY.0000077505.67574.E3
6. Goyal, M., Singh, S., Sibinga, E. M. S., Gould, N. F., Rowland-Seymour, A., Sharma, R., Berger, Z., Sleicher, D., Maron, D. D., Shihab, H. M., Ranasinghe, P. D., Linn, S., Saha, S., Bass, E. B., & Haythornthwaite, J. A. (2014). Meditation programs for psychological stress and well-being: A systematic review and meta-analysis. JAMA Internal Medicine, 174(3), 357–368. https://doi.org/10.1001/jamainternmed.2013.13018
7. Hölzel, B. K., Carmody, J., Vangel, M., Congleton, C., Yerramsetti, S. M., Gard, T., & Lazar, S. W. (2011). Mindfulness practice leads to increases in regional brain gray matter density. Psychiatry Research: Neuroimaging, 191(1), 36–43. https://doi.org/10.1016/j.pscychresns.2010.08.006
8. Innes, K. E., Bourguignon, C., & Taylor, A. G. (2005). Risk indices associated with the insulin resistance syndrome, cardiovascular disease, and possible protection with yoga: A systematic review. Journal of the American Board of Family Practice, 18(6), 491–519. https://doi.org/10.3122/jabfm.18.6.491
9. Kabat-Zinn, J. (2003). Mindfulness-based interventions in context: Past, present, and future. Clinical Psychology: Science and Practice, 10(2), 144–156. https://doi.org/10.1093/clipsy.bpg016
10. Khalsa, S. B. S. (2004). Yoga as a therapeutic intervention: A bibliometric analysis of published research studies. Indian Journal of Physiology and Pharmacology, 48(3), 269–285.
11. Lazar, S. W., Kerr, C. E., Wasserman, R. H., Gray, J. R., Greve, D. N., Treadway, M. T., McGarvey, M., Quinn, B. T., Dusek, J. A., Benson, H., Rauch, S. L., Moore, C. I., & Fischl, B. (2005). Meditation experience is associated with increased cortical thickness. NeuroReport, 16(17), 1893–1897. https://doi.org/10.1097/01.wnr.0000186598.66243.19
12. Pascoe, M. C., Thompson, D. R., Jenkins, Z. M., & Ski, C. F. (2017). Mindfulness mediates the physiological markers of stress: Systematic review and meta-analysis. Journal of Psychiatric Research, 95, 156–178. https://doi.org/10.1016/j.jpsychires.2017.08.004

13. Ross, A., & Thomas, S. (2010). The health benefits of yoga and exercise: A review of comparison studies. Journal of Alternative and Complementary Medicine, 16(1), 3–12. https://doi.org/10.1089/acm.2009.0044
14. Streeter, C. C., Whitfield, T. H., Owen, L., Rein, T., Karri, S. K., Yakhkind, A., Perlmutter, R., Prescot, A., Renshaw, P. F., Ciraulo, D. A., & Jensen, J. E. (2010). Effects of yoga versus walking on mood, anxiety, and brain GABA levels: A randomized controlled MRS study. Journal of Alternative and Complementary Medicine, 16(11), 1145–1152. https://doi.org/10.1089/acm.2010.0007
15. Bellavia, A., Larsson, S. C., Bottai, M., Wolk, A., & Orsini, N. (2013). Fruit and vegetable consumption and all-cause mortality: A dose-response analysis. The American Journal of Clinical Nutrition, 98(2), 454–459. https://doi.org/10.3945/ajcn.112.056119
16. Buettner, D., & Skemp, S. (2016). Blue Zones: Lessons from the world's longest lived. American Journal of Lifestyle Medicine, 10(5), 318–321. https://doi.org/10.1177/1559827616637066
17. Calder, P. C. (2015). Marine omega-3 fatty acids and inflammatory processes: Effects, mechanisms and clinical relevance. Biochimica et Biophysica Acta, 1851(4), 469–484. https://doi.org/10.1016/j.bbalip.2014.08.010
18. Estruch, R., Ros, E., Salas-Salvadó, J., Covas, M.-I., Corella, D., Arós, F., Gómez-Gracia, E., Ruiz-Gutiérrez, V., Fiol, M., Lapetra, J., Lamuela-Raventos, R. M., Serra-Majem, L., Pintó, X., Basora, J., Muñoz, M. A., Sorlí, J. V., Martínez, J. A., & Martínez-González, M. A. (2013). Primary prevention of cardiovascular disease with a Mediterranean diet. New England Journal of Medicine, 368(14), 1279–1290. https://doi.org/10.1056/NEJMoa1200303
19. Fontana, L., & Partridge, L. (2015). Promoting health and longevity through diet: From model organisms to humans. Cell, 161(1), 106–118. https://doi.org/10.1016/j.cell.2015.02.020
20. Holloszy, J. O., & Fontana, L. (2007). Caloric restriction in humans. Experimental Gerontology, 42(8), 709–712. https://doi.org/10.1016/j.exger.2007.03.009
21. Longo, V. D., & Mattson, M. P. (2014). Fasting: Molecular mechanisms and clinical applications. Cell Metabolism, 19(2), 181–192. https://doi.org/10.1016/j.cmet.2013.12.008
22. Mathers, J. C. (2015). Nutrition and ageing: Knowledge, gaps and research priorities. Proceedings of the Nutrition Society, 72(4), 505–512. https://doi.org/10.1017/S0029665113000396
23. Patel, S. R., Malhotra, A., White, D. P., Gottlieb, D. J., & Hu, F. B. (2006). Association between reduced sleep and weight gain in women. American Journal of Epidemiology, 164(10), 947–954. https://doi.org/10.1093/aje/kwj280
24. Rees, K., Hartley, L., Flowers, N., Clarke, A., Hooper, L., Thorogood, M., & Stranges, S. (2013). 'Mediterranean' dietary pattern for the primary prevention of cardiovascular disease. Cochrane Database of Systematic Reviews, 2013(8), CD009825. https://doi.org/10.1002/14651858.CD009825.pub2
25. Sallis, J. F., Cerin, E., Conway, T. L., Adams, M. A., Frank, L. D., Pratt, M., Salvo, D., Schipperijn, J., Smith, G., Cain, K. L., Davey, R., Kerr, J., Lai, P.-C., Mitas, J., Reis, R., Sarmiento, O. L., Schofield, G., Troelsen, J., Van Dyck, D., & Owen, N. (2016). Physical activity in relation to urban environments in 14 cities worldwide: A cross-sectional study. The Lancet, 387(10034), 2207–2217. https://doi.org/10.1016/S0140-6736(15)01284-2
26. Seals, D. R., Justice, J. N., & LaRocca, T. J. (2016). Physiological geroscience: Targeting function to increase healthspan and achieve optimal longevity. Journal of Physiology, 594(8), 2001–2024. https://doi.org/10.1113/jphysiol.2014.282665
27. Warburton, D. E. R., Nicol, C. W., & Bredin, S. S. D. (2006). Health benefits of physical activity: The evidence. CMAJ: Canadian Medical Association Journal, 174(6), 801–809. https://doi.org/10.1503/cmaj.051351

28. World Health Organization. (2020). Physical activity. https://www.who.int/news-room/fact-sheets/detail/physical-activity
29. Aggarwal, B. B., & Harikumar, K. B. (2009). Potential therapeutic effects of curcumin, the anti-inflammatory agent, against neurodegenerative, cardiovascular, pulmonary, metabolic, autoimmune and neoplastic diseases. The International Journal of Biochemistry & Cell Biology, 41(1), 40–59. https://doi.org/10.1016/j.biocel.2008.06.010
30. Bode, A. M., & Dong, Z. (2011). The amazing and mighty ginger. In I. F. F. Benzie & S. Wachtel-Galor (Eds.), Herbal medicine: Biomolecular and clinical aspects (2nd ed., pp. 131–156). CRC Press.
31. Cemek, M., Kağa, S., Şimşek, N., Büyükokuroğlu, M. E., & Konuk, M. (2008). Antihyperglycemic and antioxidative potential of Matricaria chamomilla L. in streptozotocin-induced diabetic rats. Journal of Natural Medicines, 62(3), 284–293. https://doi.org/10.1007/s11418-008-0228-1
32. Cullen, J., & Leahy, C. (2021). Cinnamon and its role in blood glucose regulation: A review of the current evidence. Journal of Herbal Medicine, 28, 100453. https://doi.org/10.1016/j.hermed.2021.100453
33. Delaquis, P. J., Stanich, K., Girard, B., & Mazza, G. (2002). Antimicrobial activity of individual and mixed fractions of dill, cilantro, coriander, and eucalyptus essential oils. International Journal of Food Microbiology, 74(1–2), 101–109. https://doi.org/10.1016/S0168-1605(01)00734-6
34. Grzanna, R., Lindmark, L., &Frondoza, C. G. (2005). Ginger—an herbal medicinal product with broad anti-inflammatory actions. Journal of Medicinal Food, 8(2), 125–132. https://doi.org/10.1089/jmf.2005.8.125
35. Jiang, T. A. (2019). Health benefits of culinary herbs and spices. Journal of AOAC International, 102(2), 395–411. https://doi.org/10.5740/jaoacint.18-0418
36. Kaefer, C. M., & Milner, J. A. (2008). The role of herbs and spices in cancer prevention. Journal of Nutritional Biochemistry, 19(6), 347–361. https://doi.org/10.1016/j.jnutbio.2007.11.003
37. Lv, J., Qi, L., Yu, C., Yang, L., Guo, Y., Chen, Y., Bian, Z., Sun, D., Du, J., Ge, P., Tang, Z., Hou, W., Li, Y., Chen, J., Chen, Z., & Li, L. (2015). Consumption of spicy foods and total and cause specific mortality: Population based cohort study. BMJ, 351, h3942. https://doi.org/10.1136/bmj.h3942
38. Mashhadi, N. S., Ghiasvand, R., Askari, G., Hariri, M., Darvishi, L., &Mofid, M. R. (2013). Anti-oxidative and anti-inflammatory effects of ginger in health and physical activity: Review of current evidence. International Journal of Preventive Medicine, 4(Suppl 1), S36–S42.
39. Rathore, S. S., Saxena, S. N., & Singh, B. (2013). Potential health benefits of major seed spices. International Journal of Seed Spices, 3(2), 1–12.
40. Singletary, K. (2010). Oregano: Overview of the literature on health benefits. Nutrition Today, 45(3), 129–138. https://doi.org/10.1097/NT.0b013e3181dec600
41. Tapsell, L. C., Hemphill, I., Cobiac, L., Sullivan, D. R., Fenech, M., Patch, C. S., Roodenrys, S., Keogh, J. B., Clifton, P. M., Williams, P. G., Fazio, V. A., & Inge, K. E. (2006). Health benefits of herbs and spices: The past, the present, the future. Medical Journal of Australia, 185(S4), S1–S24. https://doi.org/10.5694/j.1326-5377.2006.tb00548.x
42. Zheng, J., Zhou, Y., Li, S., Zhang, P., Zhou, T., Xu, D.-P., & Li, H.-B. (2016). Effects and mechanisms of fruit and vegetable juices on cardiovascular diseases. International Journal of Molecular Sciences, 18(3), 555. https://doi.org/10.3390/ijms18030555

www.ingramcontent.com/pod-product-compliance
Lightning Source LLC
LaVergne TN
LVHW070818210926
848482LV00004B/287